Schistosomiasis: Parasitology Essentials

Schistosomiasis: Parasitology Essentials

Editor: Caldwell Tidicue

www.fosteracademics.com

www.fosteracademics.com

Cataloging-in-Publication Data

Schistosomiasis : parasitology essentials / edited by Caldwell Tidicue.
   p. cm.
Includes bibliographical references and index.
ISBN 978-1-64646-570-5
1. Schistosomiasis. 2. Parasitology. 3. Parasitic diseases.
4. Communicable diseases. I. Tidicue, Caldwell.
RC182.S24 S35 2023
616.963--dc23

Foster Academics,
118-35 Queens Blvd., Suite 400,
Forest Hills, NY 11375, USA

ISBN 978-1-64646-570-5 (Hardback)

Contents

Preface

Over the recent decade, advancements and applications have progressed exponentially. This has led to the increased interest in this field and projects are being conducted to enhance knowledge. The main objective of this book is to present some of the critical challenges and provide insights into possible solutions. This book will answer the varied questions that arise in the field and also provide an increased scope for furthering studies.

Schistosomiasis refers to a group of chronic or acute diseases caused by parasitic worms called schistosomes. It is known by various names such as bilharzia, bilharziasis, snail fever or Katayama fever. The three major types of schistosomiasis are Japonica schistosomiasis, Manson's or intestinal schistosomiasis, and vesical or urinary schistosomiasis. Some common symptoms of acute schistosomiasis are abdominal pain, diarrhea, bloody stool, or blood in the urine. Liver damage, kidney failure, infertility and bladder cancer are certain complications associated with chronic schistosomiasis. The diagnosis of this disease is performed through microscopic examination of stool or urine samples for parasite eggs. Enzyme-linked immunosorbent assay, circumoval precipitation test, and alkaline phosphatase immunoassay are some other diagnostic methods that can be used to determine schistosomiasis. Imaging techniques such as X-rays, ultrasound, computed tomography (CT), and magnetic resonance imaging (MRI) are employed to investigate the severity of schistosomiasis and damage to infected organs. Its treatment involves medications such as praziquantel and oxamniquine. This book contains some path-breaking studies related to schistosomiasis. It is appropriate for medical students and researchers seeking detailed information on this parasitic disease.

I hope that this book, with its visionary approach, will be a valuable addition and will promote interest among readers. Each of the authors has provided their extraordinary competence in their specific fields by providing different perspectives as they come from diverse nations and regions. I thank them for their contributions.

Editor

Elimination of *Schistosoma japonicum* Transmission in China: A Case of Schistosomiasis Control in the Severe Epidemic Area of Anhui Province

Linhan Li [1,2,3,†], Yibiao Zhou [1,2,3,†], Tianping Wang [4], Shiqing Zhang [4], Gengxin Chen [5], Genming Zhao [1], Na He [1], Zhijie Zhang [1], Dongjian Yang [1,2,3] ⓘ, Ya Yang [1,2,3], Yu Yang [1,2,3], Hongchang Yuan [1], Yue Chen [6] and Qingwu Jiang [1,2,3,*]

1   Department of Epidemiology, School of Public Health, Fudan University, 130 Dong'an Road, Shanghai 200032, China; 16111020005@fudan.edu.cn (L.L.); ybzhou@fudan.edu.cn (Y.Z.); gmzhao@shmu.edu.cn (G.Z.); nhe@shmu.edu.cn (N.H.); zhj_zhang@fudan.edu.cn (Z.Z.); 17211020111@fudan.edu.cn (D.Y.); yayang16@fudan.edu.cn (Y.Y.); 16211020071@fudan.edu.cn (Y.Y.); hcyfduepi@163.com (H.Y.)
2   Key Laboratory of Public Health Safety, Ministry of Education, 130 Dong'an Road, Shanghai 200032, China
3   Center of Tropical Disease Research, 130 Dong'an Road, Shanghai 200032, China
4   Institute for the Prevention and Control of Schistosomiasis in Anhui Province, 337 Wuhu Road, Hefei 230061, China; wangtianping@hotmail.com (T.W.); zhangdj1994@aliyun.com (S.Z.)
5   Guichi Antischistosomiasis Station, West Qiupu Road, Chizhou 247100, China; cgx5611@163.com
6   School of Epidemiology and Public Health, University of Ottawa, 600 Peter Morand, Ottawa, ON K1G 5Z3, Canada; Yue.Chen@uottawa.ca
*   Correspondence: jiangqw@fudan.edu.cn
†   These authors contributed equally to this work.

Abstract: Over the several decades, China has been incessantly optimizing control strategies in response to the varying epidemic situations of schistosomiasis. We evaluated continuously the changing prevalence under different control strategies of two villages, Sanlian and Guifan, in China through five phases lasting 37 years. We tested residents, calculated prevalence and discussed change causes. We found the prevalence in Sanlian did not differ significant from that of Guifan ($p = 0.18$) in 1981, but decreased to 2.66%, much lower than Guifan's 11.25%, in 1984 ($p = 0$). Besides, prevalence in Guifan increased to 21.25% in 1987, while in Sanlian it rose to 20.78% until 1989. Those data confirmed that praziquantel combined with snail control could better reduce the prevalence. From 1992 to 1994, the prevalence in the two villages displayed downtrends, which showed the World Bank Loan Project worked. From 1995 to 2004, repeated oscillations with no obvious change trend was seen. Since 2005, the prevalence in both villages has shown a significant downtrend ($p < 0.05$), which suggests the integrated strategy is effective. We considered the control strategies were implemented suitably in the study area under changing social circumstances. Adjusting the strategy in consideration of social transformations is necessary and vital. The experience may be useful for policy making of other epidemic areas with an analogous situation.

Keywords: evaluation; method; policy; strategy; social; trend

1. Introduction

The archeological discovery of Schistosoma eggs in a corpse in the Changsha Mawangdui Han tomb in Hunan Province revealed that schistosomiasis has been prevalent in China for over 2000 years. Not until the American physician Logan first reported the clinical diagnosis of schistosomiasis in China [1], did Chinese people begin to consider schistosomiasis as a disease. *Schistosoma japonicum*, one of the five species of schistosome, is widely distributed in China, Indonesia, and The Philippines [2]. As it needs to go through several growth stages in water, the transmission and infection of humans is closely related to specific geographic conditions, which causes difficulties in prevalence control [3]. Schistosomiasis brings a heavy burden to China's population health, social stability, and economic development.

After the establishment of the People's Republic of China in 1949, the central government organized and delegated expert teams to conduct a national survey that found 12 provinces and 351 counties where schistosomiasis prevailed [4] with some 10.5–11.8 million people infected. Zedong Mao, the Chinese president back then, with immense political influence, wrote a famous poem "Farewell to the god of plague" and launched a massive country-wide movement to eliminate schistosomiasis [5]. With medical treatment, environmental modification, and molluscicide application, by 1980, four out of the 12 provinces and two thirds of the affected counties successfully repressed the prevalence of schistosomiasis [6]. As for the remaining eight provinces, epidemic areas were mostly distributed in marshlands and mountainous areas with complicated environmental factors that hindered control.

In order to address this predicament and search for a new and effective schistosomiasis control method, Warren and Su conducted a study in Guichi district, Anhui Province, one of the ten historically most severely affected areas in China [7] and confirmed praziquantel therapy could effectively reduce the schistosomiasis prevalence in humans. When combined with snail control in epidemic areas, the prevalence decreased even more significantly. In this study, we performed a 37-years longitudinal study from 1981 to 2017 on the basis of the study conducted by Warren and Su to understand the long-term effects of schistosomiasis transmission control strategies.

2. Materials and Methods

2.1. Study Area

The study was conducted in a marshland area including Sanlian village (30.642447, 117.346828 and Guifan village (30.574982, 117.410960), in Guichi district, Anhui Province, which is located in the middle and lower reaches of the Yangtze River Basin, the largest river in China (Figure 1).

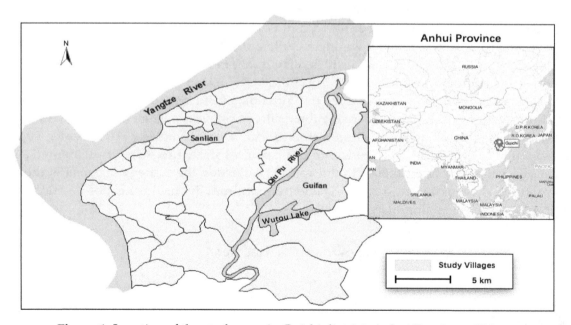

Figure 1. Location of the study area in Guichi district, Anhui Province, China.

Its humid subtropical monsoon climate has annual average temperatures of 16 degrees Celsius and annual average rainfall of 1600 mm. This provides a suitable environment for the survival of

Schistosoma japonicum. There are many small hills full of swamps, ponds and ditches in Guichi. This feature makes Guichi a typical schistosomiasis epidemic area. In addition, people in Guichi live along rivers or lakes, and their lifestyles area mainly involve farming and grazing, fishing and lake grassing. These labor activities expose local residents to be infected by schistosomiasis [7]. At the end of 2012, the total habitat area of snails in Guichi district was approximately 26.2715 km^2 [8]. Of 650,000 people in Guichi, about 400,000 people were at risk of schistosomiasis, and the endemic area covered 16 towns and 165 villages [8]. All subjects gave their informed consent for inclusion before they participated in the study. The research was approved by the Medical Ethics Committee of Fudan University School of Public Health (IRB#2011-03-0270).

2.2. Intervention Measures

Sanlian village applied molluscicide (solid pentachlorophenol) on snails' habitats every spring during 1981–1984, and simultaneously administered praziquantel to people with positive fecal examination. Guifan village only administered praziquantel to subjects with positive fecal tests. After 1984, the different control measures were all stopped, and two villages began to follow the same control strategies: (1) by local government in 1985–1991. (2) recommended by the World Bank Loan Project (WBLP) in 1992–2001. (3) by the continued WBLP measures in 2002–2004. (4) since 2005, the integrated schistosomiasis control strategy has been carried out. Table 1 provides detailed information on the intervention measures from 1981 to 2017.

2.3. Disease Diagnosis

During the study period, after the transmission season (October–November), residents aged 5 to 65 years (743 in Sanlian, 1479 in Guifan in 1981) were tested by Kato-Katz (KK) fecal test and/or indirect hemagglutination assay (IHA) [9]. After 1981, the number of examined people was about 600 to 1200 in Sanlian and Guifan, respectively. From 1981 to 1994, all subjects in the two villages were tested by the two Kato-Katz thick smears test. During the period of 1995–2004, subjects were screened by indirect hemagglutination assay method. From 2005 to 2014, all subjects were tested by three Kato-Katz thick smears test. All the subjects were screened by indirect hemagglutination assay and the seropositive were confirmed by Kato-Katz three smears test from 2015 to 2017.

2.4. Statistical Analysis

The prevalence of human infection was estimated by the formula: (1) Observed prevalence (%) = No. of egg-positive/No. of examined people × 100% (by using Kato-Katz method). (2) Observed prevalence (%) = (No. of blood-positive/No. of examined people × 100% (by using IHA test). (3) Observed prevalence (%) = (No. blood-positive/No. of examined people by using IHA test) × (No. of egg-positive/No. of examined people by using Kato-Katz method) × 100% (by using Kato-Katz and IHA).

The adjusted prevalence is the observed prevalence of human infection after taking the sensitivity and specificity of the Kato-Katz method into consideration. The adjusted formula: $p' = \frac{p_0 + \beta - 1}{\alpha + \beta - 1}$ p': adjusted prevalence, p_0: observed prevalence, α: sensitivity, β: specificity [10].

Two stool samples with three thick smears each are used as the diagnostic gold standard [11]. The sensitivities of two smears and three smears Kato-Katz methods are 64% and 75% separately. The specificities are 100% for both of them; the sensitivity and specificity of IHA and the observed prevalence measured by it are not satisfy the condition of adjusted formula [10], therefore, the results of IHA cannot be adjusted.

All data were entered and built a database with Microsoft Excel, and statistical analyses were performed with the use of SPSS (version25, IBM, New York, NY, USA) and SAS software (University Edition, The Statistical Analysis System, Raleigh, NC, USA). We used the chi-square test, including testing for trend when appropriate, to examine any difference and change over time. Two-sided p values were calculated for all comparisons [12–14].

Table 1. The varieties of control strategies of schistosomiasis from 1981–2017 in Guifan and Sanlian villages in China.

Time	Phase	Specific Methods
1981–1984	Warren's Study Control	Guifan Village: People with a positive stool examination result should receive drug chemotherapy. Sanlian Village: 1. People with positive result of stool examination should receive drug chemotherapy. 2. The areas where snail lived were sprayed with molluscicide every spring.
1985–1991	Local Government Control	1. Chemotherapy for people and cattle was the basic measure. 2. Health education for people. 3. Molluscicide was directed at the susceptible areas.
1992–2001	World Bank Loan Project	Goal: Enhanced morbidity control through praziquantel to human and bovines. Details: 1. Chemotherapy was complemented by health education. 2. Snails were controlled by environmental management. 3. Molluscicide was a key way to sustain transmission control.
2002–2004	Extended Period of WBLP Control	1. Achievements from WBLP were not reinforced. 2. The extent of chemotherapy shrinked and compliance of chemotherapy became worse. 3. Returning farmland to lake was advocated due to the molluscicide and previously reclaimed land from the lake.
2005–2017	Integrated Strategy Control	2005: 1. Chemotherapy with praziquantel for people and cattle. 2. Snail control with molluscicides. 3. Health education programmes—residents should stay away from snail-infested areas and water Since 2006: 4. All cattle were replaced with mechanized equipment. 5. Other domestic animals were fenced in. 6. Piped water and lavatories were supplied to improve sanitation.

3. Results

Infection in Humans

The trend of schistosomiasis infection rates in the residents of Sanlian and Guifan villages over the last 37 years was shown in Figure 2. In 1981, the prevalence of schistosomiasis was 32.81% in Sanlian village and 30.00% in Guifan village ($\chi^2 = 1.839$, $p = 0.175$). With the intervention measures of human chemotherapy and snail control in Sanlian village, the prevalence dropped to 2.66% in 1984, while in Guifan village with chemotherapy only, the prevalence was only reduced to 11.25% ($\chi^2 = 41.576$, $p = 0$). By 1987, the prevalence in Guifan village increased to 21.25%, while the rate in Sanlian village rose to 20.78% until 1989. Since 1987, the local government in Guifan village has strengthened its control work so the rate declined again. Since the implementation of WBLP in 1992, the prevalence in Sanlian and Guifan villages had continued to decrease from 12.51% and 14.10% in 1992 to 3.29% and 2.89% in 1994. There was a volatile stage, with no obvious change trend in both villages from 1995 to 2004. In 1998 and 1999, infection rates in Sanlian and Guifan reached their respective peaks. A comprehensive control strategy has been implemented since 2005, and the prevalence decreased from 8.12% in 2005 to 0 in 2014 in Sanlian and from 14.39% to 0.70% for the same period in Guifan. There was no infected person detected in either village from 2015 to 2017. Both prevalences had significant downtrends since 2005 (Sanlian $\chi^2 = 7.995$, $p = 0.005$; Guifan $\chi^2 = 9.433$, $p = 0.002$).

Figure 2. Prevalence of *Schistosoma japonicum* infection in humans in two villages during 1981–2017. (1) The adjusted prevalence formula: $p' = \frac{p_0 + \beta - 1}{\alpha + \beta - 1}$ p': Adjusted prevalence; p_0: Observed prevalence; α: Sensitivity; β: Specificity [10]; (2) The Kato-Katz (KK) 2 slides method was used in 1981–1994: $\alpha = 0.64$, $\beta = 1$ [11]; The indirect hemagglutination assay (IHA) method was used in 1995–2004, but IHA not meet the condition of adjusted formula [10]; The Kato-Katz 3 slides method was used in 2005–2017, $\alpha = 0.75$, $\beta = 1$ [11]; (3) Prevalence were assessed after the transmission season for each year in Sanlian and Guifan villages. (4) The I bars represent 95% confidence intervals.

4. Discussion

This study provides a long and continuous evaluation of the prevalence of schistosomiasis in China. Using disease data from 1981 to 2017, we found the changes of infection rates of humans within each historical phase were on account of different and complex causes, particularly social, economic, political, and health aspects. The schistosomiasis control strategies were suitable for the respective situations back then. Compared to most other studies concentrating on a single epidemic period or data from specific time points, infection rates and control strategies of schistosomiasis in this study are evaluated in a more comprehensive, systematic, and direct way. We confirmed that snail control and chemotherapy in combination has better effect than chemotherapy alone. In addition, we esteemed that the morbidity control measures taken in each historical period were appropriate and suited to the changing disease and social-economic status situations in China. We believed that WBLP is a successful example of disease control aided by foreign funds. Besides, we concluded the integrated strategy has greatly reduced the disease burden of schistosomiasis in China.

After different control measures were stopped in 1984, the prevalence in Sanlian village started to rise the next year, but still remained lower than that of the Guifan village until 1988. This suggests chemotherapy combined with snail control achieved robust and longer-term effects in reducing the prevalence. This conclusion corroborates control projects undertaken in other countries [15,16]. However, from 1987 to 1992, the prevalence oscillated in both villages, which was similar to other regions in China at that time. There are several possible reasons. First of all, since 1978, China's rural areas have begun to shift from a centralized system to a contracted responsibility system for joint production. The mass extermination of snails is no longer practical. Moreover, as a result of responsibility privatization and the subsequent rise of labor cost, the previous schistosomiasis control measures become too expensive. Second of all, with the reform of China's social and economic system in the 1980s, the source of schistosomiasis control budgets shifted from the previous three-level system (county, provincial, and the central governments) to the local government only, significantly intensifying the burden on local finances and therefore limiting corresponding expenditure on schistosomiasis control. Third of all, previous drug eradication of snails and environmental modification brought many problems such as environmental pollution and flooding, further increased economic burden and social impact [17]. Last but not least, praziquantel, a very effective chemotherapy drug started to be introduced to and widely used in China in the late 1980s [3], the Chinese government and the public dedicated less attention to schistosomiasis, which also partly led to the oscillation in prevalence.

In 1992, large-scale drug treatment, health education and snails control were implemented in both villages, which led to obviously prevalence declined in the next two years. In 1990s, following the WHO's recommendation that developing countries should utilize chemotherapy to achieve better morbidity control [18,19], a wide application of praziquantel, indirect hemagglutination, and the Kato-Katz method were initiated. This marked the starting point when China's schistosomiasis control strategy switched from environmental modification to praziquantel-based control. Particularly, in 1992, with the help of the WHO, China began to implement the World Bank Loan Project (No. P003624) for "Infectious and Endemic Disease Control Project" [20,21], which provided 71 million dollars to help and support the government's financial expenditure on schistosomiasis control, the application of parasite diagnostic techniques and the promotion of chemotherapeutic drugs [22]. Following a sharp decline in 1992–1994, the prevalence in the two villages rebounded in 1995 due to flooding in Guichi district. On the contrary, in 1997, the drought in Guichi decreased the risk of infection and therefore the prevalence. Similarly, prevalence peaked again in 1998 and 1999 as a result of severe flooding in China's Yangtze River Basin that year [23]. Many new snail areas also appeared after the flood and this aggravated the disease burden [24]. As shown in Figure 2, prevalence in two villages oscillated at a high level from 1995 to 2004 even with continuous praziquantel-based control, indicating human chemotherapy alone might not be sufficient to completely eliminate schistosomiasis. This was also supported by another study [25]. Fluctuation of prevalence in the late WBLP period was also confirmed by another study [26]. There are four possible reasons for the changing prevalence at that time. Firstly, the reform of government institutions and the loss of well-trained technicians caused difficulties in normal operation of schistosomiasis control and budget reduction. Secondly, with the termination of the WBLP, the public's compliance [27] with drug treatment had also decreased. Thirdly, although the prevalence and incidence of acute schistosomiasis dropped to a relatively low level in the early stage of this period [28], praziquantel could not stop transmission in high-epidemic areas and reinfection [3]. Lastly, natural factors such as floods also contributed heavily to the prevalence fluctuation.

From 2005 to 2017, the infection rates in both villages decreased significantly. This might result from four aspects. First of all, in 2004, Chinese government set up four priority control programs of communicable diseases including schistosomiasis, AIDS, tuberculosis and hepatitis B [14], and schistosomiasis received an increased attention. Second of all, Chinese government launched the "National long-term plan for control of schistosomiasis (2004–2015)" program [29] in response to the rebounded trend of prevalence, which marked the beginning of the integrated control strategy in the country. Third of all, as the government increased its public health budget for schistosomiasis, the government transfer payment program was started and the national health system was strengthened. Lastly, the comprehensive control strategy, including praziquantel treatment of human and animals, molluscide application, health education, sanitation improvement, removal of bovines, etc., were implemented in our study area in 2006 [30] which greatly helped to reduce the disease burden of schistosomiasis. This result is consistent with the conclusions of many other studies [6,30–38]. However, several issues remain as well. Firstly, the comprehensive control strategy is not able to further reduce the infection rate to less than 3% in some areas [30,39]. Secondly, although removal of agriculture main livestock, such as bovines, sheep, and horses, can reduce human prevalence to a large extent [24], the existing control measures need to be adjusted in China since 45 species of mammal can be infected by *S. japonicum* in total, including but not limited to dogs, cats, and rodents [40–42]. Thirdly, the broadly used Kato-Katz method has relatively low sensitivity, particularly for subjects with low infectiosity [43,44]. This could lead to false negative results. Recently, several studies confirmed that Helmintex method is a more sensitive egg detection procedure than Kato-Katz method and other diagnostic tests like the point-of-care immunodiagnostic for detecting schistosome cathodic circulating antigen (POC-CCA) and Saline gradient [45,46]. Perhaps widely used of Helmintex in China is feasible and necessary. Fourthly, impact of water conservancy project on schistosomiasis control still remains controversial, due to many influencing factors such as water level, temperature, and plants change [47]. Lastly, environmental change, migration of population, and effectiveness of drug treatment could also influence the transmission of *S. japonicum*. Further investigations and effective long-term policies in controlling these factors are needed.

The main limitation of our study is that the two villages are both typical bottomland areas and cannot represent all types of epidemic areas. In addition, a comparative study of the two villages was only run from 1981 to 1984. Therefore, there is no comparison group afterwards. Moreover, the study used three different diagnostic methods: two slides Kato-Katz, indirect hemagglutination assay (IHA), and three slides Kato-Katz, however, infection rate tested by IHA cannot be adjusted with its sensitivity and specificity [10].

5. Conclusions

Our results demonstrated that Guichi district has implemented suitable schistosomiasis control strategies for the respective social circumstances in different periods. This study suggested that adjusting the control strategy in according to social, economic, and political changes is necessary and vital. Schistosomiasis control in Guichi district is one of the successful examples in schistosomiasis control over the past 40 years in China. It could provide valuable experience on future policy making not only for China, but also epidemic areas with similar social conditions around the world.

Author Contributions: L.L., Y.Z., and Q.J. participated in structuring this manuscript. T.W., S.Z. and G.C. collected the data. L.L. and Y.Z. analyzed the data and wrote the first draft. G.Z., N.H., Z.Z. and H.Y. provided advices for the subject of this manuscript. L.L., Y.Z., D.Y., Y.Y. (Ya Yang) and Y.Y. (Yu Yang) searched the scientific literature. L.L., Y.Z., Y.C. and Q.J. revised the manuscript. All authors contributed to, reviewed, and approved the final draft of the paper.

References

1.   Logan, O.T. A case of dysentery in hunan province caused by the trematode *Schistosoma japonicum*. *China Mission. Med. J.* **1905**, *19*, 243–245.

2.   WHO. Schistosomiasis. Different Type of Schistosome. Available online: https://www.who.int/ schistosomiasis/epidemiology/table3/en/ (accessed on 11 October 2018).

3.   King, C.H. Toward the elimination of schistosomiasis. *N. Engl. J. Med.* **2009**, *360*, 106–109. [CrossRef] [PubMed]

4.   Mao, S.P.; Shao, B.R. Schistosomiasis control in the People's Republic of China. *Am. J. Trop. Med. Hyg.* **1982**, *31*, 92–99. [CrossRef] [PubMed]

5.   Wang, L.; Utzinger, J.; Zhou, X.N. Schistosomiasis control: Experiences and lessons from China. *Lancet* **2008**, *372*, 1793–1795. [CrossRef]

6.   Zhou, X.N.; Wang, L.Y.; Chen, M.G.; Wu, X.H.; Jiang, Q.W.; Chen, X.Y.; Zheng, J.; Utzinger, J. The public health significance and control of schistosomiasis in China—Then and now. *Acta Trop.* **2005**, *96*, 97–105. [CrossRef]

7.   Warren, K.S.; Su, D.L.; Xu, Z.Y.; Yuan, H.C.; Peters, P.A.; Cook, J.A.; Mott, K.E.; Houser, H.B. Morbidity in schistosomiasis japonica in relation to intensity of infection. A study of two rural brigades in Anhui province, China. *N. Engl. J. Med.* **1983**, *309*, 1533–1539. [CrossRef]

8.   Qian, R.F.; Han, S.M.; Ke, Y.F. The epidemic situation of schistosomiasis in Guichi District, Chizhou City, in 2008–2012. *J. Trop. Dis. Parasitol.* **2014**, *12*, 108–110. (In Chinese)

9.   Katz, N.; Chaves, A.; Pellegrino, J. A simple device for quantitative stool thick-smear technique in schistosomiasis mansoni. *Rev. Inst. Med. Trop. Sao Paulo* **1972**, *14*, 397–400.

10.   Rogan, W.J.; Gladen, B. Estimating prevalence from the results of a screening test. *Am. J. Epidemiol.* **1978**, *107*, 71–76. [CrossRef]

11.   Lin, D.D.; Liu, J.X.; Liu, Y.M.; Hu, F.; Zhang, Y.Y.; Xu, J.M.; Li, J.Y.; Ji, M.J.; Bergquist, R.; Wu, G.L.; et al. Routine Kato-Katz technique underestimates the prevalence of *Schistosoma japonicum*: A case study in an endemic area of the People's Republic of China. *Parasitol. Int.* **2008**, *57*, 281–286. [CrossRef]

12.   Bosso, L.; Lacatena, F.; Varlese, R.; Nocerino, S.; Cristinzio, G.; Russo, D. Plant pathogens but not antagonists change in soil fungal communities across a land abandonment gradient in a mediterranean landscape. *Acta Oecol.* **2017**, *78*, 1–6. [CrossRef]

13.   Steinbaum, L.; Kwong, L.H.; Ercumen, A.; Negash, M.S.; Lovely, A.J.; Njenga, S.M.; Boehm, A.B.; Pickering, A.J.; Nelson, K.L. Detecting and enumerating soil-transmitted helminth eggs in soil: New method development and results from field testing in Kenya and Bangladesh. *PLoS Negl. Trop. Dis.* **2017**, *11*, e0005522. [CrossRef]

14.   Wang, L.D.; Chen, H.G.; Guo, J.G.; Zeng, X.J.; Hong, X.L.; Xiong, J.J.; Wu, X.H.; Wang, X.H.; Wang, L.Y.; Xia, G.; et al. A strategy to control transmission of *Schistosoma japonicum* in China. *N. Engl. J. Med.* **2009**, *360*, 121–128. [CrossRef] [PubMed]

15.   Katz, N.; Rocha, R.S.; Pereira, J.P. Schistosomiasis control in Peri-Peri (Minas Gerais, Brazil) by repeated clinical treatment and molluscicide application. *Rev. Inst. Med. Trop. Sao Paulo* **1980**, *22*, 85–93, 203–211.

16.   McCullough, F.S.; Gayral, P.; Duncan, J.; Christie, J.D. Molluscicides in schistosomiasis control. *Bull. World Health Organ.* **1980**, *58*, 681–689. [PubMed]

17.   Spear, R.C.; Seto, E.; Remais, J.; Carlton, E.J.; Davis, G.; Qiu, D.; Zhou, X.; Liang, S. Fighting waterborne infectious diseases. *Science* **2006**, *314*, 1081–1083. [CrossRef] [PubMed]

18.   WHO. *The Control of Schistosomiasis: Report of a WHO Expert Committee*; World Health Organization: Geneva, Switzerland, 1985.

19.   WHO. *The Control of Schistosomiasis: Second Report of the WHO Committee*; World Health Organization: Geneva, Switzerland, 1993.

20.   Bank, T.W. Project: Infectious and Endemic Disease Control Project. Available online: http://projects. worldbank.org/P003624/infectious-endemic-disease-control-project?lang=en (accessed on 10 May 2018).

21.   Utzinger, J.; Bergquist, R.; Shu-Hua, X.; Singer, B.H.; Tanner, M. Sustainable schistosomiasis control—The way forward. *Lancet* **2003**, *362*, 1932–1934. [CrossRef]

22. Chen, X.Y.; Wang, L.Y.; Cai, J.M.; Zhou, X.N.; Zheng, J.; Guo, J.G.; Wu, X.H.; Engels, D.; Chen, M.G. Schistosomiasis control in China: The impact of a 10-year world bank loan project (1992–2000). *Bull. World Health Organ.* **2005**, *83*, 43–48.

23. Wu, X.H.; Zhang, S.Q.; Xu, X.J.; Huang, Y.X.; Steinmann, P.; Utzinger, J.; Wang, T.P.; Xu, J.; Zheng, J.; Zhou, X.N. Effect of floods on the transmission of schistosomiasis in the Yangtze River valley, People's Republic of China. *Parasitol. Int.* **2008**, *57*, 271–276. [CrossRef]

24. Yang, G.J.; Liu, L.; Zhu, H.R.; Griffiths, S.M.; Tanner, M.; Bergquist, R.; Utzinger, J.; Zhou, X.N. China's sustained drive to eliminate neglected tropical diseases. *Lancet Infect. Dis.* **2014**, *14*, 881–892. [CrossRef]

25. Zhou, Y.B.; Zhao, G.M.; Jiang, Q.W. Effects of the praziquantel-based control of schistosomiasis japonica in China. *Ann. Trop. Med. Parasitol.* **2007**, *101*, 695–703. [CrossRef] [PubMed]

26. Zhou, X.N.; Wang, L.Y.; Chen, M.G.; Wang, T.P.; Guo, J.G.; Wu, X.H.; Jiang, Q.W.; Zheng, J.; Chen, X.Y. An economic evaluation of the national schistosomiasis control programme in China from 1992 to 2000. *Acta Trop.* **2005**, *96*, 255–265. [CrossRef]

27. Jiang, Q.W.; Wang, L.Y.; Guo, J.G.; Chen, M.G.; Zhou, X.N.; Engels, D. Morbidity control of schistosomiasis in China. *Acta Trop.* **2002**, *82*, 115–125.

28. Guo, J.G.; Cao, C.L.; Hu, G.H.; Lin, H.; Li, D.; Zhu, R.; Xu, J. The role of 'passive chemotherapy' plus health education for schistosomiasis control in China during maintenance and consolidation phase. *Acta Trop.* **2005**, *96*, 177–183. [CrossRef] [PubMed]

29. Zhou, X.N.; Jiang, Q.W.; Wang, T.P.; Lin, D.D.; Wu, X.H. Status and strategy for research development of schistosomiasis control in China. *Chin. J. Schistosomiasis Control* **2005**, *17*, 1–3.

30. Zhou, Y.B.; Liang, S.; Chen, G.X.; Rea, C.; He, Z.G.; Zhang, Z.J.; Wei, J.G.; Zhao, G.M.; Jiang, Q.W. An integrated strategy for transmission control of *Schistosoma japonicum* in a marshland area of China: Findings from a five-year longitudinal survey and mathematical modeling. *Am. J. Trop. Med. Hyg.* **2011**, *85*, 83–88. [CrossRef] [PubMed]

31. Liu, R.; Dong, H.F.; Jiang, M.S. The new national integrated strategy emphasizing infection sources control for schistosomiasis control in China has made remarkable achievements. *Parasitol. Res.* **2013**, *112*, 1483–1491. [CrossRef] [PubMed]

32. Yang, Y.; Zhou, Y.B.; Song, X.X.; Li, S.Z.; Zhong, B.; Wang, T.P.; Bergquist, R.; Zhou, X.N.; Jiang, Q.W. Integrated control strategy of schistosomiasis in the People's Republic of China: Projects involving agriculture, water conservancy, forestry, sanitation and environmental modification. *Adv. Parasitol.* **2016**, *92*, 237–268.

33. Zhang, Z.; Zhu, R.; Ward, M.P.; Xu, W.; Zhang, L.; Guo, J.; Zhao, F.; Jiang, Q. Long-term impact of the world bank loan project for schistosomiasis control: A comparison of the spatial distribution of schistosomiasis risk in China. *PLoS Negl. Trop. Dis.* **2012**, *6*, e1620. [CrossRef]

34. Zhang, S.Q.; Sun, C.S.; Wang, M.; Lin, D.D.; Zhou, X.N.; Wang, T.P. Epidemiological features and effectiveness of schistosomiasis control programme in lake and marshland region in the People's Republic of China. *Adv. Parasitol.* **2016**, *92*, 39–71.

35. Sun, L.P.; Wang, W.; Hong, Q.B.; Li, S.Z.; Liang, Y.S.; Yang, H.T.; Zhou, X.N. Approaches being used in the national schistosomiasis elimination programme in China: A review. *Infect. Dis. Poverty* **2017**, *6*, 55. [CrossRef] [PubMed]

36. Sun, L.P.; Wang, W.; Zuo, Y.P.; Zhang, Z.Q.; Hong, Q.B.; Yang, G.J.; Zhu, H.R.; Liang, Y.S.; Yang, H.T. An integrated environmental improvement of marshlands: Impact on control and elimination of schistosomiasis in marshland regions along the Yangtze River, China. *Infect. Dis. Poverty* **2017**, *6*, 72. [CrossRef]

37. Wang, X.; Wang, W.; Wang, P. Long-term effectiveness of the integrated schistosomiasis control strategy with emphasis on infectious source control in China: A 10-year evaluation from 2005 to 2014. *Parasitol. Res.* **2017**, *116*, 521–528. [CrossRef] [PubMed]

38. Zhou, X.N.; Jiang, T.W.; Guo, J.G.; Wang, L.Y.; Jiang, Q.W. Project management model and its evolution in schistosomiasis control programme of China. *Chin. J. Schistosomiasis Control* **2010**, *22*, 1–4.

39. Wang, L.D.; Guo, J.G.; Wu, X.H.; Chen, H.G.; Wang, T.P.; Zhu, S.P.; Zhang, Z.H.; Steinmann, P.; Yang, G.J.; Wang, S.P.; et al. China's new strategy to block *Schistosoma japonicum* transmission: Experiences and impact beyond schistosomiasis. *Trop. Med. Int. Health* **2009**, *14*, 1475–1483. [CrossRef] [PubMed]

40. Lu, D.B.; Wang, T.P.; Rudge, J.W.; Donnelly, C.A.; Fang, G.R.; Webster, J.P. Contrasting reservoirs for *Schistosoma japonicum* between marshland and hilly regions in Anhui, China—A two-year longitudinal parasitological survey. *Parasitology* **2010**, *137*, 99–110. [CrossRef]

41. Colley, D.G.; Bustinduy, A.L.; Secor, W.E.; King, C.H. Human schistosomiasis. *Lancet* **2014**, *383*, 2253–2264. [CrossRef]

42. Zhou, Y.B.; Liang, S.; Jiang, Q.W. Factors impacting on progress towards elimination of transmission of schistosomiasis japonica in China. *Parasit. Vectors* **2012**, *5*, 275. [CrossRef]

43. Zhou, Y.B.; Yang, M.X.; Wang, Q.Z.; Zhao, G.M.; Wei, J.G.; Peng, W.X.; Jiang, Q.W. Field comparison of immunodiagnostic and parasitological techniques for the detection of schistosomiasis japonica in the People's Republic of China. *Am. J. Trop. Med. Hyg.* **2007**, *76*, 1138–1143. [CrossRef]

44. Wang, W.; Dai, J.R.; Liang, Y.S. Apropos: Factors impacting on progress towards elimination of transmission of schistosomiasis japonica in China. *Parasit. Vectors* **2014**, *7*, 408. [CrossRef]

45. Lindholz, C.G.; Favero, V.; Verissimo, C.M.; Candido, R.R.F.; de Souza, R.P.; Dos Santos, R.R.; Morassutti, A.L.; Bittencourt, H.R.; Jones, M.K.; St Pierre, T.G.; et al. Study of diagnostic accuracy of Helmintex, Kato-Katz, and POC-CCA methods for diagnosing intestinal schistosomiasis in Candeal, a low intensity transmission area in northeastern Brazil. *PLoS Negl. Trop. Dis.* **2018**, *12*, e0006274. [CrossRef]

46. Oliveira, W.J.; Magalhaes, F.D.C.; Elias, A.M.S.; de Castro, V.N.; Favero, V.; Lindholz, C.G.; Oliveira, A.A.; Barbosa, F.S.; Gil, F.; Gomes, M.A.; et al. Evaluation of diagnostic methods for the detection of intestinal schistosomiasis in endemic areas with low parasite loads: Saline gradient, Helmintex, Kato-Katz and rapid urine test. *PLoS Negl. Trop. Dis.* **2018**, *12*, e0006232. [CrossRef] [PubMed]

47. Steinmann, P.; Keiser, J.; Bos, R.; Tanner, M.; Utzinger, J. Schistosomiasis and water resources development: Systematic review, meta-analysis, and estimates of people at risk. *Lancet Infect. Dis.* **2006**, *6*, 411–425. [CrossRef]

2

Currently Available Monitoring and Surveillance Systems for *Taenia* spp., *Echinococcus* spp., *Schistosoma* spp. and Soil-Transmitted Helminths at the Control/Elimination Stage

Ganna Saelens * and Sarah Gabriël🄳

Department of Veterinary Public Health and Food Safety, Faculty of Veterinary Medicine, Ghent University, Merelbeke B-9820, Belgium; sarah.gabriel@ugent.be
* Correspondence: ganna.saelens@ugent.be

Abstract: An increasing global focus on neglected tropical diseases (NTDs) has resulted in the set up of numerous control and elimination activities worldwide. This is partly true for *Taenia solium* taeniasis/cysticercosis, the most important foodborne parasitic infection. Despite substantial progress, adequate monitoring and surveillance (M&S) are required to sustain a status of control/elimination. This is often lacking, especially for *T. solium*. Therefore, the objective was to conduct a systematic literature review of the currently available M&S systems at the control/elimination stage of the four top-ranked helminth NTDs. Specifically, *Taenia* spp., *Echinococcus* spp., *Schistosoma* spp., and soil-transmitted helminths (STHs) were considered to determine if there are any similarities between their M&S systems and whether certain approaches can be adopted from each other. The systematic review demonstrated that rigorous M&S systems have been designed for the control/elimination stage of both STHs and schistosomiasis, particularly in China. On the other hand, a concept of M&S for *Taenia* spp. and *Echinococcus* spp. has not been fully developed yet, due to a lack of epidemiological data and the fact that many endemic countries are far away from reaching control/elimination. Moreover, accurate diagnostic tools for all four diseases are still imperfect, which complicates proper M&S. Finally, there is an urgent need to develop and harmonize/standardize M&S activities in order to reliably determine and compare the epidemiological situation worldwide.

Keywords: neglected tropical diseases; monitoring and surveillance; helminth zoonoses; *Taenia* spp.; *Echinococcus* spp.; *Schistosoma* spp.; soil-transmitted helminths

1. Introduction

Neglected tropical diseases (NTDs) currently pose significant health risks to more than one billion people worldwide and cause substantial economic losses in the health and food sectors. They are traditionally believed to affect populations of developing countries with limited adequate sanitation and close contact with livestock; however, their frequencies are rising in developed, urban areas due to the influx of immigrants and increase in travel. As a result, tropical diseases have been increasingly subjected to integrated control activities in the past century, particularly in developing countries [1]. *Taenia solium*, for instance, is an NTD ranked first on the global scale of parasitic foodborne diseases with an estimated 2.5 million people all over the world carrying this pork tapeworm and 50 million people being infected with *T. solium* cysticerci [2]. Although substantial progress has been made in combating this helminthic zoonosis, it is often difficult to sustain control or elimination without adequate monitoring and surveillance (M&S) [3]. The M&S systems, although pivotal, are usually lacking in the case of *T. solium* [4]. Therefore, a first objective was to conduct a systematic review on the currently available M&S systems at the control/elimination stage of *T. solium*. Given the deficiency of these systems for *T. solium*, the review also covered the beef tapeworm *Taenia saginata* due to its close taxonomic relationship with *T. solium*. Although *T. saginata* infection is not considered an NTD, it was included to determine if there are any similarities between their M&S systems and whether certain approaches can be adopted from each other. Finally, given that the outcome for both the *Taenia* spp. was low, three other top-ranked helminthic NTDs (caused by *Echinococcus* spp., *Schistosoma* spp., and soil-transmitted helminths (STHs)) were added to look for any parallels in their M&S systems.

Before comparing the different M&S systems of *Taenia* spp., *Echinococcus* spp., *Schistosoma* spp., and STHs, it is essential to define and distinguish some epidemiological concepts for M&S data collection and management. Disease monitoring refers to the ongoing efforts of collecting, analyzing, and distributing all possible data about health, disease, and their determinants in a given population over a defined period of time [5]. Monitoring a control program, on the other hand, refers to the process of collecting and analyzing information about the effect of an intervention on the health status of a given population or environment. In other words, it ensures that the implemented interventions are effective and efficient, and is particularly important at the control stage of a disease. Monitoring is often paired with evaluation; the process that attempts to determine as systematically and objectively as possible the relevance, effectiveness, and impact of the intervention programs [6]. Although surveillance consists of a set of monitoring systems, both terms should not be confused. Specifically, disease surveillance is a more active system that only collects a minimal set of essential, spatiotemporal data designed in a way that some form of directed action can be taken whenever the data passes a certain threshold value. For instance, an effective surveillance system at the elimination stage of a disease entails the rapid detection of remaining or re-emerging pockets of transmission, the detection of possible drug resistance, the identification of low transmission/risk areas, and the comprehension of patterns in disease epidemiology (e.g., shifts in age and seasonality) [7]. In sum, when reaching the final crucial stage of transition from general disease control to effective elimination, a shift from comprehensive monitoring and evaluation for measuring morbidity and mortality toward a rigorous surveillance is required. In other words, the choice of approach depends on the stage of control/elimination achieved [2].

Given the lack of implemented M&S systems for *T. solium* and their crucial role in the sustainment of control/elimination after the implementation of control interventions, the general objective of this systematic literature review was to collect and summarize records from English scientific literature on the currently available M&S systems for *Taenia* spp., *Echinococcus* spp., *Schistosoma* spp., and STHs at the control/elimination stage. A first objective was to identify and collect data by using a combination of search terms and key elements in five search engines. A second objective was to retrieve the records relevant to this systematic review through three screening phases. A final objective was to extract and summarize specific information from the selected records in order to obtain a full picture on the existing M&S systems at the control/elimination stage. Additionally, existing gaps in these systems were identified in order to determine potential needs for improvement. In this way, this review may contribute to the establishment of rigorous M&S systems for future NTDs interventions, especially in the case of *T. solium*.

2. Methods

2.1. Review Question, Search Literature, and Literature Sources

'What are the currently available M&S systems at the control/elimination stage of four selected NTDs caused by the following parasites: *Taenia* spp., *Schistosoma* spp., *Echinococcus* spp., and STHs?'

This systematic literature review was conducted by implementing the PRISMA (Preferred Reporting Items for Systematic review and Meta-Analysis) guidelines [8]. A completed PRISMA checklist is included in the Supplementary Material to this article. Five search engines (PubMed, Web of Science, ScienceDirect, Google Scholar, and Google Search) were used to identify articles and five domains were included in this search, each with their own key elements: *Taenia* spp. (*Taenia solium* or *Taenia saginata* or tapeworm or taeniosis or taeniasis or cysticercosis), *Schistosoma* spp. (schistosome or schistosomiasis or bilharzia or bilharziasis), *Echinococcus* spp. (or echinococcosis), STHs (soil-transmitted helminths or soil-transmitted helminthiasis), and surveillance and monitoring (survey or surveil or monitor). Search terms and key elements were combined using the Boolean operators (AND, OR, NOT) resulting in the following search algorithms:

- (*Taenia solium* OR *Taenia saginata* OR tapeworm OR taeniosis OR taeniasis OR cysticercosis) AND (surveillance OR surveil OR survey OR monitoring OR monitor).
- (*Schistosoma* OR schistosome OR bilharzia OR bilharziasis) AND (surveillance OR surveil OR survey OR monitoring OR monitor).
- (*Echinococcus* OR echinococcosis) AND (surveillance OR surveil OR survey OR monitoring OR monitor).
- (STHs OR soil-transmitted helminths OR soil-transmitted helminthiasis) AND (surveillance OR surveil OR survey OR monitoring OR monitor).

2.2. Study Selection

The records included for this literature review were retrieved through three screening phases. The first screening removed duplicates (titles) after merging the results obtained from the different literature sources. A second screening phase evaluated titles and abstracts regarding the relevance to the study question, while the last phase was applied to the full texts. Four exclusion criteria were applied on the second screening phase: (i) articles written before 2004, (ii) articles not available in English, (iii) articles not containing at least one of the five domains in their titles, and (iv) articles with no available full text. The main reasons for exclusion in the last screening phase were mentioning the need for M&S and the description of M&S in general rather than at the control/elimination stage.

The final selected articles were first categorized by parasite (*Schistosoma* spp., STHs, *Taenia* spp., *Echinococcus* spp., and combinations). Next, records from each category were ordered by topic: M&S field studies, theory about M&S, purely diagnostic matter, and application of spatial technology. The last two topics are briefly discussed at the end of this review, considering the major role of diagnostic tools and spatial technology with regard to M&S.

From the final selected articles, the following data were extracted: name of parasite discussed, the timeframe, the country or region, the method of M&S, the existing gaps in the systems, and potential solutions (if any).

3. Results/Discussion

The literature search identified a total of 377 records (149 by PubMed, 108 by Web of Science, 73 by ScienceDirect, 43 by Google Scholar, and 4 by Google Search). Eighty duplicates were removed after the first screening and 62 records were removed after the second screening. A substantial number ($n = 137$) of the articles thus obtained were subsequently removed as they did not discuss M&S at the control/elimination stage, which could only be detected during the last screening of the full texts. A total of 98 articles were retained for this systematic literature review (Figure 1). The majority of the remaining records discussed post-control/elimination M&S with regard to *Schistosoma* spp. and STHs (30 and 24 records, respectively), while only 10 and 11 records discussed post-control/elimination M&S with regard to *Echinococcus* spp. and *Taenia* spp., respectively. Finally, 23 records discussed post-control/elimination M&S with regard to a combination of two or more of these NTDs.

Figure 1. PRISMA (Preferred Reporting Items for Systematic review and Meta-Analysis) flowchart diagram of the record selection process.

3.1. *Schistosoma* spp.

3.1.1. Introduction

Schistosomiasis is a parasitic, zoonotic disease caused by infection with the trematode genus *Schistosoma*. Three species are mainly accountable for public health problems worldwide: *Schistosoma mansoni*, *Schistosoma haematobium*, and *Schistosoma japonicum*. Infection results from contact with water contaminated with free-swimming cercariae that are shed from intermediate snail hosts. Subsequently, the rapid onset of acute schistosomiasis with symptoms, such as high fever, myalgia and eosinophilia, is triggered by the migration of the parasite in the body. Furthermore, a chronic schistosome infection may lead to long-term complications, such as portal hypertension, anemia, bladder cancer, and kidney failure. Additionally, various animals, such as cattle, dogs, cats, pigs, horses, and rodents, may serve as reservoir hosts for *S. japonicum* [9].

The disease represents a worldwide health problem with approximately 240 million people being infected and nearly 800 million people believed to be at risk. Nevertheless, substantial progress in reducing the burden of schistosomiasis in many countries has been achieved due to the extensive implementation of large-scale control interventions. A pioneer in the control and elimination of *S. japonicum* is the People's Republic of China (PRC) with its strong political commitment and efficient control efforts. With a variety of approaches developed over the past two decades, such as chemotherapy, snail control, health education, improved sanitation, and access to safe water, the PRC aims to achieve nationwide transmission interruption by 2020 and disease elimination by 2025 [10]. In fact, due to the implementation of these control measurements in a national schistosomiasis prevention and control plan, transmission control and interruption (i.e., elimination) have already been achieved in 135 and 313 counties, respectively. In order to sustain these accomplishments, an overall surveillance and consolidation work has been unfolded in the PRC. Therefore, the outcome of the literature search included many records regarding successful M&S systems for *S. japonicum* designed by the PRC. Finally, two records were on monitoring systems in Egypt, a country that is currently on track for complete elimination of *S. mansoni* schistosomiasis.

The scope and design of M&S systems for *Schistosoma* spp. depend on whether the stage of transmission control or transmission interruption has been reached so far. In case of control status, the emphasis is on the monitoring of local residents and livestock (i.e., identification and treatment of patients and livestock with schistosomiasis), suspected snail infestations, and factors associated with schistosomiasis. On the other hand, in case of transmission interruption, the major surveillance tasks are the detection of snails and the follow-up of risk factors and imported infection sources. Furthermore, to remain successful in the long-term, this surveillance needs to be followed by an appropriate and immediate response system at any sign of resurgence of transmission in areas where disease elimination had been declared (e.g., treatment of positive cases, examination of contact persons, and focal mollusciciding of identified freshwater bodies) [11,12].

In sum, the M&S indicators for schistosomiasis include the following: schistosomiasis cases (acute, chronic, and advanced), intermediate snail hosts (their habitat, density, and infection rate), and related epidemic factors (water level, rainfall, temperature, lifestyle of the population, and implementation of control measures). An additional indicator for *S. japonicum* is livestock as a reservoir host (i.e., mainly cattle, but also sheep, pigs, and horses). A thorough and consistent M&S system should consequently take into account each of these indicators and should be robust under spatial and temporal fluctuations. Nevertheless, some records describe a system that solely includes one or two of these indicators. Therefore, this review will first discuss each surveillance indicator separately and finally end with the records describing a combination of these indicators (Table 1).

Table 1. Summary of records describing monitoring and surveillance systems for *Schistosoma* spp. at the control/elimination stage.

Schistosoma Species	Monitoring & Surveillance (M&S) System	Time	Country	Reference
S. mansoni	Malacological survey to determine dispersal: Capture and identification of snails in a radius of 2 m at 168 selected sites, linked to data collection and analysis of water/sediment samples; landscape and climate data.	2016–2017	China	[13]
S. japonicum	Surveillance for human schistosomiasis cases: Continuous surveillance of advanced human cases in addition to immunological testing of villagers at risk and suspected patients.	1995–2002	China	[14]
All *Schistosoma* spp.	M&S for human schistosomiasis cases: Reporting of both acute and chronic cases of schistosomiasis diagnosed in hospitals to the National Infectious Diseases Reporting System by all levels of medical institutions.	1989–... [1]	China	[15]
All *Schistosoma* spp.	M&S for human schistosomiasis cases: Self-selected data entry of schistosomiasis cases in the TropNetEurop [2] database.	1999–... [1]	Europe	[16]
S. japonicum	M&S of livestock: selective treatment or isolation of the infected animal reservoir (i.e., cattle, water buffalo, goats, sheep, pigs, and dogs) to prevent further contamination of the environment.	Not yet implemented	NA	[17]
S. japonicum	M&S of *Schistosoma*-infected water using sentinel mice in cages on the water surface.	2008–... [1]	China	[18,19]
S. japonicum	M&S of *Schistosoma*-infected water: Detection of contaminated water with environmental qPCR.	2016	Madagascar	[20]
S. japonicum	National sentinel surveillance system: Surveillance of humans, cattle, and snails in 20–458 sentinel sites across the country. Treatment of positive humans and cattle, regular re-examination of advanced cases, and focal mollusciciding. Since 2015, additional water bodies and environmental surveillance (i.e., examination of wildlife feces) have been added.	1989–... [1]	China	[15,19,21,22]
S. japonicum	Provincial surveillance system (5 provinces): Surveillance of snails (frequency determined on absence/presence in the past 3–15 years). If snails were found, surveillance of humans and bovines, and treatment with praziquantel (PZQ) when positive.	1985–1995	China	[23]
S. japonicum	Routine surveys across the country: Case reports and surveys of human patients in addition to regular M&S of endemic villages (humans, snails, bovines, and other mammalian intermediate hosts) that achieved control and elimination.	2005–... [1]	China	[15,22]
S. japonicum	Risk surveillance of humans, water, free-roaming livestock, and snails based on results from previous routine surveillance.	2008–... [1]	China	[15,24,25]
S. mansoni	National elimination plan based on a monitoring and treatment system: Re-mapping residual schistosomiasis distribution in every governorate of the country with an additional mass treatment (with PZQ) policy based on the prevalence outcome. Additionally, application of molluscicides and treatment of water bodies regardless of the outcome.	2017–... [1]	Egypt	[26,27]

[1] Still ongoing, [2] The European Network on Imported Infectious Diseases Surveillance.

3.1.2. Surveillance of the Snail Intermediate Host

Considering that the transmission of schistosomiasis is particularly determined by the existence and geographic distribution of its intermediate snail host, it is crucial to determine and pursue the spatial distribution, habitat, and infection rate of these snails. Many ecological and environmental factors, such as light, water, temperature, and aquatic vegetation, may influence this distribution. Furthermore, it must be noted that each *Schistosoma* species has its own snail species as the intermediate host. In order to know if and where a suitable intermediate host is present, snail sampling at several study sites across the country should be conducted. An illustration of this is the malacological survey of *Biomphalaria straminea*, the intermediate host of *S. mansoni*, to determine its dispersal in the Guangdong province (China), where schistosomiasis has been eliminated (Figure 2). At 186 sites that were selected based on the presence of aquatic habitats and the existence of the snail species according to previous studies, snails in a radius of 2 m were captured, labeled, and anatomically identified in a laboratory. Furthermore, water and sediment samples in addition to landscape and climatic data from the study sites were collected and analyzed in order to estimate the relationship between the presence of *B. straminea* and environmental and physicochemical variables. This survey revealed the wide distribution of this snail and a correlation with water temperature and physicochemical properties of sediments (i.e., sediment zinc and water temperature were higher in places with *B. straminea*), meaning

Figure 2. Timeline of different, parallel schistosomiasis surveillance systems in the People's Republic of China with each of their surveillance indicators. TIP, transmission-interrupted province; TCP, transmission-controlled province; H, human surveillance; C, cattle surveillance; S, snail surveillance; M, other mammalian intermediate hosts surveillance (e.g., dogs); W, water bodies surveillance; E, environmental surveillance.

3.1.3. Monitoring and Surveillance for Human Schistosomiasis Cases

As indicated above, a surveillance system of the human population needs to be put in place when achieving the criteria for transmission interruption in order to prevent re-emergence. A first example of such a system is the one established in the Zhejiang province (China), a formerly highly endemic area for *S. japonicum* where elimination was achieved in 1995 after 40 years of intensive control measures. Here, villagers at risk (i.e., people living in areas still infested with the *Oncomelania* snail host, children under 14 years, people returning from schistosome-endemic areas, and boat dwellers) and suspected patients (i.e., people with symptoms of hepatic fibrosis, portal hypertension, and splenomegaly) were screened for *S. japonicum* using immunological diagnostic tests. When these were found to be positive, fecal examination with the Kato-Katz (KK) technique was followed. In case *S. japonicum* eggs were detected in the fecal samples, the patient was treated with praziquantel (PZQ) and regularly re-examined until complete cure (i.e., negative fecal examination). Additionally, advanced cases of schistosomiasis were continuously subjected to supervision and surveillance (i.e., liver function tests, laboratory examination, and health check-ups). Seven years post-transmission and after 621,431 serological screenings, the system only identified two patients between 1995 and 2002 with both the immunological tests and fecal examination. Although this had proved to be a very effective and recommended surveillance system to be pursued in the years to come, one limitation must be mentioned. Namely, out of all the 621,431 serological tests, an overall positive rate of 2.9% was found, while only two of them were positive when subjected to fecal examination. This demonstrates that the immunological processes in the host's body do not halt when the parasite is eliminated and therefore, might give false positive results. In conclusion, this surveillance system has the potential to be cost-effective; however, it warrants further research into more sensitive and specific diagnostic tools [14]. Further detailed description and incorporation of human surveillance efforts in an integrated surveillance system will be discussed below (Section 3.1.6).

A second example of M&S of humans is the establishment of the National Infectious Disease Reporting System (NIDRS) by the Centers of Disease Control and Prevention (CDC) in 1950. This system covers at present 39 infectious diseases, among them schistosomiasis, and its use was mandated by law in 1989 in the PRC (Figure 2). In this country, all levels of the staff of medical institutions are required to report both acute and chronic cases of schistosomiasis diagnosed in hospitals to the NIDRS. Contents of this report system include name, age, gender, address, contact information, occupation, history of treatment, time of diagnosis, diagnostic results, clinical symptoms, characteristics of infection site, and case classification. This reporting system not only helps the development of appropriate prevention and control programs, but is also crucial to reveal national patterns of disease transmission. Nevertheless, disparities in clinical resources (e.g., diagnostic capabilities, presence of computers, and network coverage) may result in disproportional reporting across the country [15].

A similar system was established in Europe in 1999. Due to an increasing number of immigrants, in addition to changing travel patterns, the European Network on Imported Infectious Disease Surveillance (TropNetEurop) was founded in order to facilitate a better understanding of the epidemiology of imported schistosomiasis and to improve pretravel advice. Every patient with a diagnosis of schistosomiasis is reported to TropNetEurop and further classified according to patient characteristics (immigrants, refugees, business travelers, etc.) and reason for travel. Next, individual data are stored in a database which offers a unique tool to monitor changes and to function as an early warning system. Nevertheless, schistosomiasis is a non-notifiable disease in Europe, making data entry self-selected. This inevitably results in underreporting and therefore, this network cannot provide representative data throughout Europe [16].

3.1.4. Monitoring and Surveillance of Livestock

In working from control toward the elimination of zoonotic schistosomiasis, surveillance of the animal reservoir (i.e., cattle, water buffalo, goats, sheep, pigs, and dogs) should also be included in elimination guidelines, considering that they often share the same water points. As such, cattle can infect snails present in water points used by humans, where people can then get infected. As a response, selective treatment or isolation of the infected animals has been proposed as a practical approach to prevent further contamination of the environment [17]; however, these treated animals will most likely just drink from the infected water again and/or work in infected rice fields. Therefore, an M&S system solely including livestock is not expected to be very efficient. Specifically, it should be incorporated in an integrated surveillance system which will be discussed below (Section 3.1.6).

3.1.5. Monitoring and Surveillance of *Schistosoma*-Infected Water

Another important surveillance measure is to detect water sources contaminated with miracidia and cercariae. For the detection of *S. japonicum*-infested water, an intelligent device with sentinel mice was developed. Sentinel mice are left in cages on the water surface in a way that their abdomen and tail are exposed to the water for four hours a day, two days in a month, for four months. To allow maturation of any infecting schistosome, 35 days after the last exposure, the mice are killed and dissected for the presence of eggs in the liver or worms in the portal and mesenteric veins. Although, this device has played a critical role in the surveillance of schistosomiasis in China, it is rather time-consuming and impractical on a large-scale, and poses obvious animal welfare questions. For instance, a study mentioned a 10% loss of the mice due to cages floating away and mice accidentally drowning or suffocating during feeding [18]. Furthermore, the morphology of cercariae from different species is nearly identical which makes determination at the species level without molecular tools extremely challenging, if not impossible [19]. As a result, McManus and colleagues (2018) suggested in 2018 the testing of water samples for environmental schistosome DNA to identify schistosomiasis transmission areas. A study on such a surveillance system had already been carried out in Madagascar in 2016 where an environmental DNA (eDNA) qPCR targeting one specific fragment of the *cox1* (cytochrome c oxidase subunit 1) mitochondrial gene from *S. mansoni* was developed. The results of this study indicated that this tool successfully detects *S. mansoni*-contaminated water. Furthermore, the greatest benefit of the eDNA method is the fact that it enables the collection of data from several sites within a short period of time due to the ease of collecting samples. Nevertheless, further assessment of its cost-effectiveness, potential adaptation to other *Schistosoma* species, and verification in other areas is necessary in the future. In addition, ways to differentiate between the presence of schistosome DNA and the presence of actual viable cercariae will have to be developed. Once established, the environmental qPCR could serve as a promising and feasible M&S tool [20].

3.1.6. Integrated Monitoring and Surveillance Systems for Schistosomiasis

The first integrated system of surveillance described here is a national sentinel surveillance system initiated in 1989 in China when elimination had already been reached in four provinces (Figure 2). It consisted of 20 sentinel sites dispersed over the entire country and representing the different eco-epidemiological settings. The prevalence and intensity of human infection were monitored over a 5-year period with repeated annual cross-sectional surveys and a response rate of 90%. On the other hand, the infection rate in cattle and snails was monitored longitudinally. The surveillance of human population concerned residents between 5 and 65 years of age and was executed in two different ways. The first method in 13 sites screened the people with serodiagnostic techniques (i.e., indirect hemagglutination assay (IHA) or enzyme-linked immunosorbent assay (ELISA)), while the presence of eggs in feces (i.e., the KK technique) confirmed a positive serological test. The second method in the seven remaining sites was based only on the KK technique and results were read by two laboratory technologists. In both the settings, acute and advanced cases of schistosomiasis were regularly examined and interviewed with a standardized questionnaire to reveal the spatial distribution and (environmental) risk factors. Additionally, any individual that tested positive on the KK technique was administered a single oral dose of PZQ. Subsequently, the surveillance of cattle in each of the sentinel sites occurred using the stool hatching method, while snails were collected during spring and autumn for microscopic examination and recording of various indices (i.e., habitat, density of living snails, density of infected snails, and snail infection rate). Chemotherapy with PZQ was implemented in infected livestock whenever cattle positive for schistosomiasis had been detected, and focal mollusciciding was applied in case snails had been found. At the same time, all the people and cattle in these areas were screened (and treated when positive) for schistosomiasis in case infected snails had been detected. Results from this system (between 2000 and 2003) confirmed that schistosomiasis had been successfully controlled in large areas of the PRC; however, infected snails were found in areas where transmission control had been declared [21]. As a result, China continued the ongoing efforts of snail monitoring and control, especially in areas deemed free from schistosomiasis. In 2005, the sentinel system even expanded to 80 sites across China with hilly areas now representing the most sentinel sites. Furthermore, in 2011, diagnostic protocols changed to multiple rounds of diagnoses with the addition of a miracidium hatch test on 30 g of human stool; and the coverage has extended to 458 sites, since 2014. In 2015, the examination of wildlife feces to detect environmental infection risks and the adoption of the loop-mediated isothermal amplification (LAMP) technology were further added. The latter is an effective and sensitive approach for the rapid extraction and amplification of snail genomic DNA to achieve early detection of *Schistosoma* spp. Contrary to microscopic diagnostics, prepatent snails can be discovered as of day one after exposure to miracidia with this test. Both the examination of wildlife feces and the LAMP assay are currently used to generate risk maps that can be applied to guide further local investigations and increase snail control activities in case infected snails are found [19]. In conclusion, this constantly adjusted sentinel system is still ongoing and represents the endemic status of an entire country due to consistent data collection and analysis. It must be noted that it is sometimes necessary to substitute sites in case a population exhibits fatigue from yearly surveys or when prevalence has decreased dramatically [22].

In 2005, Wu et al. described the results from a provincial surveillance system set up in five provinces of China (Fujian, Guangdong, Guangxi, Shanghai, and Zhejiang) with interrupted transmission from 1985 to 1995 (Figure 2). The frequency of snail surveys in formerly *Oncomelania hupensis*-ridden areas was determined by the absence or presence of snails in the past 3–15 years. In villages where snails had been found in the past 3 years, snail surveys were carried out annually. In villages where snails had been found in the past 3–9 years, snail surveys were carried out once every 3 years. In villages where snails had been found in the previous 10–15 years, snail surveys were carried out once every 5 years. Finally, in villages where no snails had been found in the past 15 years, snail surveys were not carried out regularly (i.e., not planned). Additionally, regular snail surveys were carried out in waterways connected with neighboring *O. hupensis*-infested areas, areas where water plants are bred, docking areas with boats, and areas with domestic animals having access to snail-infested areas. In case snails were found, all humans older than seven years and all bovines in these areas were screened first with IHA or ELISA and subsequently, in case of a positive serological test, examined with the KK technique for the presence of eggs in their stool. PZQ was administered to those with one or two positive results. Furthermore, migrants from endemic areas and suspected schistosomiasis cases (i.e., people with fever of unknown cause, symptoms of hepatosplenomegaly, and mucous or bloody stool) were submitted to either one or both of the abovementioned tests and treated with PZQ if they tested positive, and their medical history was traced. The results in 2002 demonstrated that the great achievement of disease elimination had been sustained, with only three human cases being detected since 1992. Nevertheless, as was concluded from the abovementioned national surveillance system, residual snails still existed in areas in close proximity to endemic areas and therefore, China carried on snail surveillance and control [23].

Third, routine surveys are another category of surveillance system, that began in the PRC in 2005, which includes case reports and case surveys across the country (Figure 2). Additionally, routine surveys on human and mammalian hosts in seven endemic provinces are conducted over the course of two or more years depending on the transmission status (control or elimination). At first, case reports and case surveys comprise the reporting and investigation of a schistosomiasis case within 24 h after diagnosis through NIDRS established by the CDC (Section 3.1.3), including detailed information of the case (e.g., name, age, gender, address, contact information, and occupation). Secondly, for counties from endemic provinces that achieved control and elimination, all villages are currently surveyed over a three-year period and five-year period, respectively. An exception is made for villages where information is shared from the national sentinel surveillance system. The routine surveillance involves sampling of humans (>90% of residents between 6 and 65 years old), sampling of cattle and other alternative mammalian hosts, and snail surveys in the spring. Although routine surveys provide spatial and temporal data on infection patterns, some challenges present in the national and provincial surveillance systems still need to be overcome. At first, variations were noted in sampling and screening protocols (although they were standardized by the Ministry of Health) leading to difficult comparison of data between counties. Secondly, survey efforts of the mammalian host are the responsibility of the local animal husbandry department; however, coordination between them and the public health authorities was highly inconstant. At last, participation fatigue often occurred, although this was resolved by the conduction of health education campaigns emphasizing the consequences of chronic, undetected infections and the importance of routine examinations [15,22].

A final category of surveillance is consolidated surveillance in areas where schistosomiasis has been eliminated, but where a risk of re-emergence is plausible, i.e., risk surveillance (Figure 2). The choice of risk surveillance sites relies on results from previous routine surveillance and the availability of local capacity to carry out surveillance. Risk surveillance mainly focuses on the survey of infected water with sentinel mice (see Section 3.1.5), snail investigations, human case detection, and free-roaming livestock surveillance [15]. An example of this is the risk survey conducted between 2008 and 2010 in four counties of three at-risk provinces (Jiangsu, Shandong, and Anhui) in China. Local residents aged between 6 and 65 years were serologically tested using IHA and subjected to fecal examination by KK for confirmation in case of a positive result. Snail surveillance included the capture of snail in frames placed along study sites connected to water bodies and the active search for snails in environments with mobile populations, ships, or plant matter in the water. At last, 30 farms per sentinel site were selected for survey on their livestock and dogs with the miracidium hatch method. During this survey, no snails or positive animals were found, yet 22 positive human cases were confirmed—all of them fishermen, boatmen, or immigrants (i.e., mobile population) [24]. A similar risk surveillance held between 2008 and 2012 also detected 28 positive cases in the mobile population, while no snails were found and neither local nor imported livestock was found to be infected [25]. Both of these results emphasize the important contribution of mobile population to the transmission of schistosomiasis and the importance of monitoring them.

In brief, the PRC is one of the pioneers in the control and elimination of schistosomiasis with sustained M&S taking place in different parallel systems across the country (Figure 2). Therefore, the epidemiology of schistosomiasis has shifted over time and place, as did interventions and strategies. Surveillance systems should now prioritize more the identification of remaining and/or re-emerging hot spots and the evaluation of underlying risk factors and their relation to transmission patterns. In the meantime, China's acquired experience with M&S and knowledge on diagnostic tools and techniques has the potential to be transferred to endemic countries with limited resources.

3.1.7. Monitoring and Surveillance for *Schistosoma mansoni* in Egypt

Another pioneer in the control and elimination of schistosomiasis is Egypt, due to its effective monitoring and treatment system. In 2017, this country started a national schistosomiasis elimination plan supported by the World Health Organization after 5000 years of endemicity. Since the implementation of different control strategies in 1922, schistosomiasis (*S. mansoni*) prevalence had substantially decreased to 0.2% in 2016 in most of the endemic areas. The first step from this 2016 control stage to elimination included the re-mapping of residual distribution of schistosomiasis in all endemic governorates using both the KK technique and a urine circulating cathodic antigen (CCA) test [26]. So far, 35 districts of 5 governorates have been re-mapped, while the survey of other governorates is still ongoing. Specifically, a number of schools in rural areas of the districts of each governorate were selected to provide urine and stool samples. These were collected from 100 children per school and tested for schistosomiasis with the KK technique and CCA test. Based on the outcome of the prevalence, a mass treatment policy with PZQ was implemented (i.e., (i) mass drug administration (MDA) of school children in districts with KK = 0% and CCA > 0%, (ii) MDA of all villages in districts with KK > 0% and <3% and CCA > 0%, and (iii) MDA of all rural areas in districts with KK ≥ 3% and CCA > 0%). Additionally, mass treatment of areas included the application of molluscicides and the treatment of water bodies. Further monitoring and treatment of the other governorates will enable the mapping of residual infected areas and the achievement of nationwide elimination of the parasite [27]. Although this represents an efficient system for achieving elimination as well as monitoring at the post-control stage, it must be emphasized that a rigorous post-intervention surveillance system will have to be established to maintain this elimination status. The surveillance system should specifically focus on high-risk areas/individuals, include continuous monitoring of the intermediate snail host and people, and finally, comprise an appropriate response procedure in case infected individuals/snails are found.

3.1.8. Future Challenges and Recommendations for Schistosomiasis

Although mostly occurring in developing countries, the geographical range of schistosomiasis is also spreading toward the Western world due to an increasing number of immigrants and changing pattern of travelers. Specifically, migrants/travelers who acquired the infection externally might in turn introduce local transmission of schistosomiasis in case a suitable intermediate snail host is present in non-endemic areas (e.g., Western Europe, but also in non-endemic areas in China). At the same time, a large proportion of infected people returning/migrating from *Schistosoma*-endemic areas are asymptomatic, which facilitates local transmission introduction even more [28]. Therefore, surveillance and intervention of migrants should be included and strengthened in any schistosomiasis control program, as they may form a new source of infection in non-endemic areas or areas where transmission had been controlled or even eliminated. For example, the results of a study conducted in the endemic Dongting Lake region of China demonstrated a schistosomiasis prevalence rate twice as high in immigrants as in permanent residents. These infected immigrants may move to areas where transmission control/interruption has been achieved, but where snails are still present. This may result in the re-emergence of transmission in these areas given that migration was not a feature of the national control program [29]. Consequently, surveillance systems are to be adjusted to migrants and travelers, for instance, by examination and treatment after water contact, pretravel education, and universal health coverage of the migrant population. Even when the intermediate snail host species is not present in a non-endemic area, schistosome hybridization has been shown to occur and widen the range of snail host species. Subsequently, atypical snail hosts may potentially increase the transmission risk of *Schistosoma* spp. in the non-endemic area. This was the case in Corsica, where *S. haematobium* had been introduced by people travelling from West Africa and had hybridized with the cattle schistosome (i.e., *Schistosoma bovis*). Due to this hybridization, the *Bulinus truncatus* snail, that is widely present in Corsica, became a suitable intermediate host and further aided in the rapid colonization of urogenital schistosomiasis in this country [30].

Other threats for the appearance of new foci or re-infection risk in previously controlled areas are the constantly changing ecological, environmental, and human behavioral factors due to water development projects. These are leading to a higher and changed complexity of transmission-related problems and therefore, result in additional challenges for the control and M&S of diseases. An example of this is the construction of the Three Gorges Dam, the world's largest hydropower project, in China. Along with its social and economic benefits came dramatic ecological changes resulting in the fact that *Oncomelenia* snails, the intermediate host of *S. japonicum*, could live and breed within the reservoir area. Additionally, an increase in employment (and consequently immigrants) and the transport of products to this area had the potential to aggravate the spread of schistosomiasis in this region [31]. Another example is the construction of the Diama Dam in Senegal, which instigated the spread of schistosomiasis in 1989 [32]. The latter specifically resulted in the detection of *S. haematobium* and an increase of *S. mansoni* prevalence (from 10% to >80%) in the dam region due to severe adverse effects in the local ecosystems. With this in mind, a strategic plan, including environmental assessment and surveillance of livestock (for the zoonotic *Schistosoma* spp.) and human cases in addition to monitoring the geographical distribution of the intermediate snail host, is highly recommended and essential when introducing dramatical environmental changes, such as large-scale water development projects.

Finally, although the improvement of surveillance is crucial to sustain a control/elimination status, there is currently no systematic evaluation of surveillance systems. This evaluation mainly relies on collecting and summarizing data to determine surveillance sensitivity, cost-effectiveness, functionality, and quality. Every so often, an evaluation of human and animal surveillance methods is performed in areas where schistosomiasis has re-emerged, yet these evaluations are not systematic. Therefore, in the future, a rigorous monitoring network should be established that enables a systematic evaluation of the current schistosomiasis surveillance systems in order to improve their accuracy and speed of detection [33].

3.2. Soil-Transmitted Helminths

3.2.1. Introduction

STH infections, with a focus on the four major parasite species *Ascaris lumbricoides* (roundworm), *Trichuris trichiura* (whipworm), *Necator americanus* (hookworm), and *Ancylostoma duodenale* (hookworm), cause extensive socio-economic and public health problems and mainly affect people living in areas with poor water quality, sanitation, and hygiene. In addition, travel to/migration from such areas increases the potential for dispersal of STH infections to more developed nations. Transmission occurs when eggs from infected people are passed in the feces and contaminate the soil, water sources, or vegetables. In the case of roundworms and whipworms, their eggs get ingested and adult worms develop in the intestines. On the other hand, eggs from hookworms in the soil release larvae that can actively penetrate the skin. Subsequently, people get infected by walking barefoot on the contaminated soil. Considering that these helminths impair the nutritional status of their hosts and (pre-)school-aged children predominantly carry the burden of this infection, they often present with growth retardation, impaired cognitive development, and anemia as a result [34].

Ideally, the building of decent sanitation infrastructure worldwide could interrupt the transmission of and eliminate STHs. In reality, resources required to sustain this are rarely available. Therefore, the current goal of the WHO for 2020 is to eliminate morbidity rather than the parasites themselves by the administration of large-scale periodic preventive chemotherapy and health education to all populations at risk of developing illness (i.e., (pre-)school-aged children and pregnant women) with a national coverage goal of 75% in endemic countries. Once a country has reached the stage of childhood morbidity control/elimination, the objective is to maintain and refine monitoring/surveillance and to sustain deworming programs which will be discussed below [35].

3.2.2. Monitoring and Surveillance of Soil-Transmitted Helminths

After 5–6 years of MDA with good coverage (i.e., >75% of at-risk population), a reduced prevalence and morbidity of STHs should be noticed in the target population. The questions to the public health authorities should then include whether this reduction will be permanent, whether and how the frequency of deworming interventions can be reduced, and whether sentinel site monitoring should be continued. Considering the objective of this review, we will only focus on M&S when morbidity control/elimination has been reached. The latter entails three options: (i) morbidity is under control, yet the risk of re-emergence is high (i.e., prevalence between 10% and 20%), (ii) morbidity is under control and the risk of re-emergence is low (i.e., prevalence between 2% and 10%), and (iii) elimination of morbidity (i.e., prevalence < 2%). According to the WHO, the frequency of anthelminthic treatment can be reduced to once a year for the next four years in the first case. In the second case, the frequency of anthelminthic treatment can be reduced to one round of anthelminthic treatment every two years and in the final case, preventive chemotherapy is not needed anymore. Nevertheless, in all events, continuous annual monitoring is crucial in order to inform control program managers about any possible morbidity recrudescence. If monitoring indicates that prevalence remains low (i.e., between 10% and 20%, between 2% and 10%, and < 2%, respectively, for the first, second, and third morbidity control/elimination options) for 4 years despite the reduced frequency of MDA, a further reduction is in order. In case prevalence tends to re-emerge, the original treatment frequency is warranted [36].

The abovementioned monitoring requires periodic sample collection in order to obtain epidemiological data and to assess morbidity status. To do so, several approaches have been proposed, each with its own advantages and pitfalls (Table 2).

Table 2. Summary of records describing monitoring and surveillance systems/sampling methods for soil-transmitted helminths (STHs) at the control/elimination stage.

Method of Monitoring & Surveillance/Sampling	Time	Country	Reference
National surveys (in several counties at different time intervals): The implementation of a nationwide survey every 5–7 years in people of any age to monitor the infection rate and its relation to various characteristics (e.g., age, gender, region, and urban versus rural areas).	1971– ... [1]	The Republic of Korea	[37]
Regional surveys: Fecal sample collection of school-aged children in a previously high- and previously low-endemic county in The Republic of Korea to monitor the current status of prevalence of STHs.	2017	The Republic of Korea	[38]
Integrated school-based monitoring and surveillance for both lymphatic filariasis and STHs by fecal examination of school-aged children.	2006 and 2012	Sri Lanka and Kenya	[39,40]
Lot quality assurance sampling: A minimalistic approach of sampling originally designed for manufacturing inspection. It entails the collection and assessment of a minimal number of samples and the addition of more samples until statistical significance has been reached.	Not yet implemented	Not applicable	[34]
Pooling of samples to estimate STH prevalence while minimizing the number of diagnostic procedures: 50 School-aged children of 5 schools in each district were sampled. Individual examination was compared to pooled examination (pool size = 10) and both were processed with the Kato-Katz technique.	2017	Ethiopia	[41,42]

[1] Still ongoing.

The first and the most commonly implemented approach is the simple collection of samples at sentinel sites. These predetermined sites are located in every homogenous zone of a district or country and are assumed to provide information regarding the prevalence and intensity of infection in the entire area. For example, ever since successful STH control was achieved in 2004 in The Republic of Korea through continued parasitic control projects, national surveys on the infection status of STHs have been carried out in several counties at different time intervals. Every 5–7 years since 1971, a nationwide survey is held to monitor the infection rate and its relation to various characteristics (e.g., age, gender, region, and urban versus rural areas). Each time, 300 districts from a total of 23,536 districts among the country are randomly selected to be sampled. Specifically, people of any age in the selected districts are subjected to fecal examination and subsequently, the results are compared with those from previous surveys [37]. The data showed a dramatic decrease of egg-positive rate from 84.3% in the 1st survey in 1971 to 2.6% in the 8th survey in 2012. Nevertheless, infections with *T. trichiura* are gradually increasing and thus it is deemed necessary to carefully and continuously monitor these infections. In such cases, nationwide surveys do not provide accurate data regarding parasite prevalence compared to surveys on a regional basis. Therefore, studies of inhabitants in areas where STHs are suspected to be present as endemic foci are in place. One article described a similar regional survey in a previously high- and previously low-endemic county in The Republic of Korea to monitor the current status of prevalence of STHs. From May to July 2017, 2033 fecal samples were collected at 27 elementary, 10 junior high, and 8 high schools from two counties and examined for eggs with the KK technique. Results showed very low rates (0% and 0.07% for the previously low- and high-endemic counties, respectively) [38].

A second approach that has been implemented in Sri Lanka and Kenya is the integrated school-based M&S for both lymphatic filariasis (LF) and STHs. Considering that control interventions for different NTDs often overlap (e.g., MDA of albendazole is efficient against both STHs and LF), the opportunity arises to integrate their M&S in order to reduce their costs, including costs for administration, personnel, and transport. Therefore, post-MDA M&S with transmission assessment surveys for LF can integrate the collection of stool samples for STH screening. Although this system is likely more cost-effective compared to parallel programs, it may present some problems. At first, the collection and transport schedules of blood (for LF) and stool samples require some adjustments in order to avoid intervening with each other. Furthermore, caretakers used to handle blood samples may refuse to handle stool samples. Finally, it might be required to streamline sampling strategies for both the parasitic diseases in case a different number of samples from a different number of sampling sites is required. Therefore, further research is needed to integrate the two M&S systems without compromising their integrities [39,40].

Another method for sample collection suggested by Jex and colleagues (2011) is lot quality assurance sampling (LQAS), a minimalistic approach of sampling originally designed for manufacturing inspection. The basis entails the collection of a small number of batches, their control and statistical assessment, and finally, the addition of more batches until statistical significance has been reached. In the context of disease monitoring, this is especially useful in many low-income countries where sampling size is often determined by financial and logistical constraints rather than on a scientific basis. The best sampling plan would associate the lowest sample size at the highest statistical significance, which is especially valuable when a large number of communities needs to be tested under scarce resource availability. The latter can be determined by using tables in which sample size is shown for different type I errors. Although LQAS represents a promising, effective, and cost-efficient approach for monitoring STHs and a wide range of other parasites and pathogens, it has not been implemented so far in any STH control program [34].

Pooling of samples is the final suggested system to estimate the prevalence of STHs, while minimizing the number of diagnostic tests performed. This pooling process involves the aggregation of equal proportions of a number of samples to make up one pool. Subsequently, one single test allows to measure the properties of all constituent samples and therefore, fewer tests are necessary when using a larger pool size. Furthermore, in case one pool tests negative, all the constituent samples are negative. On the other hand, in case one pool tests positive, each included sample is tested individually in order to identify the infected individuals. This system definitely represents an appealing approach that significantly gains in time (e.g., with regard to microscopic examination techniques) and budget (e.g., with regard to molecular tools) in low prevalence regions [41]. Nevertheless, according to a study from Leta and colleagues (2018) in Ethiopia, a pooled strategy reduces the detection sensitivity due to a dilution effect and only an 11% reduction in total operation costs was obtained compared to individual examination. In sum, for future application of this pooled approach, further studies are required to determine its advantages and disadvantages at different scenarios of prevalence and diagnostic tests used [42].

It can be concluded that a number of methods for the collection of epidemiological data regarding STHs are possible; however, data collected using different approaches are often hard to assess with standardized methods. Differences in sampling protocols, timing of collection, and sample sizes limit the utility of the data for cross comparison among regions. Moreover, cross comparisons often do not comply with the requirements needed to obtain statistical significance due to these differences. Therefore, validating and standardizing M&S protocols in addition to sharing of epidemiological databases need to be in place in (i.e., on a national level) and between (i.e., on a global level) STH-endemic countries.

3.3. *Echinococcus* spp.

3.3.1. Introduction

Echinococcosis is a widespread helminthic disease affecting humans and is transmitted by domestic and wild animals. The two species of the *Echinococcus* genus of major public health importance are *Echinococcus granulosus* and *Echinococcus multilocularis*, both of which cause serious morbidity and mortality in humans if left untreated. Cestode eggs excreted by the definitive hosts (primarily dogs for *E. granulosus* and foxes for *E. multilocularis*) are ingested by the intermediate hosts (herbivores for *E. granulosus* and small rodents for *E. multilocularis*) in which the hydatid/alveolar cysts develop. Subsequently, transmission is completed when the intermediate host (infected organ) is ingested by the definitive host resulting in a tapeworm infection. Humans can also act as an accidental intermediate host through contact with dogs/foxes or contamination of food and water with infective eggs from feces [43].

Despite some progress in the control of echinococcosis, effective control has not been achieved or even attempted in most endemic countries. Furthermore, positive achievements of control programs at the local level have not markedly changed the global health importance of the disease. The development of effective control strategies and the management of livestock and ecology of dog and wildlife definitive hosts remain a challenge. Therefore, many articles are concentrating more on control interventions or surveillance in countries previously thought to be free of echinococcosis. The latter resulted in a rather low outcome of the search strategy for articles focusing on post-control/elimination M&S of *Echinococcus* spp. Additionally, two articles were included focusing on surveillance in Sweden (where echinococcosis is emerging) and Japan for the reason that these systems would also be effective at the control/elimination stage (Table 3).

Table 3. Summary of records describing monitoring and surveillance systems for *Echinococcus* spp.

Echinococcus Species	Monitoring and Surveillance System	Time	Country	Reference
E. granulosis	Routine post-mortem inspection of slaughter sheep followed by mandatory sampling and cestoidal drug treatment of shepherd dogs at the farm of origin (in case of a positive result).	2007–2013	Tasmania	[44]
E. multilocularis	Annual surveillance system that includes fox sampling (300 annually) in each municipality of the country. In case of positive detection, intensification of fox sampling (to 3000 annually), collection of rodents and fox feces for analyzation, and intensification of national Norwegian surveillance system.	2000–2011	Sweden, Norway	[45–48]
E. multilocularis	Necropsy and coprological examination in addition to preventive deworming of free roaming, stray, and companion dogs.	2013–2017	Japan	[49]

3.3.2. Monitoring and Surveillance of *Echinococcus* spp.

The first, often implemented, M&S method for *E. granulosus* is the routine post-mortem meat inspection (MI) at the abattoirs. This method is applied in many countries, such as Iceland, where *E. granulosus* has been gradually controlled since 1894. It represents a useful tool to assess the national and regional animal health status and to provide farmers with feedback on the infection status of their animals as can be illustrated by the following article. The article described the abattoir surveillance system for 352,325 Tasmanian sheep throughout a 5-year recording period (2007–2013) and stated a prevalence of 0.01%, which highlighted the purposes of a hydatid cyst control program operating in this country since 1965. Subsequently, in case of positive results, mandatory sampling in addition to treatment with cestocidal drugs (of shepherd dogs) at the farm of origin was applied. Although reliability studies state that trained inspectors can correctly identify most lesions during MI, there is potential for over- or under-estimation of prevalence. This points out the need for further studies regarding meat inspector diagnostic sensitivity and differences between abattoirs. Furthermore, this passive abattoir surveillance system is rather time-consuming and highly dependent on the correct ear tag identification of individual sheep (or cattle/pigs) for accurate farm tracebacks. Therefore, this method should never be implemented as a stand-alone system, but should always be combined with other veterinary surveillance strategies and continued public awareness campaigns. Nevertheless, despite its shortcomings, the findings of this study support the purpose of ongoing routine MI and on-farm sampling and treatment activities [44].

Secondly, three articles described M&S with regard to *E. multilocularis*. Until 1980, only four European countries were known to be endemic for this fox tapeworm; however, since then *E. multilocularis* has been increasingly spreading, with its presence confirmed in foxes currently in at least 24 countries of the European Union. Among these countries is Sweden, originally free from echinococcosis (i.e., a prevalence of < 1% in the final host), where a surveillance program was initiated in 2000. The objective was to sample 300 red foxes annually from each municipality in order to estimate the prevalence and geographical extent of the infection across the country. Hunters submitted foxes (against a small remuneration), which were subsequently examined by the sedimentation and counting technique (SCT) and real-time PCR. Since the two positive findings in 2011, 140 fecal samples from hunting dogs in the four municipalities around the parish, where the positive foxes were shot, were collected and examined with a copro-antigen ELISA. Additionally, the sampling of foxes was intensified to 3000 annually and diagnosis with SCT was replaced with the more cost-effective, yet equally sensitive, segmental SCT. Rodents and fox feces were also collected for autopsy and analyses by copro-PCR, respectively [45,46]. This annual surveillance system is still ongoing and so far, four infected counties across Sweden have been revealed as having a first infected rodent. These results demonstrated that repeated monitoring of *E. multilocularis* in Sweden is definitely necessary and must even be intensified to clarify whether prevalence is increasing. Another result to the positive findings in Sweden, approximately 60 km from the Norwegian border, was the intensification of the red fox surveillance in Norway. Specifically, 500–600 fecal samples from red foxes were annually collected by hunters across the country and analyzed with copro-PCR. So far, each of these have tested negative, which supports the value of the annual surveillance system [47,48]. Finally, in Japan, the *E. multilocularis*-endemic area is restricted to the northern island of Hokkaido, where control is on its way since the enforcement of the echinococcosis control program. The risk for dog-to-human transmission by eggs excreted by stray and free-roaming dogs remains a major concern. Between 2013 and 2017, 156 shelter dogs were examined using fecal egg examinations and copro-PCR. While the prevalence of the tapeworm in companion dogs was only 0.4% in this region, a 1.9% prevalence was discovered in the shelter dogs as these are more likely to get infected by catching an intermediate rodent host. This demonstrates the purpose of continued preventive deworming of not only companion dogs, but also of stray and free-roaming dogs in order to prevent potential human infection and maintain the status of control [49].

3.4. Taenia spp.

3.4.1. Introduction

T. solium and *T. saginata*, the pork and beef tapeworm, respectively, are the most important causes of human taeniosis (TS). A cysticercus is the metacestode larval stage of these *Taenia* spp. that develops in the bovine or porcine intermediate host after ingestion of eggs (i.e., cysticercosis (CC)). These eggs are shed by the final human host, when the consumption of raw/undercooked infected pork or beef meat results in the presence of a tapeworm in the small intestine (i.e., TS). Although not a serious public threat, the financial burden of *T. saginata* due to carcass condemnation, freezing, and devaluation should not be underestimated. In the case of *T. solium*, humans may also act as an intermediate host when ingesting infective eggs. As such, cysticerci have the potential to develop in the brain (central nervous system), collectively named neurocysticercosis (NCC), with epilepsy, migraine, and other neurological manifestations as a consequence. Furthermore, not only NCC, but also porcine cysticercosis (PCC), has an enormous economic impact due to many related costs, such as hospitalization and loss of condemned carcasses [50,51]. Therefore, the increase in public awareness of these consequences has led to the implementation of prevention and control measures (such as pig confinement, vaccination, and treatment; human treatment; and health education) against *T. solium* in more and more countries. Additionally, meat inspection, which is achieved through carcass visual inspection and/or incisions, is a fundamental prevention measure for both the *Taenia* spp. and is currently included in many legislations of high- and low-income countries [52]. In sum, many countries worldwide are still considering/aiming for control/elimination of *Taenia* spp., which, once again, resulted in a low outcome of the search strategy for articles focusing on post-control/elimination M&S.

3.4.2. Monitoring and Surveillance of *Taenia solium*

Only three articles described the design of a surveillance system, all in countries where *T. solium* was formerly controlled/eliminated. Nonetheless, at least 15 articles (2 articles included in this systematic review and 13 articles not included) concluded the urgent need for a common strategy on data collection, monitoring, and reporting of *T. solium* cases, in addition to an improvement of the current human and animal surveillance systems, for example, by implementing obligatory notification of cases (Table 4).

Table 4. Summary of records describing monitoring and surveillance systems for *Taenia* spp.

Taenia spp.	Monitoring & Surveillance System	Time	Country/Region	Reference
T. solium	Observatory of Taeniasis and Cysticercosis: System consisting of several core activities mainly focusing on the detection and treatment of tapeworm carriers.	2017– ... [1]	Portugal	[53]
T. solium	The integration of multiplex bead assays for parasitic diseases into national multiple indicator surveys.	2012	Cambodia	[54]
T. solium	Ring screening and treatment system: Pig surveillance by tongue palpation. When positive, test every individual living in a 100 meter radius for taeniasis and treatment with niclosamide.	2012–2014	Northern Peru	[55]
T. saginata	Conventional, routine meat inspection of bovines over 6 weeks of age: Visual inspection and incision of predilection sites.	1964– ... [1]	Europe	[56–58]
T. saginata	Risk classification of farms/cattle and slaughterhouses based on data from history cases, serological tests, and other known risk factors. Subsequently, visual inspection of low-risk cattle and rigorous meat inspection of high-risk cattle.	Not yet implemented	United Kingdom, France, and Europe	[59–61]

[1] Still ongoing.

The first article by Fonseca and colleagues (2018) described the establishment of an integrated surveillance program applicable to industrialized countries. Due to increased travels and migration, *T. solium* TS and CC are emerging in Europe, where these diseases were formerly under control/eliminated. Additionally, data on prevalence are scarce and non-updated, both of which request for combined approaches and one health solutions. Therefore, Portugal was the first country to design a surveillance system in 2017, named the Observatory of Taeniasis and Cysticercosis. This system comprises several core activities to obtain essential information on the burden and epidemiology of CC in Portugal, namely, (i) the identification of possible geographic hotspots by systematically obtaining and analyzing data from hospitals, slaughterhouses, and human social sectors (the latter with regard to residents and migrants), (ii) the implementation of questionnaire-based surveillance targeting healthcare units and porcine distribution units to detect and monitor new human and porcine CC cases in addition to epidemiologic field surveys exploring human, animal, and environmental factors in order to identify possible human tapeworm carriers, (iii) hospital-based treatment for identified human tapeworm carriers, (iv) monitoring and supervision of the reporting process, and (v) and yearly data dissemination. This system, mainly focusing on the detection and treatment of tapeworm carriers, has just recently started and needs to be run for a minimum of five years to allow complete outcome-based evaluation; however, it may prove a valuable addition in future health programs [53].

In 2016, Priest and colleagues described the opportunities of multiplex bead assays (MBA) to monitor the impact of different NTD interventions and their post-elimination surveillance. Nowadays, multiple indicator surveys are being conducted worldwide to obtain information on a large number of diseases often using a single blood sample; however, these surveys have not been extended to include NTDs. Therefore, the Cambodian Ministry of Health conducted a national integrated biomarker survey in 2012 to gather not only information regarding immunity for poliomyelitis, measles, rubella, and tetanus, but also for several NTDs, among them *T. solium*. Samples were collected and tested by MBA for immunoglobulin G antibodies in order to generate national prevalence estimates for parasitic and viral diseases of interest. Despite its tremendous potential, multiplexing technology for integrated surveys also has its shortcomings. First, defining seropositivity cutoff values for some antigens can be challenging when banks of positively and negatively confirmed cases are not readily available. Second, cross reactivity due to previous exposure to other helminth parasites may result in false-positives, although this can be assuaged by including multiple parasite antigens in the MBA. At last, the surveys are often powered to compare regional prevalence estimates, considering the different expected levels of the diseases included. In this matter, estimates at the province or district level are missing, yet nationwide hotspots can be identified and used to target further focal screening surveys. Despite these limitations, the integration of MBAs for parasitic diseases, such as *T. solium*, into multiple indicator surveys definitely provides a useful tool for monitoring and evaluating control interventions and post-elimination surveillance for many diseases [54].

Finally, the third study implemented a ring screening and treatment system in northern Peru to reduce *T. solium* transmission in resource-poor communities. Specifically, all pigs of the intervention village (1058 residents) were surveyed for PCC by tongue inspection every four months. Whenever a heavily infected pig had been found, residents living within a 100 meter radius were tested using a copro-antigen ELISA and treated with a single oral dose of niclosamide in case of a positive result. Although the ring screening and treatment system had been used as a low-cost control measure in this study, it was stated that the ring strategy could also potentially be applied as a surveillance system at the post-control/elimination stage [55].

3.4.3. Monitoring and Surveillance of *Taenia saginata*

As is the case for *T. solium*, the control of *T. saginata* is also still far away from being realized due to a variety of factors and therefore, most articles focus on control and prevention measures rather than M&S (Table 4). Since the 64/433/EEC directive of 1964 (now EU 854/2004, and EU 625/2017), MI of all bovines over 6 weeks of age (whereby the predilections sites for CC are visually examined and/or incised to detect cysticerci) is the cornerstone for the control and surveillance of *T. saginata* in Europe. In case of general infection, the carcass is declared unfit for human consumption. In case of localized infection, the carcass must be stored at −10 °C for >14 days before release. Although widely implemented with moderate to high specificity, MI results in an underestimation of the prevalence of CC by a factor of 3–10 due to its low sensitivity [56]. Moreover, a study from Jansen and colleagues (2017) recorded an underestimation by a factor of 100 and a sensitivity of <0.76% for MI in Belgium [57]. At first, motivation and skills of the inspector play a huge role, as does the stage of degeneration of the cysticerci. Furthermore, in lightly infected animals, which is the biggest proportion of infected animals in Belgium, only a fraction of the cysts were found in the predilection sites [58].

Given the fact that current post-mortem MI is limited by its poor sensitivity, alternative methods have been studied thoroughly. In 2016, Marshall et al. suggested the implementation of risk classification of farms/cattle and slaughterhouses based on data from history cases, serological tests, and other known risk factors (e.g., gender, age, presence of contaminated pastures and water sources, and movement history) in order to improve conventional MI. For example, it was stated that young male cattle are less likely to be infected, whereas cattle derived from farms where an infected animal has resided before are at higher risk of infection [59]. Therefore, visual inspection on low-risk cattle and rigorous MI on high-risk cattle makes this surveillance system more targeted and effective compared to conventional MI [60,61].

3.5. Integrated Monitoring and Surveillance of Neglected Tropical Diseases

Although many articles mention the need for integrated M&S of several pathogens, only three records explicitly described a design of such surveillance for the helminthic zoonoses discussed above (Table 5).

Table 5. Summary of records describing integrated monitoring and surveillance systems at the control/elimination stage of *Taenia* spp., *Echinococcus* spp., *Schistosoma* spp., and soil-transmitted helminths (STHs).

Parasite Species	Monitoring & Surveillance System	Time	Country/Region	Reference
Taenia saginata and *Echinococcus granulosus*	A retrospective approach of spatial analysis for the integrated surveillance of both bovine cysticercosis and cystic echinococcosis combined with further actions based on the outcome.	2006–2010	Veneto (northeastern Italy)	[62]
Schistosoma spp. and STHs	Integrated cross-sectional surveys with anamnestic questionnaire for monitoring STHs and schistosomiasis.	2010	Taboo (south-central Côte d'Ivoire)	[63]
Schistosoma spp. and STHs	Screening for STHs, schistosomiasis, and polio using the global polio laboratory network.	2016–2017	Ghana	[64]

One author suggested an integrated M&S system of both *T. saginata* and *E. granulosus* in hypo-endemic countries based on the identification of risk areas by a spatial analysis. A study on this was carried out in the Veneto region (northeastern Italy), where the prevalence of bovine CC and cystic echinococcosis (CE) is generally low. The data (age, sex, location, etc.) on local farm cattle slaughtered between 2006 and 2010 were integrated with passive abattoir surveillance data on the bovine CC/CE status of each animal using geographical information systems. Subsequently, the aggregation of this data was investigated using a scan statistic with a Bernoulli probability model in order to locate the most likely bovine CC and CE clusters. Its reliability with regard to CE was confirmed by an epidemiological survey collecting and analyzing dog fecal samples from all farm dogs located in a cluster area. Additionally, based on the identification of the clusters, detailed epidemiological surveys on positive farms in these areas could contribute to the clarification of risk factors maintaining this disease and the identification of the most probable introduction route of *T. saginata* or *E. granulosus* into the farms. Concerning surveillance response, further actions can be taken based on the outcome to break the parasite's life cycle (e.g., deworming of dogs, examination and/or anthelminthic treatment of farmers, intensified on-farm control, and a more rigorous MI of farm animals derived from such clusters in order to substantially increase the sensitivity of detection). It can be concluded from this study that a retrospective approach of the spatial analysis for integrated surveillance is very effective, especially for these two parasitic diseases considering their mandatory abattoir surveillance [62].

The second article described the implementation of cross-sectional surveys in Taboo (south-central Côte d'Ivoire), where morbidity control of STHs and schistosomiases was achieved due to preventive chemotherapy. Additionally, an anamnestic questionnaire was administered with the ultimate goal to estimate the individuals' helminth infection status and subsequently apply a more cost-effective targeted treatment. Seven percent of all the households in the study area were selected for a random sampling procedure (i.e., stool and urine for microscopical examination with KK and CCA tests) and completing a questionnaire on risk factors and signs and symptoms pertaining to different NTDs, among them STHs and schistosomiasis. Subsequently, multivariable logistic regression was used to reveal associations between the infection status of different helminths and the diagnostic variables (i.e., risk factors, signs, and symptoms). Disappointingly, results showed that risk factors, signs and symptoms should not be considered as strong diagnostic variables as they did not perform well in predicting schistosomiasis and STH infections. Therefore, the question arises to how one might identify groups that need treatment when targeting multiple NTDs. Despite the shortcomings of anamnestic questionnaires for both STH and schistosomiasis, efforts have already been made to integrate monitoring for these two parasitic diseases and this opens the way for the development of more comprehensive approaches for M&S of several NTDs [63].

Finally, the third article studied the potential of a polio surveillance system for the screening of STHs and schistosomiasis at the same time. Since the WHO set out to eradicate polio worldwide in 1988, the global polio laboratory network (GPLN) was established with 16 GPLN labs across Africa receiving an average of 22,017 fecal samples per year. Despite its major contribution to the eradication of polio, samples collected here are only screened for polio, while many diseases tend to be co-endemic in the poorest communities. Therefore, the Ghanaian National Polio Laboratory explored whether it is possible to identify polio as well as STHs and schistosomiasis from the collected fecal materials. The samples were linked to the age and region from the participant and tested for the different helminth types using a multiplex PCR assay. The findings of this study showed that it would indeed be sensible to expand the existing surveillance platform of polio to other diseases and include new diagnostic techniques, such as multiplex PCR. Nevertheless, the samples in this study were not representative for the different regions of Ghana as they originated from individuals presenting specific symptoms of polio. With a change in sample submission policy, the GPLN surveillance platform would be suitable for pilot screening of other NTDs and cost-effective compared to a de novo set up of standard surveillance platforms for each parasite separately [64].

3.6. Future Challenges and Recommendations

3.6.1. The Case for Strengthening Diagnostic Capacity

As the prevalence of many NTDs decreases, accurate and sensitive diagnosis is vital for M&S, especially in low-endemic regions to assess the impact of control programs, to identify risk areas, and to detect re-introduction or new transmission areas [11,65]. Nevertheless, a fast and standardized diagnostic method suitable for large-scale sampling is often lacking. For instance, the SCT for the diagnosis of echinococcosis was long seen as the golden standard for detection in the final host, yet it represented a labor-intensive and time-consuming method [66]. Furthermore, many diagnostic techniques rely on the determination of eggs in urine for urogenital schistosomiasis (*S. haematobium*) [67] and the microscopic detection and counting of eggs in stool samples, such as the KK technique for intestinal schistosomiasis (*S. mansoni* and *S. japonicum)* and STHs [68,69]. These techniques are highly specific (except for *Taenia* spp.), easy to perform, and relatively inexpensive. Nevertheless, issues with sensitivity are well-known and may result in an underestimation of the prevalence, particularly in countries that have reached the control/elimination stage. As a result, the obtaining of an additional fecal sample (i.e., duplicate KK technique) has been suggested, as this substantially improves the diagnostic sensitivity (23–100%) despite the increase in cost (31%) [68]. On the other hand, the FLOTAC technique (i.e., another fecal egg count technique) offers a higher sensitivity than a triplicate KK examination as it uses a much larger amount of stool, thereby increasing the chance of detection [70]. Nonetheless, all the above-mentioned techniques have the major limitation that they require trained personnel to identify eggs and tapeworms at species level and to distinguish eggs from other microscopic features.

During the past 15–20 years, substantial progress has been made with immunological methods detecting circulating antigens and antibodies of several NTDs. Two examples of such immunological diagnostic tools are the up-converting phosphor lateral flow assay detecting the *Schistosoma* CCA in body fluids and the point-of-care CCA test detecting a different *Schistosoma* antigen in urine [71–73]. Both the tools display advantages over microscopic detection and have proven to be rapid, cost-efficient monitoring tools to indicate worm burden. Other promising and often implemented immunological diagnostic tools are the copro-antigen ELISA for the detection for *Echinococcus* spp., and (cocktail-)ELISA, magnetic affinity ELISA, IHA, and dot immunogold filtration assay for the diagnosis of schistosomiasis. Finally, several rapid diagnostic tests targeting the antigens of or antibodies against foodborne helminthic zoonoses have been developed (e.g., the rES33 magnetic immune-chromatographic test and the up-converting phosphor reporter rT24H lateral flow assay for *T. solium*, the HP10 lateral flow assay for *Taenia* spp. and *E. granulosus*, and HCF-rEM18-immunochromatography for *Echinococcus* spp.). These qualitative or semi-quantitative diagnostic medical devices have been designed to give fast results without the involvement of any automated procedures. Despite their potential use as tools in the M&S of control programs, especially when integrated with conventional tests, many of these rapid tests have not yet undergone any field performance evaluation [74]. With some validation and optimization, these tools definitely present a huge step forward in the M&S for zoonotic parasites in multiple host species [75–79].

Although there is increased development of immunological diagnostic tests, it must be noted that their sensitivity does not yet reach that of molecular diagnostics [80,81]. As a solution, the replacement by highly sensitive and specific molecular diagnostic tools has been suggested to tackle this problem of sensitivity and to perform insightful epidemiological studies [82]. Nevertheless, their use is currently still hampered due to the need for trained personnel, expensive laboratory equipment, and cold-chain storage, often not available in endemic countries with low-resource settings. For example, PCR is the gold standard for several pathogens in terms of specificity and sensitivity, but is relatively expensive compared to the KK method [75,80,83–88]. Another recently developed, promising, sensitive, and specific molecular diagnostic tool is the 28S lateral flow recombinase polymerase assay for schistosomiasis, which requires less equipment, specialized personnel, and technical support, but still needs some further optimization and validation before it can be implemented in the field [88,89]. Finally, current studies evaluating LAMP assays for the early detection of *Schistosoma* and *Echinococcus* DNA in stool and serum samples reveal easy to perform, specific, and sensitive diagnostic tests [74,90–92]. In summary, molecular diagnostics are currently unlikely to be implemented in large-scale control programs considering their cost; however, with some field-friendly adaptations and standardization of these tests, they are definitely applicable as a future field diagnostic and surveillance tool for low transmission areas [66,78,81,93].

In conclusion, the constantly growing control efforts against NTDs urgently require research and further investment into improved and standardized diagnostic tools, especially at the stage of control/elimination. When applying some adjustments with regard to standardization and validation, the recently developed tests discussed above definitely offer field-deployable potential for the future [74]. Furthermore, their potentially higher costs may be outweighed by their long-term benefits [69,94,95].

3.6.2. The Emergence of Drug Resistance

Although no evidence of drug resistance has yet been confirmed, its risk is emerging considering the large-scale implementation of broad-spectrum anthelminthic drugs for STHs and schistosomiasis. So far, many studies regarding the efficacy of drugs have been performed; however, all of which are highly heterogenous in their reporting of results, design set-up, and implementation, making it difficult to draw any conclusions [96]. Therefore, the establishment of a standard operating procedure for the periodic monitoring of anthelminthic efficacy is in place. For example, the application of statistical modeling on a shared database containing individual patient data on drug efficacy against not only STHs and schistosomiasis, but also other NTDs, shows great potential for public health end-users to identify atypical responses potentially indicative of emerging drug resistance [97,98].

3.6.3. The Introduction of Spatial Technology

As mentioned above, (re-)emergence of many parasitic diseases is frequently associated with human factors, such as travel/migration, trade, and global population expansion. Furthermore, due to the often complex ecology involving multiple hosts and transmission routes, many diseases are affected by the advent of climate change and therefore, tend to expand their geographical distribution in the future. Finally, to achieve nationwide disease elimination, rapid detection of remaining sources of infection in low-endemic areas is essential. Although mass surveys would provide valuable data in this context, these are often not evident in financial and practical terms. Therefore, changes in the current applied M&S strategies are definitely required. This generates a chance for the introduction of spatial technology in M&S systems in order to improve survey quality and meet the requirements of current monitoring work [99].

Spatial technology includes any of the formal techniques which study the description and examination of diseases and their geographical variations by using data collected during previous surveys, i.e., geographical information systems (GIS), remote sensing (RS), global positioning system (GPS), Google Earth (GE), and spatiotemporal statistics and models [100]. The combination of land surface information (soil type, altitude, vegetation index, etc.) derived from RS and GE, weather conditions, GPS coordinates, and direct data from M&S sites (e.g., infection rate) can be used to spatially analyze complex geospatial data and to construct maps showing not only high-risk areas, but also the scope of disease/intermediate host distribution. These maps can be considered as an innovative tool to further guide risk-based surveillance strategies [18,101–104]. Finally, the application of the aforementioned tools combined with statistical or mathematical modeling provides important advances to explore spatiotemporal transmission dynamics, trends in habitat range, and risk/environmental factors of diseases in the past, present, and future [105–108]. This can consequently guide surveillance systems and point out areas that still acquire continuous monitoring. Nevertheless, these rapid and cost-efficient tools can be used at any stage of a control program (e.g., to establish baseline estimations, predict the spatial parasite distributions, and select treatment strategies), especially in regions with limited available epidemiological data.

For the M&S of schistosomiasis at the post-control/elimination stage, 15 articles obtained in this review indeed mentioned the use of spatial technology, out of which the majority focused on using it for monitoring snail density [12,15,18,99–101,103–111]. At present, snail surveys are extremely time-consuming as they are conducted manually and their quality can be influenced by many factors, such as temperature, light, and vegetation. Spatial technology takes into account the interplay between the snail intermediate host and environmental factors and therefore, helps the targeting of surveys. Nevertheless, it must be noted that transmission does not solely depend on the distribution of snails. Therefore, more studies are required that also put emphasis on the infection status of snails and other important reservoirs (such as bovines, dogs, people, and water bodies) that include certain human behavior as a risk factor and investigate access to water of each intermediate host.

Similarly, at least five records suggested the application of spatial technology at the post-control/elimination stage of STHs [34,112–115], while four articles did this for both *E. multilocularis* and *E. granulosus*. Specifically, for echinococcosis, an opportunity for landscape epidemiology was recommended by these articles with regard to surveillance. This landscape epidemiology investigates environmental and anthropogenic factors (e.g., temperature, rain fall, urbanization, deforesting, and agricultural practices) and makes integrated use of spatial technology in order to define the link between these variables and disease risk and to design more accurate predictive transmission models and updated risk maps [110,116]. The latter may subsequently guide decision makers to target serological screening of emerging transmission foci identified by these predictive modeling tools. This presents a cost-effective alternative to mass screening in order to detect early cases and has already been successfully implemented in Finland, Ireland, and the United Kingdom [117,118].

Although the implementation of spatial technology for the M&S of many diseases is increasingly being propagated, this spatiotemporal epidemiology is, however, a sophisticated profession in terms of training, expertise, and experience in both mathematical and computational knowledge and often requires expensive specialized software. Fortunately, this is gradually being countered by the provision of free software for mapping, the use of Internet for dissemination of information, and free access to satellite imagery of GE. At last, even the most updated form of spatial technology still requires surveillance data from the field in order to dispense any trustworthy information and conclusions.

These data are often lacking with deficient quality or heterogeneity due to varied sampling and diagnostic protocols [119]. As can be seen, spatial technology definitely offers powerful capabilities that facilitate the M&S of diseases, yet more research is required to tackle its related costs and to further guide on-site data collection.

3.6.4. The lack of data for *Taenia* spp. and *Echinococcus* spp.

It can be concluded that many countries are far from reaching a control, let along elimination, status for both *Taenia* spp. and *Echinococcus* spp. This resulted in limited records describing a functioning, validated M&S system at the post-control/elimination stage of these parasites. Moreover, the few methods described above were derived from scattered infrequent surveys as existing epidemiological data on regular national surveillance is lacking. This is especially the case for *T. solium* spp. as this is a non-notifiable disease in most countries and PCC prevalence is based on the underestimating MI [120]. Also, echinococcosis remains a huge challenge considering the asymptomatic infection in livestock and dogs, the involvement of many types of wildlife species in the transmission of *E. multilocularis*, and the fact that it is not prioritized by local veterinary services and public health institutions. Therefore, systematic national and sub-national data collection systems covering all parts of an endemic country are first recommended to reveal the true prevalence profiles before one can even consider sustained control/elimination [58].

3.7. Limitations of Systematic Literature Review

This systematic literature review has potential limitations. First of all, the process of literature search and study identification was conducted by only one reader, which could have given rise to bias at the study and outcome level. For the same reason, incomplete retrieval of the identified research might have occurred at the review level. Finally, there was no inclusion of grey literature and the review only focused on English literature, which inherently may have resulted in missed information. Despite these limitations, it is believed that their impact on the quality of this review is little given the descriptive presentation of the results and considering that this is the first review, to the best of our knowledge.

4. Conclusions and Global Lessons

Although combined health efforts in the past two decades have led to significant improvements in the battle against *T. solium*, it still poses a major public health threat worldwide. Furthermore, as control and elimination programs are progressing, the sustainability of achieved control and elimination remains their ultimate challenge, which continuously requires rigorous M&S. The latter are essential and integral components of any control program as they provide the ability to take pragmatic action against (re-)emergence, to deliver reliable information on prevalence, incidence, spatiotemporal distribution, and burden of diseases, to identify disease transmission hotspots and risk areas, to evaluate the applied program, etc. Nevertheless, a concept of M&S at the post-control/elimination stage of *T. solium* has not been (fully) developed and validated as can be concluded from this review. Subsequently, when looking into *T. saginata* due to its similarities with *T. solium*, and *Echinococcus* spp., the same conclusion could be drawn. Moreover, reliable estimates on global distribution and transmission of any of these parasitic species are still absent, which needs to be tackled urgently before implementing post-control/elimination M&S strategies. While there still remains much to be done in terms of control of *Taenia* spp. and *Echinococcus* spp., substantial progress has been achieved in China, particularly with regard to STHs and schistosomiasis. How exactly these strategies may be translated to other countries must be explored.

When developing an appropriate M&S framework, it is also important to determine how many animals/people, at how many sites, at what frequency, and at which site need to be collected in order to gain a realistic idea on the disease status and to rapidly detect new cases. Sample size calculations depend on a number of determinants (e.g., variance, prevalence, and consequences of the disease) and may increase so dramatically that they quickly become unrealistic in practical and financial terms. Further research into the development of alternative statistical frameworks for sample size calculations is therefore needed to solve this problem. Additionally, instead of random selection of inspection sites, local knowledge and understanding of site-specific heterogeneities should be embedded in a sampling framework, which provides a unique opportunity for spatial technology. Taken together, sampling should be a semi-structured activity, taking transmission status and the everchanging environment also into account [121,122].

Furthermore, the design of M&S systems for various NTDs vary considerably due to their distinct life cycles and epidemiological features. Still, control and elimination strategies, especially those for STHs and schistosomiasis (e.g., large-scale MDA), have striking similarities which provide opportunities for the possible integration of M&S. Ideally, such integration would include the harmonization of sampling strategies, fieldwork protocols, and diagnostic approaches, which most likely would result in increased population compliance, simplification of survey procedures, and most importantly, reduced costs. Specifically, these diseases tend to be co-endemic in the poorest communities, which would benefit from these financial advantages [123]. Nevertheless, a challenge in the integration of M&S is the establishment of a sampling strategy for diseases that do not perfectly overlap within districts or countries. Consequently, the issue arises in calculating a sample size large enough to obtain a required significance level. Other challenges that need to be addressed are the fact that M&S indicators are often measured in different populations (e.g., school-aged children for STHs vs. communities for schistosomiasis) and the little overlap in diagnostic procedures or sample matrix. In sum, although full integration of all elements of M&S for several NTDs is not feasible, opportunities should be considered for at least some integrated strategies [124].

Next, all the four helminthic zoonoses discussed above are among the most serious helminth zoonoses threatening public health worldwide (except for *T. saginata*); however, diagnostic tools to detect them are still imperfect. Accurate diagnostics are crucial both upstream (e.g., survey and design) and downstream (e.g., targeting, monitoring, evaluation, and surveillance) of control programs. This is especially the case in low-prevalence and low-endemic areas that are approaching elimination, thanks to the continuous implementation of control measures. Furthermore, expanding treatment programs will increase the pressure on drugs for resistance development, which requires monitoring during any operational program, especially those of STH's. In order to do so, new and sensitive diagnostic tools are once again an urgent need [125].

Finally, considering that not only the NTDs discussed here, but also many other NTDs, have animal origins, a more effective collaboration between medical and veterinary services is required. Currently, many M&S systems consist of separate animal- and human-orientated components, which bring along the challenge to build bridges between human and veterinary medicine in the routes to control/elimination sustainability [126]. Furthermore, both M&S require strong leadership, international cooperation, and the allocation of adequate resources, infrastructure, and qualified staff for the collection, analysis, and reporting of data. Unfortunately, in developing countries, where most of these diseases circulate, these are often poor to non-existent due to budget shortages. Last, but not the least, there is an urgent need to harmonize/standardize M&S activities in order to reliably determine the epidemiological situation worldwide and compare results from different countries. A major step forward in this would be the establishment of a global, constantly updated, NTD database providing open access to every georeferenced survey data.

Author Contributions: Conceptualization, G.S. and S.G.; methodology, G.S. and S.G.; validation, S.G.; formal analysis, G.S.; investigation, G.S.; data curation, G.S. and S.G.; writing—original draft preparation, G.S.; writing—review and editing, G.S. and S.G.; visualization, G.S. and S.G.; supervision, S.G. All authors have read and agreed to the published version of the manuscript.

References

1. Zhou, X.N.; Bergquist, R.; Tanner, M. Elimination of tropical disease through surveillance and response. *Infect. Dis. Poverty* **2013**, *2*, 1:1–1:5. [CrossRef]

2. Dorny, P.; Flisser, A.; Geerts, S.; Kyvsgaard, N.C.; McManus, D.; Nash, T.; Pawlowski, Z.; World Organisation for Animal Health (OIE). WHO/FAO/OIE Guidelines for the Surveillance, Prevention and Control of Taeniosis/Cysticercosis. Available online: https://www.who.int/taeniasis/resources/9290446560/en/ (accessed on 16 October 2019).

3. Bergquist, R.; Yang, G.J.; Knopp, S.; Utzinger, J.; Tanner, M. Surveillance and response: Tools and approaches for the elimination stage of neglected tropical diseases. *Act. Trop.* **2015**, *141*, 229–234. [CrossRef] [PubMed]

4. Murrell, K.D. Zoonotic foodborne parasites and their surveillance. *Rev. Sci. Tech.* **2013**, *32*, 559–569. [CrossRef] [PubMed]

5. Christensen, J. Epidemiological concepts regarding disease monitoring and surveillance. *Act. Vet. Scand.* **2001**, *94*, S1. [CrossRef] [PubMed]

6. Gyorkos, T.W. Monitoring and evaluation of large-scale helminth control programmes. *Act. Trop.* **2003**, *86*, 275–282. [CrossRef]

7. Tambo, E.; Ai, L.; Zhou, X.; Chen, J.H.; Hu, W.; Bergquist, R.; Guo, J.G.; Utzinger, J.; Tanner, M.; Zhou, X.N. Surveillance-response systems: The key to elimination of tropical diseases. *Infect. Dis. Poverty* **2014**, *5*, 49:1–49:12. [CrossRef]

8. PRISMA-P Group; Moher, D.; Shamseer, L.; Clarke, M.; Ghersi, D.; Liberati, A.; Petticrew, M.; Shekelle, P.; Stewart, L.A. Preferred reporting items for systematic review and meta-analysis protocols (PRISMA-P) 2015 statement. *Syst. Rev.* **2015**, *4*, 1:1–1:9. [CrossRef]

9. Colley, D.G.; Bustinduy, A.L.; Secor, W.E.; King, C.H. Human schistosomiasis. *Lancet* **2014**, *383*, 2253–2264. [CrossRef]

10. Sun, L.P.; Wang, W.; Zuo, Y.P.; Zhang, Z.Q.; Hong, Q.B.; Yang, G.J.; Zhu, H.R.; Liang, Y.S.; Yang, H.T. An integrated environmental improvement of marshlands: Impact on control and elimination of schistosomiasis in marshland regions along the Yangtze River, China. *Infect. Dis. Poverty* **2017**, *6*, 1:1–1:10. [CrossRef]

11. Rollinson, D.; Knopp, S.; Levitz, S.; Stothard, J.R.; Tchuem Tchuenté, L.A.; Garba, A.; Mohammed, K.A.; Schur, N.; Person, B.; Colley, D.G.; et al. Time to set the agenda for schistosomiasis elimination. *Act. Trop.* **2013**, *128*, 423–440. [CrossRef]

12. Bergquist, R.; Zhou, X.N.; Rollinson, D.; Reinhard-Rupp, J.; Klohe, K. Elimination of schistosomiasis: The tools required. *Infect. Dis. Poverty* **2017**, *6*, 158:1–158:9. [CrossRef] [PubMed]

13. Yang, Y.; Huang, S.Y.; Pei, F.Q.; Chen, Y.; Jiang, Q.W.; Deng, Z.H.; Zhou, Y.B. Spatial distribution and habitat suitability of *Biomphalaria straminea*, intermediate host of *Schistosoma mansoni*, in Guangdong, China. *Infect. Dis. Poverty* **2018**, *7*, 109:1–109:10. [CrossRef] [PubMed]

14. Wu, W.L.; Wang, J.R.; Wen, L.Y.; Huang, Y.Y.; Xu, X.F.; Yu, W.M. Surveillance and control of post-transmission schistosomiasis in Jiaxing prefecture, Zhejiang province, China. *Act. Trop.* **2005**, *96*, 282–287. [CrossRef] [PubMed]

15. Zhang, L.J.; Li, S.Z.; Wen, L.Y.; Lin, D.D.; Abe, E.M.; Zhu, R.; Du, Y.; Lv, S.; Xu, J.; Webster, B.L.; et al. The establishment and function of schistosomiasis surveillance system towards elimination in The People's Republic of China. *Adv. Parasit.* **2016**, *92*, 117–141. [CrossRef]

16. Grobusch, M.P.; Mühlberger, N.; Jelinek, T.; Bisoffi, Z.; Corachán, M.; Harms, G.; Matteelli, A.; Fry, G.; Hatz, C.; Gjørup, E.; et al. Imported schistosomiasis in Europe: Sentinel surveillance data from TropNetEurop. *J. Travel Med.* **2006**, *10*, 164–167. [CrossRef] [PubMed]

17. Angeles, J.M.M.; Leonardo, L.R.; Goto, Y.; Kirinoki, M.; Villacorte, E.A.; Hakimi, H.; Moendeg, K.J.; Lee, S.; Rivera, P.T.; Inoue, N.; et al. Water buffalo as sentinel animals for schistosomiasis surveillance. *Bull. World Health Organ.* **2015**, *93*, 511–512. [CrossRef]

18. Sun, L.P.; Liang, Y.S.; Wu, H.H.; Tian, Z.X.; Dai, J.R.; Yang, K.; Hong, Q.B.; Zhou, X.N.; Yang, G.J. A Google Earth-based surveillance system for schistosomiasis japonica implemented in the lower reaches of the Yangtze River, China. *Parasit. Vectors* **2011**, *4*, 223:1–223:8. [CrossRef]

19. Sun, L.P.; Wang, W.; Hong, Q.B.; Li, S.Z.; Liang, Y.S.; Yang, H.T.; Zhou, X.N. Approaches being used in the national schistosomiasis elimination programme in China: A review. *Infect. Dis. Poverty* **2017**, *6*, 55:1–55:9. [CrossRef]

20. McManus, D.P.; Gordon, C.; Weerakoon, K.G.A.D. Testing of water samples for environmental DNA as a surveillance tool to assess the risk of schistosome infection in a locality. *Int. J. Infect. Dis.* **2018**, *76*, 128–129. [CrossRef]

21. Zhao, G.M.; Zhao, Q.; Jiang, Q.W.; Chen, X.Y.; Wang, L.Y.; Yuan, H.C. Surveillance for schistosomiasis japonica in China from 2000 to 2003. *Act. Trop.* **2005**, *96*, 288–295. [CrossRef]

22. Liang, S.; Yang, C.; Zhong, B.; Guo, J.; Li, H.; Carlton, E.J.; Freeman, M.C.; Remais, J.V. Surveillance systems for neglected tropical diseases: Global lessons from China's evolving schistosomiasis reporting systems, 1949–2014. *Emerg. Themes Epidemiol.* **2014**, *11*, 19:1–19:14. [CrossRef] [PubMed]

23. Wu, X.H.; Ming-Gang, C.; Jiang, Z. Surveillance of schistosomiasis in five provinces of China which have reached the national criteria for elimination of the disease. *Act. Trop.* **2005**, *96*, 276–281. [CrossRef] [PubMed]

24. Qian, Y.J.; Li, S.Z.; Xu, J.; Yang, K.; Huang, Y.X.; Cao, Z.G.; Miu, F.; Dang, H.; Zhang, L.J.; Wang, Q.; et al. Potential schistosomiasis foci in China: A prospective study for schistosomiasis surveillance and response. *Act. Trop.* **2015**, *141*, 342–348. [CrossRef] [PubMed]

25. Dang, H.; Xu, J.; Li, S.Z.; Cao, Z.G.; Huang, Y.X.; Wu, C.G.; Tu, Z.W.; Zhou, X.N. Monitoring the transmission of *Schistosoma japonicum* in potential risk regions of China, 2008–2012. *Int. J. Environ. Res. Public Health* **2014**, *11*, 2278–2287. [CrossRef]

26. Abou-El-Naga, I.F. Towards elimination of schistosomiasis after 5000 years of endemicity in Egypt. *Act. Trop.* **2018**, *181*, 112–121. [CrossRef] [PubMed]

27. Haggag, A.A.; Rabiee, A.; Abd Elaziz, K.M.; Gabrielli, A.F.; Abdel Hay, R.; Ramzy, R.M.R. Mapping of *Schistosoma mansoni* in the Nile Delta, Egypt: Assessment of the prevalence by the circulating cathodic antigen urine assay. *Act. Trop.* **2017**, *167*, 9–17. [CrossRef] [PubMed]

28. GeoSentinel Surveillance Network; Schwartz, E.; Von Sonnenburg, F.; Reed, C.; Weld, L.H.; Nicolls, D.J.; Kozarsky, P.E. Characteristics of schistosomiasis in travelers reported to the GeoSentinel Surveillance Network 1997–2008. *Am. J. Trop. Med. Hyg.* **2008**, *79*, 729–734. [CrossRef]

29. Cao, C.; Bao, Z.; Li, S.; Wei, W.; Yi, P.; Yu, Q.; Zhu, H.Q.; Xu, J.; Guo, J.G.; Feng, Z. Schistosomiasis in a migrating population in the lake region of China and its potential impact on control operation. *Act. Trop.* **2015**, *145*, 88–92. [CrossRef]

30. Boissier, J.; Grech-Angelini, S.; Webster, B.L.; Allienne, J.F.; Huyse, T.; Mas-Coma, S.; Toulza, E.; Barré-Cardi, H.; Rollinson, D.; Kincaid-Smith, J.; et al. Outbreak of urogenital schistosomiasis in Corsica (France): An epidemiological case study. *Lancet Infect. Dis.* **2016**, *16*, 971–979. [CrossRef]

31. Zeng, H.; Yang, X.; Meng, S.; Wang, H.; Tang, X.; Tang, W.; Zeng, S.; Jeschke, S.; Wang, Y. Awareness and knowledge of schistosomiasis infection and prevention in the "Three Gorges Dam" reservoir area: A cross-sectional study on local residents and health personnel. *Act. Trop.* **2011**, *120*, 238–244. [CrossRef]

32. Shaikh, N.; Rahman-Shepherd, A.; Dar, O. Schistosomiasis in the Senegal River basin. *Lancet Planet. Health* **2018**, *2*, S27. [CrossRef]

33. Carlton, E.J.; Bates, M.N.; Zhong, B.; Seto, E.Y.W.; Spear, R.C. Evaluation of mammalian and intermediate host surveillance methods for detecting schistosomiasis re-emergence in southwest China. *PLoS Negl. Trop. Dis.* **2011**, *5*, e987. [CrossRef] [PubMed]

34. Jex, A.R.; Lim, Y.A.L.; Bethony, J.M.; Hotez, P.J.; Young, N.D.; Gasser, R.B. Soil-transmitted helminths of humans in southeast Asia—Towards integrated control. *Adv. Parasit.* **2011**, *74*, 231–265. [CrossRef]

35. Montresor, A. World Health Organization 2012. Eliminating Soil-Transmitted Helminthiases as a Public Health Problem in Children: Progress Report 2001–2010 and Strategic Plan 2011–2020. Available online: https://apps.who.int/iris/bitstream/handle/10665/44804/9789241503129_eng.pdf?sequence=1 (accessed on 19 October 2019).

36. Montresor, A. World Health Organization 2011. In *Helminth Control in School-Age Children: A Guide for Managers of Control Programmes*, 2nd ed.; World Health Organization: Geneva, Switzerland, 2011. Available online: https://apps.who.int/iris/bitstream/handle/10665/44671/9789241548267_eng.pdf?sequence=1 (accessed on 19 October 2019).

37. Kim, T.S.; Cho, S.H.; Huh, S.; Kong, Y.; Sohn, W.M.; Hwang, S.S.; Chai, J.Y.; Lee, S.H.; Park, Y.K.; Oh, D.K.; et al. A nationwide survey on the prevalence of intestinal parasitic infections in The Republic of Korea, 2004. *Korean J. Parasitol.* **2009**, *47*, 37–47. [CrossRef]

38. Bahk, Y.Y.; Park, Y.K.; Na, B.K.; Sohn, W.M.; Hong, S.J.; Chai, J.Y.; Kim, T.S. Survey on intestinal helminthic infection status of students in two counties, Hadong-gun and Goseong-gun, Korea. *Korean J. Parasitol.* **2018**, *56*, 335–339. [CrossRef]

39. Gunawardena, S.; Gunawardena, N.K.; Kahathuduwa, G.; Karunaweera, N.D.; de Silva, N.R.; Ranasinghe, U.B.; Samarasekara, S.D.; Nagodavithana, K.C.; Rao, R.U.; Rebello, M.P.; et al. Integrated school-based surveillance for soil-transmitted helminth infections and lymphatic filariasis in Gampaha District, Sri Lanka. *Am. J. Trop. Med. Hyg.* **2014**, *90*, 661–666. [CrossRef]

40. Smith, J.L.; Sturrock, H.J.W.; Assefa, L.; Nikolay, B.; Njenga, S.M.; Kihara, J.; Mwandawiro, C.S.; Brooker, S.J. Factors associated with the performance and cost-effectiveness of using lymphatic filariasis transmission assessment surveys for monitoring soil-transmitted helminths: A case study in Kenya. *Am. J. Trop. Med. Hyg.* **2015**, *92*, 342–353. [CrossRef]

41. Truscott, J.E.; Dunn, J.C.; Papaiakovou, M.; Schaer, F.; Werkman, M.; Littlewood, D.T.J.; Walson, J.L.; Anderson, R.M. Calculating the prevalence of soil-transmitted helminth infection through pooling of stool samples: Choosing and optimizing the pooling strategy. *PLoS Negl. Trop. Dis.* **2019**, *13*, e0007196. [CrossRef]

42. Leta, G.T.; French, M.; Dorny, P.; Vercruysse, J.; Levecke, B. Comparison of individual and pooled diagnostic examination strategies during the national mapping of soil-transmitted helminths and *Schistosoma mansoni* in Ethiopia. *PLoS Negl. Trop. Dis.* **2018**, *12*, e0006723. [CrossRef]

43. Eckert, J.; Deplazes, P. Biological, epidemiological, and clinical aspects of echinococcosis, a zoonosis of increasing concern. *Clin. Microbiol. Rev.* **2004**, *17*, 107–135. [CrossRef]

44. Phythian, C.; Jackson, B.; Bell, R.; Citer, L.; Barwell, R.; Windsor, P. Abattoir surveillance of *Sarcocystis* spp., *Cysticercosis ovis* and *Echinococcus granulosus* in Tasmanian slaughter sheep, 2007–2013. *Aust. Vet. J.* **2018**, *96*, 62–68. [CrossRef] [PubMed]

45. Lind, E.O.; Juremalm, M.; Christensson, D.; Widgren, S.; Hallgren, G.; Erik, A.A.; Uhlhorn, H.; Lindberg, A.; Cedersmyg, M.; Wahlström, H. First detection of *Echinococcus multilocularis* in Sweden, February to March 2011. *Eurosurveillance* **2011**, *16*, 696–705. [CrossRef]

46. Wahlström, H.; Enemark, H.L.; Davidson, R.K.; Oksanen, A. Present status, actions taken and future considerations due to the findings of *E. multilocularis* in two Scandinavian countries. *Vet. Parasitol.* **2015**, *213*, 172–181. [CrossRef] [PubMed]

47. Madslien, K.; Øines, Ø.; Handeland, K.; Urdahl, A.M.; Albin-Amiot, C.; Jore, S.; Norwegian Veterinary Institute. The Surveillance Programme for *Echinococcus Multilocularis* in Red Foxes (*Vulpes Vulpes*) in Norway in 2014. Available online: https://www.vetinst.no/en/surveillance-programmes/echinococcus-in-red-foxes (accessed on 29 August 2019).

48. European Food Safety Authority. Annual Assessment of *Echinococcus multilocularis* Surveillance Reports Submitted in 2018 in the Context of Commission Regulation (EU) No 1152/2011. Available online: https://www.efsa.europa.eu/en/efsajournal/pub/5486 (accessed on 29 August 2019).

49. Irie, T.; Mukai, T.; Yagi, K. *Echinococcus multilocularis* surveillance using copro-DNA and egg examination of shelter dogs from an endemic area in Hokkaido, Japan. *Vector-Borne Zoonot. Dis.* **2018**, *18*, 390–392. [CrossRef]

50. Hobbs, E.C.; Mwape, K.E.; Devleesschauwer, B.; Gabriël, S.; Chembensofu, M.; Mambwe, M.; Phiri, I.K.; Masuku, M.; Zulu, G.; Colston, A.; et al. *Taenia solium* from a community perspective: Preliminary costing data in the Katete and Sinda districts in Eastern Zambia. *Vet. Parasitol.* **2018**, *251*, 63–67. [CrossRef] [PubMed]

51. Trevisan, C.; Sotiraki, S.; Laranjo-González, M.; Dermauw, V.; Wang, Z.; Kärssin, A.; Cvetkovikj, A.; Winkler, A.S.; Abraham, A.; Bobic, B.; et al. Epidemiology of taeniosis/cysticercosis in Europe, a systematic review: Eastern Europe. *Parasit. Vectors* **2018**, *11*, 569:1–569:11. [CrossRef]

52. Okello, A.L.; Thomas, L.F. Human taeniasis: Current insights into prevention and management strategies in endemic countries. *Risk Manag. Health Policy* **2017**, *10*, 107–116. [CrossRef]

53. Fonseca, A.G.; Torgal, J.; de Meneghi, D.; Gabriël, S.; Coelho, A.C.; Vilhena, M. One Health-ness evaluation of cysticercosis surveillance design in Portugal. *Front. Public Health* **2018**, *6*, 74:1–74:10. [CrossRef]

54. Priest, J.W.; Jenks, M.H.; Moss, D.M.; Mao, B.; Buth, S.; Wannemuehler, K.; Soeung, S.C.; Lucchi, N.W.; Udhayakumar, V.; Gregory, C.J.; et al. Integration of multiplex bead assays for parasitic diseases into a national, population-based serosurvey of women 15–39 years of age in Cambodia. *PLoS Negl. Trop. Dis.* **2016**, *10*, e0004699. [CrossRef]

55. Cysticercosis Working Group in Peru; O'Neal, S.E.; Moyano, L.M.; Ayvar, V.; Rodriguez, S.; Gavidia, C.; Wilkins, P.P.; Gilman, R.H.; Garcia, H.H.; Gonzalez, A.E. Ring-screening to control endemic transmission of *Taenia solium*. *PLoS Negl. Trop. Dis.* **2014**, *8*, e3125. [CrossRef]

56. Abuseir, S.; Epe, C.; Schnieder, T.; Klein, G.; Kühne, M. Visual diagnosis of *Taenia saginata* cysticercosis during meat inspection: Is it unequivocal? *Parasitol. Res.* **2006**, *99*, 405–409. [CrossRef] [PubMed]

57. Jansen, F.; Dorny, P.; Berkvens, D.; Van Hul, A.; Van den Broeck, N.; Makay, C.; Praet, N.; Eichenberger, R.M.; Deplazes, P.; Gabriël, S. High prevalence of bovine cysticercosis found during evaluation of different *post-mortem* detection techniques in Belgian slaughterhouses. *Vet. Parasitol.* **2017**, *244*, 1–6. [CrossRef] [PubMed]

58. Dorny, P.; Praet, N. *Taenia saginata* in Europe. *Vet. Parasitol.* **2007**, *149*, 22–24. [CrossRef] [PubMed]

59. Dupuy, C.; Morlot, C.; Demont, P.; Ducrot, C.; Calavas, D.; Callait-Cardinal, M.P.; Gay, E. Construction of standardized surveillance indicators for bovine cysticercosis. *Prev. Vet. Med.* **2014**, *115*, 288–292. [CrossRef] [PubMed]

60. Marshall, L.R.; Prakashbabu, B.C.; Ferreira, J.P.; Buzdugan, S.N.; Stärk, K.D.C.; Guitian, J. Risk factors for *Taenia saginata* cysticercus infection in cattle in the United Kingdom: A farm-level case-control study and assessment of the role of movement history, age and sex. *Prev. Vet. Med.* **2016**, *135*, 1–8. [CrossRef]

61. Blagojevic, B.; Robertson, L.J.; Vieira-Pinto, M.; Johansen, M.V.; Laranjo-González, M.; Gabriël, S. Bovine cysticercosis in the European Union: Impact and current regulations, and an approach towards risk-based control. *Food Cont.* **2017**, *78*, 64–71. [CrossRef]

62. Cassini, R.; Mulatti, P.; Zanardello, C.; Simonato, G.; Signorini, M.; Cazzin, S.; Tambalo, P.; Cobianchi, M.; Pietrobelli, M.; Capelli, G. Retrospective and spatial analysis tools for integrated surveillance of cystic echinococcosis and bovine cysticercosis in hypo-endemic areas. *Geospat. Health* **2014**, *8*, 509–515. [CrossRef]

63. Fürst, T.; Ouattara, M.; Silué, K.D.; N'Goran, D.N.; Adiossan, L.G.; Bogoch, I.I.; N'Guessan, Y.; Koné, S.; Utzinger, J.; N'Goran, E.K. Scope and limits of an anamnestic questionnaire in a control-induced low-endemicity helminthiasis setting in South-Central Côte d'Ivoire. *PLoS ONE* **2013**, *8*, e64380. [CrossRef]

64. Cunningham, L.J.; Odoom, J.; Pratt, D.; Boatemaa, L.; Asante-Ntim, N.; Attiku, K.; Banahene, B.; Osei-Atweneboana, M.; Verweij, J.J.; Molyneux, D.; et al. Expanding molecular diagnostics of helminthiasis: Piloting use of the GPLN platform for surveillance of soil transmitted helminthiasis and schistosomiasis in Ghana. *PLoS Negl. Trop. Dis.* **2018**, *12*, e0006129. [CrossRef]

65. Spear, R.C.; Seto, E.Y.W.; Carlton, E.J.; Liang, S.; Remais, J.V.; Zhong, B.; Qiu, D. The challenge of effective surveillance in moving from low transmission to elimination of schistosomiasis in China. *Int. J. Parasit.* **2011**, *41*, 1243–1247. [CrossRef]

66. Isaksson, M.; Hagström, Å.; Armua-Fernandez, M.T.; Wahlström, H.; Ågren, E.O.; Miller, A.; Holmberg, A.; Lukacs, M.; Casulli, A.; Deplazes, P.; et al. A semi-automated magnetic capture probe-based DNA extraction and real-time PCR method applied in the Swedish surveillance of *Echinococcus multilocularis* in red fox (*Vulpes vulpes*) faecal samples. *Parasit. Vectors* **2014**, *7*, 583:1–583:10. [CrossRef] [PubMed]

67. French, M.D.; Rollinson, D.; Basáñez, M.G.; Mgeni, A.F.; Khamis, I.S.; Stothard, J.R. School-based control of urinary schistosomiasis on Zanzibar, Tanzania: Monitoring micro-haematuria with reagent strips as a rapid urological assessment. *J. Pediatr. Urol.* **2007**, *3*, 364–368. [CrossRef] [PubMed]

68. Liu, C.; Lu, L.; Zhang, L.; Bai, Y.; Medina, A.; Rozelle, S.; Smith, D.S.; Zhou, C.; Zang, W. More poop, more precision: Improving epidemiologic surveillance of soil-transmitted helminths with multiple fecal sampling using the Kato–Katz Technique. *Am. J. Trop. Med. Hyg.* **2017**, *97*, 870–875. [CrossRef] [PubMed]

69. Turner, H.C.; Bettis, A.A.; Dunn, J.C.; Whitton, J.M.; Hollingsworth, T.D.; Fleming, F.M.; Anderson, R.M. Economic considerations for moving beyond the Kato-Katz Technique for diagnosing intestinal parasites as we move towards elimination. *Trends Parasitol.* **2017**, *33*, 435–443. [CrossRef]

70. Knopp, S.; Rinaldi, L.; Khamis, I.S.; Stothard, J.R.; Rollinson, D.; Maurelli, M.P.; Steinmann, P.; Marti, H.; Cringoli, G.; Utzinger, J. A single FLOTAC is more sensitive than triplicate Kato–Katz for the diagnosis of low-intensity soil-transmitted helminth infections. *Trans. R. Soc. Trop. Med. Hyg.* **2009**, *103*, 347–354. [CrossRef]

71. Koukounari, A.; Donnelly, C.A.; Moustaki, I.; Tukahebwa, E.M.; Kabatereine, N.B.; Wilson, S.; Webster, J.P.; Deelder, A.M.; Vennervald, B.J.; van Dam, G.J. A latent Markov modelling approach to the evaluation of circulating cathodic antigen strips for schistosomiasis diagnosis pre- and post-praziquantel treatment in Uganda. *PLoS Comput. Biol.* **2013**, *9*, e1003402. [CrossRef]

72. Adriko, M.; Standley, C.J.; Tinkitina, B.; Tukahebwa, E.M.; Fenwick, A.; Fleming, F.M.; Sousa-Figueiredo, J.C.; Stothard, J.R.; Kabatereine, N.B. Evaluation of circulating cathodic antigen (CCA) urine-cassette assay as a survey tool for *Schistosoma mansoni* in different transmission settings within Bugiri District, Uganda. *Act. Trop.* **2014**, *136*, 50–57. [CrossRef]

73. Knopp, S.; Corstjens, P.L.A.M.; Koukounari, A.; Cercamondi, C.I.; Ame, S.M.; Ali, S.M.; de Dood, C.J.; Mohammed, K.A.; Utzinger, J.; Rollinson, D.; et al. Sensitivity and specificity of a urine circulating anodic antigen test for the diagnosis of *Schistosoma haematobium* in low endemic settings. *PLoS Negl. Trop. Dis.* **2015**, *9*, e0003752. [CrossRef]

74. Mubanga, C.; Mwape, K.E.; Phiri, I.K.; Trevisan, C.; Zulu, G.; Chabala, C.; van Damme, I.; Schmidt, V.; Dorny, P.; Gabriël, S. Progress on the development of rapid diagnostic tests for foodborne neglected zoonotic helminthiases: A systematic review. *Act. Trop.* **2019**, *194*, 135–147. [CrossRef]

75. Angeles, J.M.; Goto, Y.; Kirinoki, M.; Leonardo, L.; Tongol-Rivera, P.; Villacorte, E.; Inoue, N.; Chigusa, Y.; Kawazu, S. Human antibody response to thioredoxin peroxidase-1 and tandem repeat proteins as immunodiagnostic antigen candidates for *Schistosoma japonicum* infection. *Am. J. Trop. Med. Hyg.* **2011**, *85*, 674–679. [CrossRef]

76. Zhou, X.N.; Xu, J.; Chen, H.G.; Wang, T.P.; Huang, X.B.; Lin, D.D.; Wang, Q.Z.; Tang, L.; Guo, J.G.; Wu, X.H.; et al. Tools to support policy decisions related to treatment strategies and surveillance of schistosomiasis Japonica towards elimination. *PLoS Negl. Trop. Dis.* **2011**, *5*, e1408. [CrossRef] [PubMed]

77. Yu, Q.; Yang, H.; Feng, Y.; Yang, X.; Zhu, Y. Magnetic affinity enzyme-linked immunoassay based on recombinant 26 kDa glutathione-S-transferase for serological diagnosis of schistosomiasis japonica. *Act. Trop.* **2012**, *124*, 199–202. [CrossRef] [PubMed]

78. Morel, N.; Lassabe, G.; Elola, S.; Bondad, M.; Herrera, S.; Marí, C.; Last, J.A.; Jensen, O.; Gonzalez-Sapienza, G. A monoclonal antibody-based copro-ELISA kit for canine echinococcosis to support the PAHO effort for hydatid disease control in South America. *PLoS Negl. Trop. Dis.* **2013**, *7*, e1967. [CrossRef] [PubMed]

79. Moendeg, K.J.; Angeles, J.M.M.; Goto, Y.; Leonardo, L.R.; Kirinoki, M.; Villacorte, E.A.; Rivera, P.T.; Inoue, N.; Chigusa, Y.; Kawazu, S. Development and optimization of cocktail-ELISA for a unified surveillance of zoonotic schistosomiasis in multiple host species. *Parasitol. Res.* **2015**, *114*, 1225–1228. [CrossRef] [PubMed]

80. Caldeira, R.L.; Jannotti-Passos, L.K.; Dos Santos Carvalho, O. Use of molecular methods for the rapid mass detection of *Schistosoma mansoni* (Platyhelminthes: Trematoda) in *Biomphalaria* spp. (Gastropoda: Planorbidae). *J. Trop. Med.* **2017**, *2017*, 1–6. [CrossRef] [PubMed]

81. Ni, X.W.; McManus, D.P.; Lou, Z.Z.; Yang, J.F.; Yan, H.B.; Li, L.; Li, H.M.; Liu, Q.Y.; Li, C.H.; Shi, W.G.; et al. A comparison of Loop-Mediated Isothermal Amplification (LAMP) with other surveillance tools for *Echinococcus granulosus* diagnosis in canine definitive hosts. *PLoS ONE* **2014**, *9*, e100877. [CrossRef] [PubMed]

82. Gordon, C.A.; Gray, D.J.; Gobert, G.N.; McManus, D.P. DNA amplification approaches for the diagnosis of key parasitic helminth infections of humans. *Mol. Cell. Probes* **2011**, *25*, 143–152. [CrossRef]

83. Mohammed, A.S.; Daubenberger, C.; Benninghoff, M.; Knopp, S.; Schindler, T.; Rothen, J.; Lweno, O.; Mohammed, A.S.; Singo, R.; Benninghoff, M.; et al. Diagnostic accuracy of Kato–Katz, FLOTAC, Baermann, and PCR Methods for the detection of light-intensity hookworm and *Strongyloides stercoralis* infections in Tanzania. *Am. J. Trop. Med. Hyg.* **2014**, *90*, 535–545. [CrossRef]

84. Gordon, C.A.; Acosta, L.P.; Gobert, G.N.; Olveda, R.M.; Ross, A.G.; Williams, G.M.; Gray, D.J.; Harn, D.; Li, Y.; McManus, D.P. Real-time PCR demonstrates high prevalence of *Schistosoma japonicum* in the philippines: Implications for surveillance and control. *PLoS Negl. Trop. Dis.* **2015**, *9*, e0003483. [CrossRef]

85. Hessler, M.J.; Cyrs, A.; Krenzke, S.C.; Mahmoud, E.S.; Sikasunge, C.; Mwansa, J.; Lodh, N. Detection of duo-schistosome infection from filtered urine samples from school children in Zambia after MDA. *PLoS ONE* **2017**, *12*, e0189400. [CrossRef]

86. Weerakoon, K.G.; Gordon, C.A.; Williams, G.M.; Cai, P.; Gobert, G.N.; Olveda, R.M.; Ross, A.G.; Olveda, D.U.; McManus, D.P. Droplet digital PCR diagnosis of Human schistosomiasis: Parasite cell-free DNA detection in diverse clinical samples. *J. Infect. Dis.* **2017**, *216*, 1611–1622. [CrossRef] [PubMed]

87. Xu, J.; Duan, Z.L.; Guan, Z.N.; Wang, Y.Y.; Lin, C.; Zhang, T.T.; Zhang, H.Q.; Qian, X.; Xia, C.M. Early detection of circulating DNA of *Schistosoma japonicum* in sentinel mice models. *Exp. Parasitol.* **2017**, *176*, 82–88. [CrossRef] [PubMed]

88. He, P.; Gordon, C.A.; Williams, G.M.; Li, Y.; Wang, Y.; Hu, J.; Gray, D.J.; Ross, A.G.; Harn, D.; McManus, D.P. Real-time PCR diagnosis of *Schistosoma japonicum* in low transmission areas of China. *Infect. Dis. Poverty* **2018**, *7*, 8:1–8:11. [CrossRef] [PubMed]

89. Corstjens, P.L.A.M.; Hoekstra, P.T.; de Dood, C.J.; van Dam, G.J. Utilizing the ultrasensitive Schistosoma up-converting phosphor lateral flow circulating anodic antigen (UCP-LF CAA) assay for sample pooling-strategies. *Infect. Dis. Poverty* **2017**, *6*, 155:1–155:13. [CrossRef] [PubMed]

90. Poulton, K.; Webster, B. Development of a lateral flow recombinase polymerase assay for the diagnosis of *Schistosoma mansoni* infections. *Anal. Biochem.* **2018**, *546*, 65–71. [CrossRef] [PubMed]

91. Hamburger, J.; Abbasi, I.; Kariuki, C.; Wanjala, A.; Mzungu, E.; Mungai, P.; King, C.H. Evaluation of Loop-Mediated Isothermal Amplification suitable for molecular monitoring of schistosome-infected snails in field laboratories. *Am. J. Trop. Med. Hyg.* **2013**, *88*, 344–351. [CrossRef]

92. Fernández-Soto, P.; Gandasegui, A.J.; Sánchez, H.A.; López, A.J.; Vicente, S.B.; Muro, A. A Loop-Mediated isothermal amplification (LAMP) assay for early detection of *schistosoma mansoni* in stool samples: A diagnostic approach in a murine model. *PLoS Negl. Trop. Dis.* **2014**, *8*, e3126. [CrossRef]

93. Huang, Y.; Yang, W.; Qiu, J.; Chen, X.; Yang, Y.; Qiu, D.; Xiao, N.; Xiao, Y.; Heath, D. A modified coproantigen test used for surveillance of *echinococcus* spp. in Tibetan dogs. *Vet. Parasitol.* **2007**, *149*, 229–238. [CrossRef]

94. Dunn, J.C.; Turner, H.C.; Tun, A.; Anderson, R.M. Epidemiological surveys of, and research on, soil-transmitted helminths in Southeast Asia: A systematic review. *Parasit. Vectors* **2016**, *9*, 31:1–31:13. [CrossRef]

95. Hoekendijk, D.J.L.; Hill, P.C.; Sowerby, S.J. Rationale for quality assurance in fecal egg monitoring of soil-transmitted helminthiasis. *Am. J. Trop. Med. Hyg.* **2016**, *95*, 502–504. [CrossRef]

96. Tchuem Tchuenté, L.A. Control of soil-transmitted helminths in sub-Saharan Africa: Diagnosis, drug efficacy concerns and challenges. *Act. Trop.* **2011**, *120*, S4–S11. [CrossRef] [PubMed]

97. Halder, J.B.; Benton, J.; Julé, A.M.; Guérin, P.J.; Olliaro, P.L.; Basáñez, M.G.; Walker, M. Systematic review of studies generating individual participant data on the efficacy of drugs for treating soil-transmitted helminthiases and the case for data-sharing. *PLoS Negl. Trop. Dis.* **2017**, *11*, e0006053. [CrossRef] [PubMed]

98. Walker, M.; Mabud, T.S.; Olliaro, P.L.; Coulibaly, J.T.; King, C.H.; Raso, G.; Scherrer, A.U.; Stothard, J.R.; Sousa-Figueiredo, J.C.; Stete, K.; et al. New approaches to measuring anthelminthic drug efficacy: Parasitological responses of childhood schistosome infections to treatment with praziquantel. *Parasit. Vectors* **2016**, *9*, 41:1–41:15. [CrossRef] [PubMed]

99. Yang, Y.; Cheng, W.; Wu, X.; Huang, S.; Deng, Z.; Zeng, X.; Yuan, D.; Yang, Y.; Wu, Z.; Chen, Y.; et al. Prediction of the potential global distribution for *Biomphalaria straminea*, an intermediate host for *Schistosoma mansoni*. *PLoS Negl. Trop. Dis.* **2018**, *12*, e0006548. [CrossRef] [PubMed]

100. Wang, X.Y.; He, J.; Yang, K.; Liang, S. Applications of spatial technology in schistosomiasis control programme in The People's Republic of China. *Adv. Parasitol.* **2016**, *92*, 143–163. [CrossRef] [PubMed]

101. Zhang, Z.; Carpenter, T.E.; Chen, Y.; Clark, A.B.; Lynn, H.S.; Peng, W.; Zhou, Y.; Zhao, G.; Jiang, Q. Identifying high-risk regions for schistosomiasis in Guichi, China: A spatial analysis. *Act. Trop.* **2008**, *107*, 217–223. [CrossRef]

102. Nihei, N.; Komagata, O.; Kobayashi, M.; Saitoh, Y.; Mochizuki, K.; Nakamura, S. Spatial analysis and remote sensing for monitoring systems of *Oncomelania nosophora* following the eradication of schistosomiasis japonica in Yamanashi Prefecture, Japan. *Jpn. J. Infect. Dis.* **2009**, *62*, 125–132. [CrossRef]

103. Nihei, N.; Kajihara, N.; Kirinoki, M.; Chigusa, Y.; Matsuda, H.; Saitoh, Y.; Shimamura, R.; Kaneta, H.; Nakamura, S. Establishment of a GIS monitoring system for schistosomiasis japonica in Kofu, Japan. *Ann. Trop. Med. Parasit.* **2006**, *100*, 143–153. [CrossRef]

104. Tong, Q.B.; Chen, R.; Zhang, Y.; Yang, G.J.; Kumagai, T.; Furushima-Shimogawara, R.; Lou, D.; Yang, K.; Wen, L.Y.; Lu, S.H.; et al. A new surveillance and response tool: Risk map of infected *Oncomelania hupensis* detected by Loop-mediated isothermal amplification (LAMP) from pooled samples. *Act. Trop.* **2015**, *141*, 170–177. [CrossRef]

105. Zhang, Z.; Clark, A.B.; Bivand, R.; Chen, Y.; Carpenter, T.E.; Peng, W.; Zhou, Y.; Zhao, G.; Jiang, Q. Nonparametric spatial analysis to detect high-risk regions for schistosomiasis in Guichi, China. *Trans. R. Soc. Trop. Med. Hyg.* **2009**, *103*, 1045–1052. [CrossRef]

106. Scholte, R.G.C.; Gosoniu, L.; Malone, J.B.; Chammartin, F.; Utzinger, J.; Vounatsou, P. Predictive risk mapping of schistosomiasis in Brazil using bayesian geostatistical models. *Act. Trop.* **2014**, *132*, 57–63. [CrossRef] [PubMed]

107. Xu, J.F.; Lv, S.; Wang, Q.Y.; Qian, M.B.; Liu, Q.; Bergquist, R.; Zhou, X.N. Schistosomiasis japonica: Modelling as a tool to explore transmission patterns. *Act. Trop.* **2015**, *141*, 213–222. [CrossRef] [PubMed]

108. Hu, Y.; Ward, M.P.; Xia, C.; Li, R.; Sun, L.; Lynn, H.; Gao, F.; Wang, Q.; Zhang, S.; Xiong, C.; et al. Monitoring schistosomiasis risk in East China over space and time using a Bayesian hierarchical modeling approach. *Sci. Rep.* **2016**, *6*, 24173:1–24173:9. [CrossRef] [PubMed]

109. Schur, N.; Utzinger, J.; Vounatsou, P. Modelling age-heterogeneous *Schistosoma haematobium* and *S. mansoni* survey data via alignment factors. *Parasit. Vectors* **2011**, *4*, 142:1–142:10. [CrossRef] [PubMed]

110. Yang, K.; Sun, L.P.; Huang, Y.X.; Yang, G.J.; Wu, F.; Hang, D.R.; Li, W.; Zhang, J.F.; Liang, Y.S.; Zhou, X.N. A real-time platform for monitoring schistosomiasis transmission supported by google earth and a web-based geographical information system. *Geospat. Health* **2012**, *6*, 195–203. [CrossRef] [PubMed]

111. Feng, Y.; Liu, L.; Xia, S.; Xu, J.F.; Bergquist, R.; Yang, G.J. Reaching the surveillance-response stage of schistosomiasis control in The People's Republic of China. *Adv. Parasitol.* **2016**, *92*, 165–196. [CrossRef]

112. Brooker, S.; Clements, A.C.A.; Bundy, D.A.P. Global epidemiology, ecology and control of soil-transmitted helminth infections. *Adv. Parasit.* **2006**, *62*, 221–261. [CrossRef]

113. Lai, Y.S.; Zhou, X.N.; Utzinger, J.; Vounatsou, P. Bayesian geostatistical modelling of soil-transmitted helminth survey data in The People's Republic of China. *Parasit. Vectors* **2013**, *6*, 359:1–359:16. [CrossRef]

114. Scholte, R.G.C.; Schur, N.; Bavia, M.E.; Carvalho, E.M.; Chammartin, F.; Utzinger, J.; Vounatsou, P. Spatial analysis and risk mapping of soil-transmitted helminth infections in Brazil, using Bayesian geostatistical models. *Geospat. Health* **2013**, *8*, 97–110. [CrossRef]

115. Karagiannis-Voules, D.A.; Biedermann, P.; Ekpo, U.F.; Garba, A.; Langer, E.; Mathieu, E.; Midzi, N.; Mwinzi, P.; Polderman, A.M.; Raso, G.; et al. Spatial and temporal distribution of soil-transmitted helminth infection in sub-Saharan Africa: A systematic review and geostatistical meta-analysis. *Lancet Infect. Dis.* **2015**, *15*, 74–84. [CrossRef]

116. Atkinson, J.A.; Gray, D.J.; Clements, A.C.A.; Barnes, T.S.; McManus, D.P.; Yang, Y.R. Environmental changes impacting *Echinococcus* transmission: Research to support predictive surveillance and control. *Glob. Chang. Biol.* **2013**, *19*, 677–688. [CrossRef] [PubMed]

117. Conraths, F.J.; Deplazes, P. *Echinococcus multilocularis*: Epidemiology, surveillance and state-of-the-art diagnostics from a veterinary public health perspective. *Vet. Parasitol.* **2015**, *213*, 149–161. [CrossRef] [PubMed]

118. Cadavid, A.M.; Yang, Y.R.; McManus, D.P.; Gray, D.J.; Giraudoux, P.; Barnes, T.S.; Williams, G.M.; Soares, R.J.; Hamm, A.S.; Clements, A.C.A. The landscape epidemiology of echinococcoses. *Infect. Dis. Poverty* **2016**, *5*, 13:1–13:13. [CrossRef]

119. Schur, N.; Hürlimann, E.; Garba, A.; Traoré, M.S.; Ndir, O.; Ratard, R.C.; Tchuem Tchuenté, L.A.; Kristensen, T.K.; Utzinger, J.; Vounatsou, P. Geostatistical model-based estimates of schistosomiasis prevalence among individuals aged ≤20 years in West Africa. *PLoS Negl. Trop. Dis.* **2011**, *5*, e1194. [CrossRef]

120. Handali, S.; Pawitan, Y. Verifying elimination programs with a special emphasis on cysticercosis endpoints and postelimination surveillance. *J. Parasitol. Res.* **2012**, *2012*, 6. [CrossRef]

121. Basáñez, M.G.; McCarthy, J.S.; French, M.D.; Yang, G.J.; Walker, M.; Gambhir, M.; Prichard, R.K.; Churcher, T.S. A research agenda for helminth diseases of humans: Modelling for control and elimination. *PLoS Negl. Trop. Dis.* **2012**, *6*, e1548. [CrossRef]

122. Stothard, J.R.; Campbell, S.J.; Osei-Atweneboana, M.Y.; Durant, T.; Stanton, M.C.; Biritwum, N.K.; Rollinson, D.; Ombede, D.R.E.; Tcheum-Tchuenté, L.A. Towards interruption of schistosomiasis transmission in sub-Saharan Africa: Developing an appropriate environmental surveillance framework to guide and to support 'end game' interventions. *Infect. Dis. Poverty* **2017**, *6*, 10:1–10:4. [CrossRef]

123. Solomon, A.W.; Engels, D.; Bailey, R.L.; Blake, I.M.; Brooker, S.; Chen, J.X.; Chen, J.H.; Churcher, T.S.; Drakeley, C.J.; Edwards, T.; et al. A diagnostics platform for the integrated mapping, monitoring, and surveillance of neglected tropical diseases: Rationale and target product profiles. *PLoS Negl. Trop. Dis.* **2012**, *6*, e1746. [CrossRef]

124. Baker, M.; Mathieu, E.; Fleming, F.; Deming, M.; King, J.; Garba, A.; Koroma, J.B.; Bockarie, M.; Kabore, A.; Sankara, D.P.; et al. Mapping, monitoring, and surveillance of neglected tropical diseases: Towards a policy framework. *Lancet* **2010**, *375*, 231–238. [CrossRef]

125. Albonico, M.; Levecke, B.; LoVerde, P.T.; Montresor, A.; Prichard, R.; Vercruysse, J.; Webster, J.P. Monitoring the efficacy of drugs for neglected tropical diseases controlled by preventive chemotherapy. *J. Glob. Antimicrob. Resist.* **2015**, *3*, 229–236. [CrossRef]

126. Singer, B.H.; de Castro, M.C. Bridges to sustainable tropical health. *Proc. Natl. Acad. Sci. USA* **2007**, *104*, 16038–16043. [CrossRef] [PubMed]

3

Baseline Mapping of Schistosomiasis and Soil Transmitted Helminthiasis in the Northern and Eastern Health Regions of Gabon, Central Africa: Recommendations for Preventive Chemotherapy

Rodrigue Mintsa Nguema [1,2,3,*], Jacques F. Mavoungou [1], Krystina Mengue Me Ngou-Milama [3,4], Modeste Mabicka Mamfoumbi [2], Aubin A. Koumba [1], Mariama Sani Lamine [5], Abdoulaye Diarra [5,†], Ghislaine Nkone Asseko [5], Jean R. Mourou [2], Marielle K. Bouyou Akotet [2], Hélène Moné [6], Gabriel Mouahid [6] and Julienne Atsame [3]

[1] Research Institute in Tropical Ecology, National Center for Scientific and Technological Research, Libreville BP 13354, Gabon; mavoungoujacques@yahoo.fr (J.F.M.); aubinho25@yahoo.fr (A.A.K.)
[2] Department of Parasitology-Mycology, Faculty of Medicine, University of Health Sciences of Libreville, Libreville BP 4009, Gabon; mabikmamfoumbi@yahoo.fr (M.M.M.); mangondu20@yahoo.fr (J.R.M.); mariellebouyou@gmail.com (M.K.B.A.)
[3] Control Program of Parasitic Diseases, Libreville BP 2434, Gabon; ngoukrystina@yahoo.fr (K.M.M.N.-M.); julienneatsame@yahoo.fr (J.A.)
[4] National Laboratory of Public Health, Libreville BP 10736, Gabon
[5] Word Health Organization Country Office Gabon, Libreville BP 820, Gabon; salamarine_06@yahoo.fr (M.S.L.); diarraa@who.int (A.D.); nkoneassokog@who.int (G.N.A.)
[6] IHPE, Univ Montpellier, CNRS, UM, IFREMER, Univ Perpignan Via Domitia, Perpignan F-66860, France; mone@univ-perp.fr (H.M.); mouahid@univ-perp.fr (G.M.)
* Correspondence: rodriguemintsa@yahoo.fr
† Current Address: WHO Country Office Union des Comores, P.O. Box 435, Moroni, Union des Comores.

Abstract: In order to follow the Preventive Chemotherapy (PC) for the transmission control as recommended by WHO, Gabon initiated in 2014 the mapping of Schistosomiasis and Soil Transmitted Helminthiasis (STH). Here, we report the results of the Northern and Eastern health regions, representing a third of the land area and 12% of its total population. All nine departments of the two regions were surveyed and from each, five schools were examined with 50 schoolchildren per school. The parasitological examinations were realized using the filtration method for urine and the Kato-Katz technique for stool samples. Overall 2245 schoolchildren (1116 girls and 1129 boys), mean aged 11.28 ± 0.04 years, were examined. Combined schistosomiasis and STH affected 1270 (56.6%) with variation between regions, departments, and schools. For schistosomiasis, prevalence were 1.7% across the two regions, with no significant difference ($p > 0.05$) between the Northern (1.5%) and the Eastern (1.9%). Schistosomiasis is mainly caused by *Schistosoma haematobium* with the exception of one respective case of *S. mansoni* and *S. guineensis*. STH are more common than schistosomiasis, with an overall prevalence of 56.1% significantly different between the Northern (58.1%) and Eastern (53.6%) regions ($p = 0.034$). *Trichuris trichiura* is the most abundant infection with a prevalence of 43.7% followed by *Ascaris lumbricoides* 35.6% and hookworms 1.4%. According to these results, an appropriate PC strategy is given. In particular, because of the low efficacy of a single recommended drug on *T. trichiura* and hookworms, it is important to include two drugs for the treatment of STH in Gabon, due to the high prevalence and intensities of *Trichuris* infections.

Keywords: schistosomiasis; soil-transmitted-helminthiasis; mapping; preventive chemotherapy; transmission control; Gabon; Central Africa

1. Introduction

Combined schistosomiasis and Soil Transmitted Helminthiasis (STH) are the most prevalent infectious diseases in the world. They are the cause of serious global public health problems and impose a great burden on poor populations in the developing world [1]. Indeed, with the exclusion of malaria, the World Health Organization (WHO) further estimated that schistosomiasis and STH were responsible for more than 40% of the disease burden due to tropical diseases [2].

Schistosomiasis is acknowledged to be distributed in Africa, Asia, and South America with about 200 million infected people [3]. The WHO regards the disease as a Neglected Tropical Disease (NTD), with an estimated 732 million persons being vulnerable to infection worldwide in renowned transmission areas [4]. The Sub-Sahara African region remains the most affected with still high prevalence with about 192 million people infected [5]. In Gabon, with confirmed occurrence of *Schistosoma guineensis*, formely *S. intercalatum* lower Guinea strain, [6,7] and *S. haematobium*, with some cases of *S. mansoni*, it is estimated that a total of 310,391 people require preventive chemotherapy (PC) [8]. However, these 2010 estimates likely need revising.

Soil Transmitted Helminthiasis corresponds to a group of parasitic diseases that are caused by nematode worms that are transmitted to humans by faecally contaminated soil. The three major human diseases are caused by *Ascaris lumbricoides*, *Trichuris trichiura*, and hookworms (*Necator americanus* and *Ancylostoma duodenale*). The latest estimates indicate that more than two billion people are infected by at least one species worldwide and more frequently in areas where sanitation and water supply are insufficient [9]. STH infections are most common in children and such children have malnutrition, growth stunting, intellectual retardation, and cognitive and educational deficits [10]. It is estimated that over 35.4 million African school-aged children (SAC) are infected by *A. lumbricoides*, 40.1 million with *T. trichiura*, and 41.1 million with hookworms [11]. Since many children have multiple infections, it is estimated that 89.9 million are infected by at least one STH species [11]. In 2009, according to the burden of STH per country in the WHO African Region, 145,518 preschool (1−5 years) and 349,386 SAC (6−14 years), with a need of revising, were requiring PC in Gabon [9]. Indeed, the situation of STH in Gabon remains of concern and the latest local studies that were carried out showed that the prevalence is low in the sub-urban area (Melen, Libreville) and moderate in the rural area (Ekouk, 80 km of Libreville) [12].

Despite the burden that they cause in world public health, schistosomiasis and STH are considered as NTD's. Since the World Health Assembly in 2001, access to essential medicines for schistosomiasis and STH in endemic areas for the treatment of both clinical cases and groups at high risk for morbidity was recommended and endorsed by World Health Assembly resolution WHA54.19. The resolution urges member states to ensure access to essential drugs against schistosomiasis and STH in all health services in endemic areas for the treatment of clinical cases and groups at high risk of morbidity such as women and children. The declared that the aim of this resolution was to achieve at least the 75% coverage target of regular administration of anthelminthic drugs and up to 100% of all SAC at risk of morbidity by 2010 [13]. The strategy that was adopted by WHO since 2006 advocates integrated PC using a school-based approach with the concept of coordinated use of anthelminthic medicines against schistosomiasis and STH given the consideration that the diseases are largely co-endemic and that these medicines can safely be co-administered [14]. The 2010 target was not achieved, only 200 million SAC of the 600 million in need received treatment in 2010 [9]. The current goal is to revitalize the control strategy for achieving the 75% coverage target by 2020. PC for the populations at-risk in endemic areas was adopted once or twice a year, depending on risk levels, over a five-year period. Preschool and SAC in endemic areas were the primary target of PC interventions. Therefore, the target population was expanded to include all adults in high-risk areas. Communities can be classified into low-risk (<10% for schistosomiasis and <20% for STH), moderate-risk (≥10% for schistosomiasis and ≥20% for STH but <50% for both), and high-risk (≥50% for both) areas. These prevalence based on the SAC sampling are essential to adapt the frequency of PC (including SAC and at risk adults in the whole communities) according to the WHO disease specific thresholds [15].

Thus, the first step for establishing the PC strategy for schistosomiasis and STH is the knowledge of the geographic distribution of prevalence and the degree of overlap of the diseases in endemic areas [16]. The distribution of schistosomiasis and STH is particularly sensitive to environmental changes whose heterogeneity reflects numerous human and ecological factors, including changes of human origin and focal transmission [17]. For these purposes, there is a need to identify restricted areas where infection remains a public health problem for an integrated control identifying the broad scale patterns. A successful role for GIS applications in investigating the spatial epidemiology of the major human helminths was well recognized and helping to this purpose [18]. In 2009, 20 of the 32 African endemic countries had initiated the mapping of schistosomiasis and STH in order to implement the PC interventions [9]. In Gabon, schistosomiasis and STH are known to occur in many areas [8,9]; however, there has not been any sustained effort to control the diseases, apart from the establishment of the National Program for Control of Parasitic Disease in 1999, and to date, no major action had been taken at the national level by this program.

Until early 2014, PC interventions for schistosomiasis and STH had not been started in Gabon. To be in line of the WHO's target for the control of schistosomiasis and STH, Gabon initiated, in April 2014, the evaluation of the prevalence levels of schistosomiasis and STH throughout its territory. The aim was to report the outcome of schistosomiasis and STH at several levels in order to provide recommendations that are related to the implementation of PC interventions according to the WHO requirement. The present paper publishes the results regarding the Northern and Eastern health regions of Gabon.

2. Materials and Methods

2.1. Authorization and Ethical Assessment

Gabon aligns with the NTD coordinated mapping guidelines of WHO [15]. The implementation of the present study will enable the rapid scaling up of national mass treatment interventions and achieve the WHO targets that are set for 2020. An agreement was obtained for the implementation of this study as a public health exercise assumed for the Ministry of Health. Surveys were conducted in schools with the approval of the Ministry of National Education, school inspectors, directors, and teachers. Informed written consent was sought from the directors of selected schools as the legal guardian of all study schoolchildren. The school director receives prior verbal consent of the parents or guardians of schoolchildren after having explained to them the study and its objectives, with a translation in local language when necessary. Each individual that was involved in the study was registered in a data file and assigned to an anonymous identification number. At the end of the trial, infected persons were provided with appropriate chemotherapy, before the beginning of PC interventions, according to the WHO recommendations.

2.2. Study Area

Gabon is part of Central Africa. The Ministry of Public Health divides the country into 10 health regions and 52 departments. The health regions analyzed in this paper represent a third of the land of Gabon and include nine health departments, with five (Woleu, Ntem, Haut-Ntem, Haut-Okano and Okano) in the North region and four (Ivindo, Lopé and Mvoung and Zadié) in the East region (Figure 1). The General Direction for Statistic (GDS) estimated the total Gabonese population at 1,811,079 inhabitants, of which 34.7% were pre and SAC, and an urbanization rate of 87% [19]. However, predominantly urban population live in only 1% of the total space of the country, whereas the majority of territory (99% of superficies) is rural and hosts only 13% of population of the county. The study area comprises a total population of 218,279 inhabitants (154,986 and 63,293 in the North and East health regions, respectively).

Figure 1. Study area showing the nine health departments surveyed: in the Northen region (gray): Woleu, Ntem, Haut-Ntem, Haut-Okano, Okano and in the Eastern region (white): Ivindo, Lopé, Mvoung, and Zadié.

2.3. Study Type, Period and Population

A cross-sectional prospective study was carried out from January to February 2015. It included both male and female schoolchildren aged 10 to 14 years in priority (where the infection rates will be the highest and where WHO base their guidelines from) in the selected schools. Each included schoolchild must have provided both stool and urine, otherwise they were excluded from the survey.

2.4. Selection and Location of Schools

Each health department was considered as an ecologically homogeneous area. Five schools were selected randomly among those available for each department. Schools were either urban or rural and either public or private. The geographical coordinates of each school were recorded while using a Garmin GPS (Global Positioning System) (Table S1).

2.5. Schoolchildren Sampling

In each school, select 50 schoolchildren (25 girls and 25 boys) aged 10 to 14 years from the upper class, for a total of 250 schoolchildren in each health department. For the sampling, align all schoolchildren in the age group of interest from the upper class in two rows according to their gender (girl and boy). In each row (gender), select 25 schoolchildren.

If the row contains more than 25 schoolchildren, then a systematic random sampling method is used. For example, say there are 100 schoolchildren in the row, divide the total number of schoolchildren (100) by the number of schoolchildren you want in the sample (25), the answer is 4. This means that you are going to select every fourth schoolchildren from the row. Choose randomly a number between 1 and 4. This is your random starting point. Say your random starting point is

"3", this means you select schoolchild 3 in the row as your first schoolchild, and then every fourth schoolchild down the row (3, 7, 11, 15, 19, etc.) until you have 25 schoolchildren.

If the row contains exactly 25 schoolchildren, no random sampling is necessary; all 25 schoolchildren are directly selected.

If the row contain less than 25 schoolchildren, select them and complete the sample with schoolchildren in the age group of interest from the next upper class using a random sampling method, as described above.

2.6. Sample Collection and Parasitological Examination

Stool and urine samples of each individual were collected from 9.00 to 11.00 h am in a 100 and 50 mL of plastic screw-cap vial respectively and forwarded for examination in the laboratories equipped for the circumstance at the department level. Small cakes have been distributed to encourage them. Those who did not provide both samples despite any efforts were replaced according to the schoolchildren sampling protocol. For schools with fewer than 50 schoolchildren, enrollment is completed among the other schools that were selected in the same district. For each selected schoolchild, the urine and stool samples were collected, along with information on gender and age.

Urine was analyzed for the presence and the number of *S. haematobium* eggs, using a slightly modified Nucleopore syringe urine filtration method [20], filtering a 10 mL unique aliquot from each urine sample [21]. When the volume of the sample was less than 10 mL, it was measured before filtration and the number of eggs per 10 mL was estimated. Intensity of *S. haematobium* infection was expressed as the number of eggs per 10 mL of urine (eggs/10 mL). Stool samples were examined for the presence and the number of both STH and intestinal *Schistosoma* (*S. mansoni* and *S. guineensis*) eggs while using the Kato-Katz technique [22]. A single thick smear equivalent to 41.7 mg of stool was analyzed for each stool sample. The method used is that described in the Kato-Katz kit (VESTERGAARD FRANDSEN). Eggs were immediately examined and counted by microscopy to avoid egg lysis of hookworm eggs. Individual intensity of infection was expressed as eggs per gram of feces (epg).

2.7. Data Analysis

All the collected data: age, gender, and parasitological results, were reported on an Excel sheet. Prevalence of infection (percentage of infected schoolchildren among those examined) was estimated for each parasite, for each parasite group: schistosomiasis and STH and for the combined schistosomiasis and STH, at the overall, regional, departmental, school, school category (public/private), school location (urban/rural), and gender levels. The 95% confidence intervals (CI) for prevalence were calculated using the exact method in the software R version 3.2.2. Arithmetic mean intensities of infection (number of egg per infested schoolchild) with standard deviations (SD) for each parasite species were estimated, including only the positives schoolchildren [23]. The Chi squared or Fisher exact tests were used to compare the prevalence differences in relation to the region, gender, school category (private/public), and school area (urban/rural), while the non-parametric Wilcoxon or Mann-Whitney rank sum test were used to compare differences in mean intensities of infection using R version 3.2.2 or SPSS 10.0 for Windows software. The significance of tests was defined at $p < 0.05$. Prevalence generated in each department were used to produce the prevalence maps of distribution for each species using software ArcGis version 10.1.

3. Results

3.1. Characteristics of Sampling

A total of 45 schools were examined, 25 for North and 20 for East region, 27 for urban versus 18 for rural area and 27 for public versus 18 for private category. A total of 2245 schoolchildren (1116 girls and 1129 boys) and the mean number of schoolchildren per school was 49.9 ± 3.9. The number of examined schoolchildren is 1236 (632 girls and 604 boys) in the North region and 1009 (484 girls and 525 boys) in the East region. 1754 schoolchildren were from urban versus 491 from rural area and 1420 public versus 825 private. Age of schoolchildren ranged from 4 to 17 years with median age of 11 years. The total average ages of examined schoolchildren were 11.28 ± 0.04; 11.39 ± 0.05 in the Northern and 11.26 ± 0.09 in the Eastern region.

3.2. Prevalence

3.2.1. Combined Schistosomiasis and Soil Transmitted Helminthiasis

Of the 2245 schoolchildren surveyed, 1270 (56.57%; 95% CI 54.49–58.63%) were affected by schistosomiasis (at least one species) and/or STH (at least one species) (Table 1). Schoolchildren from the North region: 723 (58.50%; 95% CI 55.3–60.9%) were significantly more infected than those from the East region: 548 (54.31%; 95% CI 50.5–56.7%), (X-squared=4.5129, df = 1; p = 0.04169). At the department level, prevalence was from 44.4% (WLE department) to 73.6% (HKO department) in the Northern region and from 46.56% (LPE department) to 67.45% (ZAD department) in the Eastern. Prevalence was significantly different between departments (X-squared = 84.672, df = 8, p < 0.0001). All of the schools were infected with prevalence ranging from 28.6% at school 3 of WLE to 92.9% at school 3 of NTM in the North region and from 8.3% at school 4 of MVG department to 88.2% at school 4 of IVD in the East region (Table S2). There were significant differences between schools (X-squared = 325.31, df = 44, p < 0.0001). Gender and school category had no influence on prevalence of the combined schistosomiasis and/or STH (p > 0.05), while STH infections in rural schoolchildren (72.10%; 95% CI 67.90–76.02%) were significantly more prevalent than the urbans (51.60; 95% CI 49.23–53.96%), (X-squared = 64.633, df = 1, p < 0.00001).

Of the total 1270 affected schoolchildren, 718 had one species, 537 two species, 15 three species, and no schoolchild had four, five, six or more parasites concomitantly. For those affected with schistosomiasis only one had two species, and for those with STH, 528 had two species, eight had three species, and the rest had one species (Table 2).

Table 1. Percentage of infected schoolchildren (prevalence) [95% confidence intervals], at overall level, at regional level, according to gender, school area, and school category.

	N	Schistosomiasis			Soil Transmitted Helminthiasis			SCH	STH	SCH-STH
		S. haematobium	S. mansoni	S. guineensis	A. lumbricoides	T. trichiura	Hookworms			
Overall	2245	1.65 [1.16–2.27]	0.04 [0.0–0.25]	0.04 [0.0–0.25]	35.59 [33.61–37.59]	43.74 [41.68–45.82]	1.43 [0.98–2.01]	1.69 [1.2–2.32]	56.08 [54.0–58.15]	56.57 [54.49–58.63]
By region										
Northern	1236	1.46 [0.87–2.29]	0.08 [0.0–0.45]	0.08 [0.0–0.45]	29.13 * [26.60–31.75]	52.83 * [50.0–55.65]	1.62 [0.99–2.49]	1.54 [0.93–2.39]	58.09 * [55.29–60.86]	58.5 * [55.69–61.26]
Eastern	1009	1.88 [1.14–2.93]	0.00 [0.0–0.37]	0.00 [0.0–0.37]	43.51 [40.42–46.63]	32.61 [29.72–35.60]	1.19 [0.62–2.07]	1.88 [1.14–2.93]	53.62 [50.48–56.73]	54.2 [51.08–57.32]
By gender										
Girl	1116	1.25 [0.69–2.1]	0.00 [0.0–0.33]	0.09 [0.0–0.5]	34.14 [31.36–37.01]	42.47 [39.55–45.43]	0.81 [0.37–1.53]	1.34 [0.75–2.2]	54.84 [51.87–57.79]	55.11 [52.13–58.05]
Boy	1129	2.04 [1.30–3.04]	0.09 [0.0–0.49]	0.00 [0.0–0.49]	37.02 [34.20–39.92]	45.00 [42.07–47.95]	2.04 * [1.30–3.04]	2.04 [1.30–3.04]	57.31 [54.36–60.21]	58.02 [55.08–60.91]
By school area										
urban	1754	1.48 [0.97–2.16]	0.06 [0.0–0.32]	0.06 [0.0–0.32]	30.84 * [28.69–33.06]	40.59 [38.28–42.93] *	1.37 [0.88–2.03]	1.54 [1.02–2.23]	51.60 [49.23–53.96] *	52.17 [49.80–54.48] *
rural	491	2.24 [1.12–3.97]	0.00 [0.0–0.75]	0.00 [0.0–0.75]	52.55 [48.02–57.04]	54.99 [50.47–59.45]	1.63 [0.71–3.19]	2.24 [11.24–3.97]	72.10 [67.90–76.02]	72.51 [68.33–76.41]
By school category										
Public	1420	1.97 [1.31–2.84]	0.07 [0.0–0.39]	0.07 [0.0–0.39]	36.76 [34.25–39.33]	45.35 [43.74–47.98] *	1.62 [1.03–2.42]	2.04 [1.37–2.92]	57.61 [54.99–60.19]	58.24 [55.62–60.82] *
Private	825	1.09 [0.50–2.06]	0.00 [0.0–0.45]	0.00 [0.0–0.45]	33.58 [30.36–36.91]	40.97 [37.59–44.41]	1.09 [0.50–2.06]	1.09 [0.50–2.06]	53.46 [49.98–56.90]	53.82 [50.35–57.26]

* $p < 0.05$ (Chi squared test). SCH = combined Schistosomiasis (together *S. haematobium*, *S. mansoni* and *S. guineensis*); STH = combined soil transmitted helminthiasis (together *A. lumbricoides*, *T. trichiura* and Hookworms). SCH-STH = presence at least one schistosomiasis and/or soil transmitted helminthiasis.

Table 2. Proportion of polyparasitism for schistosomiaisis, soil transmitted helminthiasis (STH) and combined (schistosomiais-STH). N is the total number of examined schoolchildren.

Number of Species	N	Schistosomiasis	STH	Schistosomiasis-STH
1		37	723	718 *
2		1	528	537
3		0	8	15
4	2245	0	0	0
5		0	0	0
6		0	0	0
>6		0	0	0
Negative		2207	986	975

* In the STH column some of those also have schistosomiasis, so this decreases the number with 1 species in the SCH-STH column.

3.2.2. Combined Schistosomiasis

Including all three species, overall 38 cases (1.7%) were positive for schistosomiasis in 21 schools of the 45 surveyed, with no significant difference ($p > 0.05$) between the North, 19 cases (1.5%; 95% CI 0.9–2.4%), and the East region, 19 cases (1.88%; 95% CI 1.1–2.9%), (Table 1). Gender, school area and school category had no influence on prevalence of the combined schistosomiasis ($p > 0.05$). At the department level, prevalence was all <10%. It varied from 0.8% at WLE to 2.6% at HKO department in the North region ($p > 0.05$) and from 0.0% at ZAD to 4.4% at MVG department in the East region (X-squared = 22.032, df = 8, $p = 0.004857$). At the school level, prevalence was all < 10% (0% in 25 schools), with the exception of school 5 in MVG department, it was 15.8% (X-squared = 84.762, df = 44, $p = 0.0002171$).

3.2.3. Schistosomiasis Haematobium

It is the most frequent schistosomiasis that was found to be prevalent in 20 schools from the 45 studied (Table S2). Overall, *S. haematobium* affected 37 (1.45%; 95% CI 1.16–2.27%) schoolchildren with 18 (1.46%. 95% CI 0.87–2.29%) in the North and 19 (1.88%; 95% CI 1.14–2.93%) in the East region ($p > 0.05$). Gender, school area, and school category had no influence on prevalence of *S. haematobium* ($p > 0.05$). At the department level (Figure 2), the prevalence of *S. haematobium* was all <10%, from 0.8% (HNT department) to 2.4% (NTM department) in the North region and from 0% (ZAD department) to 4.36% (MVG department) in the East region, (X-squared = 21.741, df = 8, $p = 0.00542$). At the school level, prevalence varied from 0 (in 25 schools) to15.8% (six cases in school 5 in the MVG department) (X-squared = 85.959, df = 44, $p = 0.0001583$).

3.2.4. Other Schistosomiasis

S. guineensis and *S. mansoni* are very unusual, only one case of each respectively was listed in the North region. The *S. mansoni* case was encountered in school 4 of NTM department, while the *S. guineensis* case was in school 1 of HKO department (Table S2). All the distribution maps of schistosomiasis are presented in the Figure 2.

(A)

(B)

Figure 2. *Cont.*

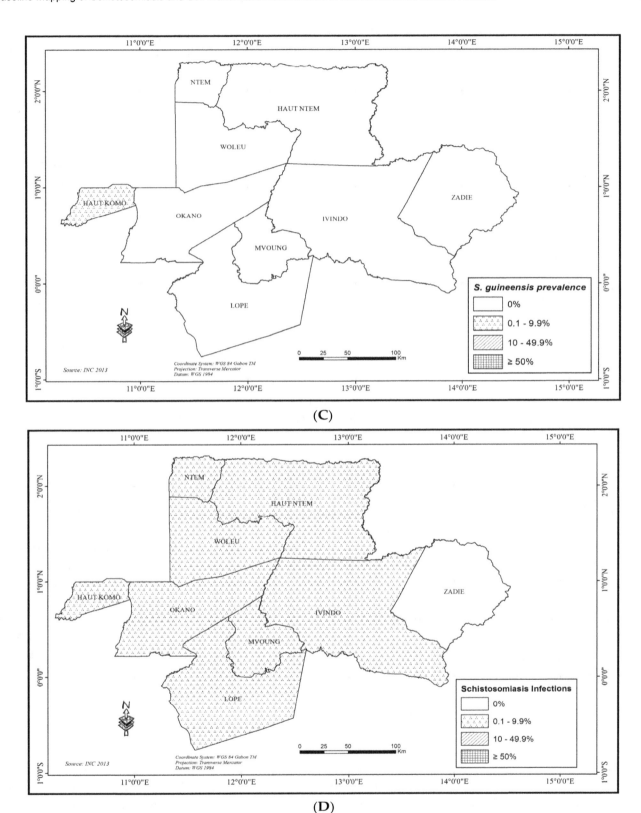

Figure 2. Map of prevalence levels for Schistosomiasis at department scale: (**A**) *Schistosoma haematobium*; (**B**) *S. mansoni*; (**C**) *S. guineensis*; and, (**D**) Combined schistosomiasis.

3.2.5. Combined Soil Transmitted Helminthiasis (STH)

Including all the STH, a total of 1259 (56.08%; 95% CI 54.0–58.15%) schoolchildren were affected by STH (Table 1). At the regional level, the North health region (58.09%; 95% CI 55.29–60.86%) was more affected than Eastern (53.62%; 95% CI 50.48–56.73%), (X-squared = 4.3331, df = 1, p = 0.03738). At the department level, significant differences were found (X-squared = 85.435, df = 8, p < 0.0001). Prevalence varied from 44.736% (WLE department) to 73.16% (HKO department) in the North and from 46.56% (LPE department) to 67.45% (LPE department) in the East region. At the school level, there were heterogeneity between schools (X-squared = 326.25, df = 44, p < 0.00001). One school had a prevalence of STH < 20%, 14 schools had a prevalence ≥20%, but <50% and 29 had a prevalence ≥50% (Table S2). Gender and school category had no influence on overall prevalence of STH (p > 0.05) while according to school area: schoolchildren of rural schools (72.1% [67.90–76.02]) had significantly higher prevalence than those of urban schools (51.6%; 95% CI 49.23–53.96%), X-squared = 64.633, df = 1, p < 0.0001.

3.2.6. *Ascaris lumbricoides*

A. lumbricoides was identified in 44 of the 45 schools studied for a total of 799 (35.59% (95% CI 33.61–37.59%)) schoolchildren affected (Table 1). According to the health region, East (43.51% (95% CI 40.42–46.63%)) was more affected than North (29.13% (95% CI 26.60–31.75%)), (X-squared = 50.126, df = 1, p < 0.0001). Gender and school category had no influence on overall prevalence of *A. lumbricoides* (p > 0.05) while rural schools (52.55% (95% CI 48.02–57.04%)) were more affected by *A. lumbricoides* than urban schools (30.84% (95% CI 28.69–33.06%)), (X-squared = 77.872, df = 1, p < 0.0001). At the department level (Figure 3), prevalence ranged from 12.9% in the WLE department to 58.04% in ZAD, (X-squared = 160.82, df = 8, p < 0.0001). Significant heterogeneity (X-squared = 382.81, df = 44, p < 0.0001) existed between schools: one is non-infected (0%), nine schools had a low prevalence (<20%), 19 had a moderate prevalence (≥20% but <50%), and 16 had a high prevalence (≥50%) (Table S2).

3.2.7. *Trichuris trichiura*

T. trichiura was prevalent in all schools surveyed and it was the more frequently found species with a total of 982 (43.7% (95% CI 41.68–45.8%)) infected schoolchildren. According to health region, a higher prevalence was found in the North (52.8% (95% CI 50–55.7%)) as compared to the East (32.6% (95% CI 29.7–35.6%)), (X-squared = 91.521, df = 1, p < 0.0001). There was a significant difference between rural (55%; 95% CI 50.5–59.5%) and urban schools (40.6%; 95% CI 38.3–42.9%), (X-squared = 31.729, df = 1, p < 0.0001)); and, between public (45.4%; 95% CI 43.7–48%) and private schools (41%; 95% CI 37.6–44.4%), (X-squared = 3.8965, df = 1, p < 0.0001) for the overall prevalence of *T. trichiura*. There was no significant difference of overall prevalence of *T. trichiura* according to gender (p > 0.05). At the department level, (Figure 3) the prevalence of *T. trichiura* varied from 27.13% in LPE to 67.53% in HKO department with significant heterogeneity (X-squared = 142.85, df = 8, p < 0.0001). At the school level, six schools had a prevalence of *T. trichiura* <20%, 21 schools had a prevalence ≤20% but <50%, and 18 had a prevalence ≥50% (Table S2). There was a significant difference in the distribution of *T. trichiura* among schools (X-squared = 340.14, df = 44, p < 0.0001).

3.2.8. Hookworms

Hookworms were present in 12 of the 45 studied schools with an overall prevalence of 1.43% (95% CI 1–2%): 1.6% (95% CI 0.99–2.49%) in the North region, 1.2% (95% CI 0.6–2.1%) in the East region. There was no significance difference between regions, school areas, and school categories (p>0.05), while there was a significant difference in overall prevalence of hookworm between girls (1.3%; 95% CI: 0.8–2.2%) and boys (2%; 95% CI: 1.3–3%) (X-squared = 5.2061, df = 1, p = 0.02251). At the department level (Figure 3), the prevalence was from 0 (for three departments) to a maximum of 6% in the WLE department with significant difference between departments (X-squared = 53.552, df = 8, p < 0.0001). Prevalence of hookworm in schools ranged from 0% (33 of the 45 schools surveyed) to 14.3% (Table S2). There were significant differences between schools (X-squared = 159.25, df = 44, p < 0.0001). Geographical distribution of the STH is presented in Figure 3.

(A)

(B)

Figure 3. *Cont.*

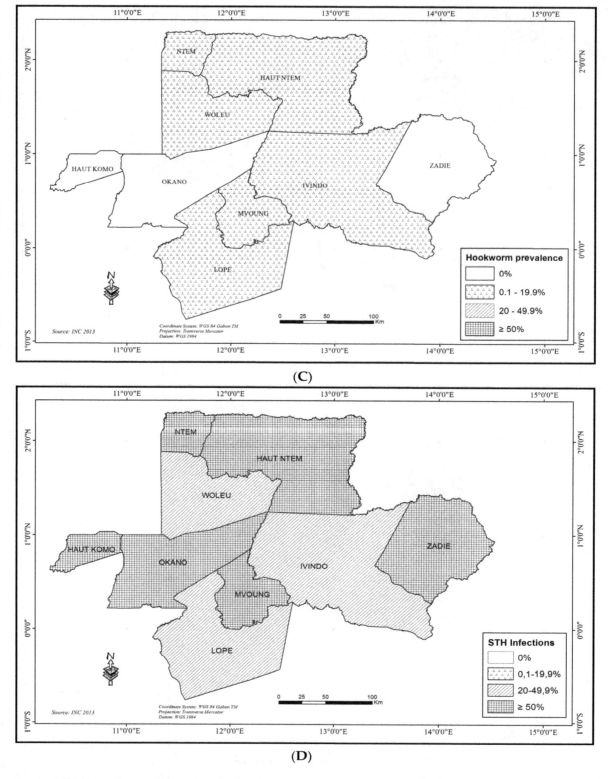

Figure 3. Map of prevalence levels for Soil Transmitted Helminthiasis at the department scale: (**A**) *Ascaris lumbricoides*; (**B**) *Trichurus trichuira*; (**C**) Hookworm; and, (**D**) Combined STH.

3.3. Intensity of Infection

3.3.1. Schistosomiasis

For the 37 schoolchildren that were infected with *S. haematobium*, the mean intensity of infections was 101.9 ± 41.1 eggs per 10 mL of urine with a significant difference between the North (18.3 ± 8.2 epg) and the East region (181.1 $\pm$ 85.6 epg), (W = 246, p = 0.02176) (Table 3). On the 20 schools prevalent with *S. haematobium*, light-intensity infections (<50 eggs/10 mL) occurred in 12 schools (11 in the North region and one in the East Region) and heavy-intensity infections ($\geq$50 eggs/10 mL) occurred in eight schools (one in the North region and seven in the East Region) (Table S3). The maximum individual egg counts was 1534 eggs/10 mL of urine; 73% of infected schoolchildren had low-intensity infections and 27% had heavy-intensity infections. Overall, there is no significant difference between the genders, the school areas, and the school categories (p > 0.05).

Intensity of infections was 72 epg for the only case of *S. mansoni* and 240 epg for the only case of *S. guineensis* (Table 3).

3.3.2. *Ascaris lumbricoides*

Overall mean intensity of infection was moderate: 9586.6 $\pm$ 618.3 epg and significantly different between the two regions: 11,433.6 $\pm$ 1061.7 epg for the North and 8071.9 $\pm$ 707.3 epg for the East region (W = 69,804, p = 0.004523) (Table 3). Of the 44 schools prevalent with *A. lumbricoides*, light-intensity infections (1–4999 epg) occurred in 10 schools (four in the North region and six in the East region), moderate-intensity infections (5000–49,999 epg) occurred in 33 schools (20 in the North region and 13 in the East region), and heavy-intensity infections ($\geq$50,000 epg) occurred in one school (in the North region) (Table S3). The maximum individual egg counts was 176,640, whereas 59.1% of infected schoolchildren had low-intensity infections, 37.5% with moderate-intensity infection, and 3.4% with heavy-intensity infections. Overall, gender, school area, and school category had no influence on the *A. lumbricoides* intensity of infection (p > 0.05).

3.3.3. *Trichuris trichiura*

The overall mean intensity of infection was moderate: 1143.2 $\pm$ 97 with a significant difference between the North (1395.2 $\pm$ 126.6 epg) and the East region (642.9 $\pm$ 140.2 epg), (W = 76,502, p = 1.551 $\times$ 10^{-13}) (Table 3). Intensities of infection were classified in the light-intensity infections class (1–999 epg) for 30 schools (13 in the North region and 17 in the East region), in the moderate-intensity infections class (1000–9999) for 15 schools (12 in the North region and three in the East region). No school had the heavy intensity infections ($\geq$10,000 epg) (Table S3). The maximum individual egg count was 37,440; 77.8% of the infected schoolchildren had low-intensity infections, 20.1% moderate-intensity infections, and 2.1% heavy-intensity infections. Overall, gender and school area had no influence on the *T. trichiura* intensity of infection (p > 0.05), while intensities of infection were higher in public schools (1193.5 $\pm$ 113.1 epg) than in private schools (1047.3 $\pm$ 182.1 epg) (W = 98,024, p-value = 0.01032) in the same class of intensity.

3.3.4. Hookworm

The overall mean intensity of infection was light: 618.0 $\pm$ 499.6 epg; 130.8 $\pm$ 31.1 epg in the North region and 1430.0 $\pm$ 1369.1 epg in the East region (Table 3). No significant difference was found between regions, gender, school areas, and school categories. The maximum individual egg count was 15,840 eggs and 96.9% of the schoolchildren had light-intensity infections (Table S3).

Table 3. Mean intensity of infection ± standard deviation at overall, by region, gender, school area, and school category. (N).

	Schistosomiasis			Soil Transmittted Helminthiasis		
	S. haematobium	*S. mansoni*	*S. guineensis*	*A. lumbricoides*	*T. trichiura*	**Hookworms**
Overall	101.9 ± 45.1 (37)	72 (1)	240 (1)	9586.6 ± 618.3 (799)	1143.2 ± 97.0 (982)	618.0 ± 499.6 (32)
By region						
North	18.3 ± 8.2 (18)	72 (1)	240 (1)	11433.6 ± 1061.7 (360)	1395.2 ± 126.6 (653)	130.8 ± 31.1 (20)
East	181.1 ± 85.6 (19)	-	-	8071.9 ± 707.3 (439)	642.9 ± 140.2 (329)	1430.0 ± 1369.1 (12)
By gender						
Girl	65.3 ± 32.4 (14)	-	240 (1)	10131.3 ± 1053.6 (381)	1152.6 ± 147.4 (474)	1861.3 ± 1853.7 (9)
Boy	124.2 ± 70.9 (23)	72 (1)	-	9018.1 ± 688.7 (418)	1130.1 ± 127.7 (508)	131.5 ± 35.0 (23)
By school area						
urban	109.5 ± 61.0 (26)	72 (1)	240 (1)	9144.6 ± 665.8 (541)	1139.9 ± 113.9 (712)	791.0 ± 669.2 (24)
rural	174.7 ± 55.3 (11)	-	-	10513.4 ± 1313.1 (258)	1151.7 ± 185.9 (270)	99.0 ± 46.9 (8)
By school category						
Public	73.3 ± 26.3 (28)	72 (1)	240 (1)	8874.4 ± 624.4 (522)	1193.5 ± 113.1 (644)	97.0 ± 18.9 (23)
Private	504.9 ± 178.5 (9)	-	-	10928.7 ± 1340.5 (277)	1047.3 ± 182.1 (338)	1949.3 ± 1843.5 (9)

3.4. Community Diagnosis and Recommended Treatment Strategies

According to our results on the prevalence and the intensity of infection, the recommended treatment strategies by department were summarized in Table 4.

Table 4. Diagnosis of health department and recommended treatment strategies.

Department	Category	MDA Interventions in Schools (Enrolled and Non-Enrolled)	Drug
Schistosomiasis infections			
Woleu Ntem Haut-Ntem Haut-Okano Okano Ivindo Lopé Mvoung	Low prevalence	MDA of SAC twice during primary schooling (once on entry, again on leaving)	Praziquantel
Zadié	Not endemic	No required MDA. Treatment of individual confirmed cases	
Soil Transmitted Helminthiasis infections			
Woleu	Moderate prevalence and moderate intensity	Annual MDA	
Ntem Haut-Ntem Haut-Komo Okano	High prevalence	Biannual MDA	Mebendazole + Levamisole
Ivindo Lopé	Moderate prevalence and moderate intensity	Annual MDA	
Mvoung Zadié	High prevalence	Biannual MDA	

MDA = mass drug administration; SAC = school-aged children.

4. Discussion

Our study showed that schistosomiasis and STH remain common in schoolchildren of both North and East health regions of Gabon with heterogenic proportions. Of the 2245 examined schoolchildren, 1270 (56.6%) were diagnosed by at least one schistosomiasis and/or STH. Infections were more influenced by both regions and school area. Indeed, schoolchildren in the North region (58.5%) were more affected than those in the East region (54.2%) and rural schoolchildren (72.10%) were more affected than urban schoolchildren (51.6%). Gender (girl/boy) and school category (public/private) had no influence on the burden of combined schistosomiasis or combined STH. However, hookworms affect more the boys than the girls and *T. trichiura* affect more the public than the private schoolchildren burden was most supported by STH than by schistosomiasis that is very low.

For schistosomiasis, the present study indicates that the infection is low endemic in the surveyed area, with the prevalence being 1.7% (all three species). Exhaustive results indicate that distribution of schistosomiasis is heterogeneous with an overall low endemicity for all the three species in the whole of the study area. Schistosomiasis haematobium was the most frequent and was diagnosed with at least one case in 20 schools from the 45 studied and from these 20 schools only one school was moderately endemic with a prevalence at 15.8%. Overall infection of *S. haematobium* was low (1.7%) in both the North (1.5%) and the East regions (1.9%). At the departmental level, prevalence was from 0.8% to 2.4% in the North region and from 0 to 4.4% in the Eastern region. Schistosomiasis *mansoni* and *guineensis* were rare in the surveyed areas with only one case of *S. mansoni* and *S. guineensis* respectively from the total schoolchildren examined. Data obtained here contrast with the results available for other areas and for the overall estimations in Gabon. Indeed, Mintsa *et al.* reported prevalence for *S. haematobium* at 17% and 26% in Melen, Libreville and Ekouk (80 km to Libreville), respectively [24], Gabon. Even wider, the estimation of prevalence of schistosomiasis in Gabon was about 45% [3]. Outside Gabon, in Central Africa, prevalence of schistosomiasis is generally high. For instance, in Cameroon, some localities in the East, West, and Central regions had prevalence of between 20 and 50%, and for some of them >50% [25]. In the Littoral, North-West and South-West Cameroon regions [26], prevalence were also much higher than those recorded in our study. This contrast confirms the patching distribution of schistosomiasis. Some parameters can explain the patching distribution of schistosomiasis and they include human and ecological factors [27], temperature, and rainfall [28]. The use of GIS for epidemiological survey in Tanzania showed that schistosomiasis was not endemic in areas where the temperature was below 20 °C [18,29]. By contrast, in Cameroon, prevalence is >10% for the areas where temperature is >40 °C and precipitation <1500 mm [30]. These differences can be attributed to both distribution of the intermediate snail host species in Africa [31] and their optimal conditions for development in West Africa [32]. In our study sites, temperature is >30 °C and precipitation >1000 mm, this should be in favor of high prevalence. Besides temperature and rainfall, relief [33], demography and living conditions [34] can also play a role in the distribution of schistosomiasis. Otherwise, the low presence *S. guineensis* can also be attributed to the possibilities of hybrid species which are mentioned in the country and are very indistinguishable using microscopy [24]. The hypothesis of the hybridization zones between *S. guineensis* and *S. haematobium* has been suggested in two provinces of western Gabon, Moyen-Ogooué [35] and Estuaire [36]. Hydridization between *S. guineensis* and *S. haematobium* led to the extinction of *S. guineensis* in favor of *S. haematobium*, as at Loum in Cameroon [37]. The low prevalence of *S. mansoni* in this study is not surprising because its distribution in the country is uncertain [38].

In addition to the low prevalence recorded in this study, schistosomiasis was characterized by low intensity of infections. Indeed, 73% of schoolchildren that were infected by *S. haematobium* had a light (<50 eggs/10 mL urine) intensity of infection, and 27% a heavy one (≥50 eggs/10 mL urine). These results are lower than those that were recorded at baseline results in the Barombi Kotto focus, Cameroon where the total intensity of infection was 212.1 e/10 mL urine in schoolchildren of ages between 3 and 22 years [23] and in the Sahel region, Burkina Faso [39]. The intensity of infection to *Schistosoma* is often correlated to the morbidity in SAC and other susceptible groups [40,41] and it plays an important role for the estimation of prevalence with consequences for the treatment strategy in PCT [38,42]. Although the microscopic techniques that were used in our study (urine filtration for *S. haematobium* diagnosis and Kato-Katz for *S. mansoni* and *S. guineensis* diagnosis) are the most recommended by WHO [43] and the most widely used diagnostic approaches in epidemiological surveys, their sensitivity is very discussed in foci with low intensity of infection because of day to day egg variations [44]. Hence, multiple Kato-Katz thick smears are required to enhance sensitivity [45], but this poses operational challenges and strains financial resources. As an alternative to these conventional diagnostic methods, novel tools showing a very high diagnostic accuracy have recently been developed. They include the detection of monoclonal antibody-based circulating antigens CCA and CAA [46] and the molecular approaches [47]. For example, it has been shown that estimation of prevalence with Kato-Katz technique underestimates the prevalence of active *S. japonicum* infections in China by a factor of 10 compared with the UCP-LF CAA assay [48]. Similarly, estimation of *S. haematobium* prevalence was several-fold higher with UCP-LF CAA assay than the one detected with a single urine filtration [49]. Since 2008, a more sophisticated Point-Of-Care (POC) test detecting *Schistosoma* CCA in urine has been developed and is now commercially available and is recommended by the authors for *S. mansoni* diagnosis [50,51]. A POC-CCA test revealed higher sensitivity than triplicate Kato-Katz, and it produced similar prevalence as nine Kato-Katz in many field survey evaluations [21,52]. The use of CCAs or CAAs might thereby affect the results and the recommendations for treatment strategies

Our results showed that STH were highly endemic. Overall, 56.1% of the schoolchildren examined were affected by the combined STH (together *A. lumbricoides*, *T. trichiura*, and Hookworms). This confirms the important level of STH in Central Africa, as in Cameroun [53]. Factors that may explain high levels of STH infections include lacks of sanitation and access to drinking water [9]. Our results indicate that the North region (58.1%) was most prevalent that the East (53.1%) and schoolchildren from rural schools (72.1%) were more affected than those from urban schools (51.6%).Various factors, such as genetics, poly-parasitism, demography, and urbanization, may explain these differences [11]. The most common STH was *T. trichiura* (43.7%), followed by *A. lumbricoides* (35.6%), with heterogeneous distributions between departments (Figure 3) and between schools. Indeed, *T. trichiura* and *A. lumbricoides* were moderately prevalent ($\geq$20 and <50%) in 21 and 19 schools, respectively, and both were very highly prevalent ($\geq$50%) in 16 schools. In contrast to the high prevalence of *A. lumbricoides* and *T. trichiura*, the prevalence of hookworm was low, 1.4% at overall, 1.6% in the North, and 1.2% in the East region. These results confirm the well documented observation that the prevalence of *T. trichiura* and *A. lumbricoides* were always higher than prevalence of hookworms [12,25,26]. Besides prevalence, the intensity of infection is a good indicator for epidemiology of STH. Indeed, most of the morbidity is accounted for by infected individuals who are the most heavily infected [54]. Our results showed a moderate-intensity infections for *T. trichiura*. (1143.2 epg overall) and *A. lumbricoides* (overall 9586.6 epg) and light-intensity infection for hookworms (overall 618 epg). However, 2.1% and 3.4% of schoolchildren had heavy-intensity of infections for *T. trichiura* and *A. lumbricoides*, respectively, attesting the burden of these STH in the surveyed foci.

One of the objectives of our study was to address recommendations for SCH and STH preventive chemotherapy in Gabon. Following WHO guidelines, based on prevalence and intensity of infections, the program is classifying communities according to three strategies: (1) a high prevalence ($\geq$50% for both Schistosomiasis and STH) or heavy-intensity infections, schoolchildren are treated every year, and high risk groups, such as fishermen, are treated; (2) a moderate prevalence ($\geq$10% for Schistosomiasis and $\geq$20% for STH, but <50% for both schistosomiasis and STH) and light-intensity infections, schoolchildren are treated once every two years; and (3) a low prevalence (<10% for Schistosomiasis and <20% for STH) and light-intensity infections, chemotherapy is made available in health facilities for treatment of suspected cases [15]. For schistosomiasis, considering the low prevalence recorded in our study, we recommend PC of SAC twice during primary schooling (once on entry, again on leaving) for eight departments and individual treatment for the confirmed cases in the Zadié department. We also recommend the diagnosis of other communities at high risk (such as pre-schoolchildren, pregnant women, and special occupation groups) and chemotherapy will be made available in health facilities for treatment of suspected cases according to OMS guidelines [15]. WHO recommended the drug Praziquantel (PZQ) with a dosage of 40mg/Kg for the treatment of schistosomiasis in PTC. Impact of treatment varies according to region and treatment strategy. An annual treatment strategy has significantly reduced prevalence of schistosomiasis 1, 2, and 3 years post-treatment in West Africa, i.e., Burkina Faso [38], Niger [55], Ghana [56]; East Africa i.e., Uganda [57], and in Central Africa, i.e., Cameroun [23,26]. For STH, we recommend a biannual PC strategy including pre and SAC, women of child bearing age including pregnant women in the 2nd and 3rd trimesters and lactating women and adults at high risk in certain occupations (e.g. tea-pickers and miners) for the six departments (Ntem, Haut-Ntem, Haut-Komo, Okano, Mvoung and Zadié), where the prevalence was high ($\geq$50%) and an annual PC strategy for the three departments (Woleu, Ivindo, Lopé) with moderate prevalence. Four anthelminthics are currently on the WHO model list of essential medicines for the treatment and control of STH: albendazole, mebendazole, levamisole, and pyrantel-pamoate [15]. Impact of these different drugs on STH are discussed by Keizer and Utzinger [58]. For these authors, oral single-doses of these drugs show high cure rates against *A. lumbricoides*, but not always against *T trichiura* and hookworms. Combination of mebendazole and levamisole shows the best cure rate against STH [59]. Furthermore, considering the total costs per child treated against schistosomiasis and STH, including drug and delivery, US$ 0.32 in Burkina Faso [35], the PC should integrate and progress with both schistosomiasis and STH.

Supplementary Materials: Table S1: list of schools surveyed per region and department with their respective geographical position. Non-italic = public school; italics = private school. In bold = urban school; normal = rural school, Table S2: Number of infected schoolchildren (prevalence in %) for each parasite according to school and department investigated. N is the number of schoolchildren examined. * $p < 0.05$ (Fisher-Exact-test); * is followed by school number or by department name with a significant difference, Table S3: Intensity of infection (mean ± standard deviation) for each parasite according to school and department investigated. N is the number of schoolchildren examined. * $p < 0.05$ (Mann-Whitney test); * is followed by the school number or department code with significant difference. L, M and H indicate class intensity of infection. L = light-intensity infection, M = moderate-intensity infections, H = heavy-intensity infections according to each species.

Author Contributions: Conceptualization: R.M.N., K.M.M.N.-M., J.A. and M.S.L. Data curation: R.M.N., J.F.M. and K.M.M.N.-M. Formal analysis: R.M.N., J.F.M., A.A.K., H.M. and G.M. Funding acquisition and relevant documents: J.A., A.D., and G.N.A. Investigation: R.M.N., K.M.M.N.-M., J.A. and M.M.M. Methodology: R.M.N., K.M.M.N.-M., M.S.L. and J.A. Project administration: R.M.N., K.M.M.N.-M., A.D., G.N.A. and J.A. Resources: J.A., K.M.M.N.-M., M.M.M., J.R.M. and M.K.B.A. Software: R.M.N., A.A.K., H.M. and G.M. Supervision: J.A., M.S.L., M.M.M. and J.R.M. Validation: M.S.L., G.N.A., M.K.B.A., G.M., H.M. and J.A. Visualization: R.M.N., G.M. and H.M. Original draft preparation: R.M.N. and J.F.M. Review and editing: All the authors.

Acknowledgments: The authors are grateful to the both Regional Directors of Health: Dr. Guikombi Jean Réné in the North and Ms. Mbeng Mba Félicité in the East for planning and communication work in the field. We want to thank all the participants in this study, particularly the schoolchildren and their parents, the directors and teachers of the schools surveyed. We are very grateful to Lilody Ikoutsi Gertrude, Ollomo Nziengui Fabrice, Oniane Nicole, Emane Alain Georges, Nzamba Boulingui Antoine Chyder, Minko mi Engone Gui, and Inguimba Elvis for the technical supports and assistance.

References

1. Hotez, P.J.; Kamath, A. Neglected tropical diseases in sub-Saharan Africa: Review of their prevalence, distribution, and disease burden. *PLoS Negl. Trop. Dis.* **2009**, *3*, e412. [CrossRef] [PubMed]

2. World Health Organization. Schistosomiasis and soil-transmitted helminth infections—preliminary estimates of the number of children treated with albendazole or mebendazole. *Wkly. Epidemiol. Rec.* **2006**, *81*, 145–163.

3. Steinmann, P.; Keiser, J.; Bo, R.; Tanner, M.; Utzinger, J. Schistosomiasis and water resources development: Systematic review, meta-analysis, and estimates of people at risk. *Lancet Infect. Dis.* **2006**, *6*, 411–425. [CrossRef]

4. WHO. *World Health Organization Schistosomiasis Fact Sheet*; World Health Organization: Geneva, Switzerland, 2014.

5. Adenowoa, A.F.; Oyinloyea, B.E.; Ogunyinkaa, B.I.; Kappo, A.P. Impact of human schistosomiasis in sub-Saharan Africa. *Braz. J. Infect. Dis.* **2015**, *19*, 196–205. [CrossRef] [PubMed]

6. Kane, R.A.; Southgate, V.R.; Rollinson, D.; Littlewood, D.T.J.; Lockyer, A.E.; Pagès, J.R.; Tchuem Tchuente, L.A.; Jourdane, J. A phylogeny based on three mitochondrial genes supports the division of *Schistosoma intercalatum* into two separate species. *Parasitology* **2003**, *127*, 131–137. [CrossRef] [PubMed]

7. Pagès, J.R.; Jourdane, J.; Southgate, V.R.; Tchuem Tchuente, L.A. Reconnaissance de deux espèces jumelles au sein du taxon *Schistosoma intercalatum* Fisher, 1934, agent de la schistosomose humaine rectale en Afrique. Description de *Schistosoma guineensis* n. sp. In *Taxonomy, Ecology and Evolution of Metazoan Parasites*; tome II; Combes, C., Jourdane, J., Eds.; Presses Universitaire de Perpignan: Perpignan, France, 2003; pp. 139–146.

8. WHO. *Schistosomiasis: Progress Report 2001–2011 and Strategic Plan 2012–2020*; WHO/HTM/NTD/PTC; World Health Organization: Geneva, Switzerland, 2013; p. 2.

9. WHO. *Soil-Transmitted Helminthiases: Eliminating Soil-Transmitted Helminthiases as a Public Health Problem in Children: Progress Report 2001–2010 and Strategic Plan 2011–2020*; WHO/HTM/NTD/PTC; World Health Organization: Geneva, Switzerland, 2012; p. 4.

10. WHO. *Deworming for Health and Development*; Report of the Third Global Meeting of the Partners for Parasite Control; World Health Organization: Geneva, Switzerland, 2005.

11. Brooker, S.; Clements, A.C.A.; Bundy, D.A.P. Global epidemiology, ecology and control of soil-transmitted helminth infections. *Adv. Parasitol.* **2006**, *62*, 221–261. [PubMed]

12. Mabika-Mamfoumbi, M.; Moussavou-Boussougou, M.N.; Nzenze-Afene, S.; Owono-Medang, M.; Bouyou-Okotet, M.; Kendzo, E.; Kombila, M. Prevalence evaluation of intestinal parasites in rural and sub-urban area in Gabon. *Bull. Med. Owendo* **2009**, *12*, 85–88.

13. Schistosomiasis and Soil-Transmitted Helminth Infections. Fifty-fourth World Health Assembly: Resolution WHA54.192001. 2001. Available online: http://apps.who.int/gb/archive/pdf_files/WHA54/ea54r19.pdf (accessed on 12 April 2018).

14. Namwanje, H.; Kabatereine, N.; Olsen, A. A randomised controlled clinical trial on the safety of co-administration of albendazole, ivermectin and praziquantel in infected schoolchildren in Uganda. *Trans. R. Soc. Trop. Med. Hyg.* **2011**, *105*, 181–188. [CrossRef] [PubMed]

15. WHO. *Preventive Chemotherapy in Human Helminthiasis: Coordinated Use of Anthelminthic Drugs in Control Interventions*; World Health Organization: Geneva, Switzerland, 2006.

16. Kolaczinski, J.; Kabatereine, N.B.; Onapa, A.; Ndyomugyengi, R.; Kakmebo, A.S.; Brooker, S. Neglected tropical diseases in Uganda: The prospect and challenge of integrated control. *Trend Parasitol.* **2007**, *23*, 485–493. [CrossRef] [PubMed]

17. Hunter, J.M.; Rey, L.; Chu, K.Y.; Adekolu-John, E.O.; Mott, K.E. *Parasitic Diseases in Water Resources Development: The Need for Intersectoral Collaboration*; World Health Organization: Geneva, Switzerland, 1993.

18. Brooker, S.; Micheal, E. The potential of geographical information systems and remote sensing in the epidemiology and control of human helminths infections. *Adv. Parasitol.* **2000**, *47*, 246–288.

19. Direction Générale de la Statistique. Résultats globaux du Recensement Général de la Population et des Logements de 2013 du Gabon (RGPL-2013). Libreville, Publication de la Direction Générale de la Statique (DGS). 2015. Available online: https://www.mays-mouissi.com/wp-content/uploads/2016/07/Recensement-general-de-la-population-et-des-logements-de-2013-RGPL.pdf (accessed on 01 December 2017).

20. Peters, P.A.; Mahmoud, A.A.; Warren, K.S.; Ouma, J.H.; Siongok, T.K. Field studies of a rapid, accurate means of quantifying *Schistosoma haematobium* eggs in urine samples. *Bull. World Health Organ.* **1976**, *54*, 159–162. [PubMed]

21. Coulibaly, J.T.; Knopp, S.; N'Guessan, N.A.; Silue, K.D.; Furst, T.; Lohourignon, L.K.; Brou, J.K.; N'Gbesso, Y.K.; Vounatsou, P.; N'Goran, E.K.; et al. Accuracy of Urine Circulating Cathodic Antigen (CCA) Test for *Schistosoma mansoni* diagnosis in different settings of Côte d'Ivoire. *PLoS Negl. Trop. Dis.* **2011**, *5*, e1384. [CrossRef] [PubMed]

22. Katz, N.; Chaves, A.; Pellegrino, J. A simple device for quantitative stool thick-smear technique in *Schistosomiasis mansoni*. *Rev. Inst. Med. Trop. Sao Paulo* **1972**, *14*, 397–400. [PubMed]

23. Nkengazong, L.; Njiokou, F.; Asonganyi, T. Two years impact of single praziquantel treatment on infection of urinary schistosomiasis in the Barombi Kotto focus, Cameroon. *Int. J. Biosci.* **2013**, *3*, 98–107.

24. Mintsa Nguema, R.; Mengue Ngou-Milama, K.; Kombila, M.; Rechard-Lenoble, D.; Tisseyre, P.; Ibikounlé, M.; Moné, H.; Mouahid, G. Morphometric and molecular characterizations of schistosome populations in Estuaire province Gabon. *J. Helminthol.* **2010**, *84*, 81–85. [CrossRef] [PubMed]

25. Tchuem Tchuenté, L.A.; Kamwa Ngassam, R.I.; Sumo, L.; Ngassam, P.; Dongmo Noumedem, C.; Luogbou Nzu, D.D.; Dankoni, E.; Kenfack, C.M.; Gipwe, N.F.; Akame, J.; et al. Mapping of Schistosomiasis and Soil-Transmitted Helminthiasis in the Regions of Centre, East and West Cameroon. *PLoS Negl. Trop. Dis.* **2012**, *6*, e1553. [CrossRef] [PubMed]

26. Tchuem Tchuenté, L.A.; Dongmo Noumedem, C.; Ngassam, P.; Mérimé Kenfack, C.; Feussom Gipwe, N.; Dankoni, E.; Merrime Kenfack, C.; Feussom Gipwe, N.; Akame, J.; Tarini, A.; et al. Mapping of schistosomiasis and soil transmitted helminthiasis in the regions of Littoral, North-West, South and South-West Cameroon and recommendations for treatment. *BMC Infect. Dis.* **2013**, *13*, 602. [CrossRef] [PubMed]

27. Woolhouse, M.E.J.; Chandiwana, S.K. Spatial and temporal heterogeneity in the population dynamics of *Bulinus globosus* and *Biomphalaria pfeifferi* and in the epidemiology of their infection with Schistosomes. *Parasitology* **1989**, *98*, 21–34. [CrossRef] [PubMed]

28. Brooker, S. Schistosomes, snails and satellites. *Acta Trop.* **2002**, *82*, 207–214. [CrossRef]

29. Brooker, S.; Hay, S.I.; Issae, W.; Hall, A.; Kihamia, C.M.; Lwambo, N.J.S.; Wint, W.; Rogers, D.J.; Bundy, D.A.P. Predicting the distribution of urinary schistosomiasis in Tanzania using satellite sensor data. *Trop. Med. Int. Health* **2001**, *6*, 998–1007. [CrossRef] [PubMed]

30. Brooker, S.; Hay, S.I.; Tchuem Tchuenté, L.A.; Ratard, R. Modelling human helminth distributions for planning disease control in Cameroon. *Photogramm. Eng. Remote Sens.* **2002**, *68*, 175–179.

31. Brown, S.D. *Freshwater Snail of Africa and Their Medical Importance*; Taylor and Francis: London, UK, 1994.

32. Greer, G.J.; Mimpfoundi, R.; Malek, E.A.; Joky, A.; Ngonseu, E.; Ratard, R.C. Human schistosomiasis in Cameroon II. Distribution of the snail hosts. *Am. J. Trop. Med. Hyg.* **1990**, *6*, 573–580. [CrossRef]

33. Kabatereine, N.B.; Brooker, S.; Tukahebwa, E.M.; Kazibwe, F.; Onapa, A. Epidemiology and geography of *Schistosoma mansoni* in Uganda: Implications for planning control. *Trop. Med. Int. Health* **2004**, *9*, 372–380. [CrossRef] [PubMed]

34. WHO. *Report on the WHO Informal Consultation on Schistosomiasis Control*; World Health Organization: Geneva, Switzerland, 1999; p. 2.

35. Burchard, G.D.; Kern, P. Probable hybridization between *S. intercalatum* and *S. haematobium* in Western Gabon. *Trop. Geogr. Med.* **1985**, *37*, 119–123. [PubMed]

36. Richard-Lenoble, D.; Kombila, M.; Duong, T.H.; Gendrel, D. Bilharziose à *Schistosoma intercalatum*, bilharziose récente et oubliée. *Rev. Pratc.* **1993**, *43*, 432–439.

37. Webster, B.L.; Tchuem Tchuenté, L.A.; Jourdane, J.; Southgate, V.R. The interaction of *Schistosoma haematobium* and *S. guineensis* in Cameroon. *J. Helminthol.* **2005**, *79*, 193–197. [CrossRef] [PubMed]

38. Mintsa Nguema, R.; Mve Ondo, B.; Mabika Mamfoumbi, M.; Koumba, A.A.; Bouyou Akotet, M.K.; Kombila, M. Recent Examination for Assessing Epidemiological Status of Schistosoma *Mansoni* in Plaine Orety, Urban Area of Libreville, Gabon, Central Africa. *CAJPH* **2018**, *4*, 81–85. [CrossRef]

39. Toure, S.; Zhang, Y.; Bosque-Oliva, E.; Ky, C.; Ouedraogo, A.; Koukounariet, A.; Gabrielli, A.F.; Sellin, B.; Websterb, J.P.; Fenwickb, A. Two-year impact of single praziquantel treatment on infection in the national control programme on schistosomiasis in Burkina Faso. *Bull. World Health Organ.* **2008**, *86*, 780–787. [CrossRef] [PubMed]

40. Smith, D.H.; Warren, K.S.; Mahmoud, A.A.F. Morbidity in *Schistosomiasis Mansoni* in relation to intensity of infection: Study of a community in Kisumu, Kenya. *Am. J. Trop. Med. Hyg.* **1979**, *28*, 220–229. [PubMed]

41. Genming, Z.; Brinkmann, U.K.; Qingwu, J.; Shaoji, Z.; Zhide, L.; Hongchang, Y. The relationship between morbidity and intensity of *Schistosomiasis japonicum* infection of a community in Jiangxi Province, China. *Southeast. Asian J. Trop. Med. Public Health* **1977**, *28*, 245–250.

42. Utzinger, J.; Becker, S.L.; van Lieshout, L.; van Dam, G.J.; Knopp, S. New diagnostic tools in schistosomiasis. *Clin. Microbiol. Infect.* **2015**, *21*, 529–542. [CrossRef] [PubMed]

43. WHO. *Basic Laboratory Methods in Medical Parasitology*; World Health Organization: Geneva, Switzerland, 1991.

44. Braun-Munzinger, R.A.; Southgate, B.A. Repeatability and reproducibility of egg counts of *Schistosoma haematobium* in urine. *Trop. Med. Parasitol.* **1992**, *43*, 149–154. [PubMed]

45. Lamberton, P.H.L.; Kabatereine, N.B.; Oguttu, D.W.; Fenwick, A.; Webster, J.P. Sensitivity and specificity of multiple Kato-Katz thick smears and a Circulating Cathodic Antigen test for *Schistosoma mansoni* Diagnosis Pre-and Post-repeated-Praziquantel treatment. *PLoS Negl. Trop. Dis.* **2014**, *8*, e3139. [CrossRef] [PubMed]

46. Van Lieshout, L.; Polderman, A.M.; Deelder, A.M. Immunodiagnosis of schistosomiasis by determination of the circulating antigens CAA and CCA, in particular in individuals with recent or light infections. *Acta Trop.* **2000**, *77*, 68–80. [CrossRef]

47. Obeng, B.B.; Aryeetey, Y.A.; de Dood, C.J.; Amoah, A.S.; Larbi, I.A.; Deelder, A.M.; Yazdanbakhsh, M.; Hartgers, F.C.; Boakye, D.A.; Verweij, J.J.; et al. Application of a circulating-cathodic-antigen (CCA) strip test and real-time PCR, in comparison with microscopy, for the detection of *Schistosoma haematobium* in urine samples from Ghana. *Ann. Trop. Med. Parasitol.* **2008**, *102*, 625–633. [CrossRef] [PubMed]

48. Van Dam, G.J.; Xu, J.; Bergquist, R.; de Dood, C.J.; Utzinger, J.; Qin, Z.Q.; Guanb, W.; Fengb, T.; Yug, X.L.; Zhoug, J.; et al. An ultra-sensitive assay targeting the circulating anodic antigen for the diagnosis of *Schistosoma japonicum* in a low-endemic area, People's Republic of China. *Acta Trop.* **2015**, *141*, 190–197. [CrossRef] [PubMed]

49. Knopp, S.; Corstjens, P.L.A.M.; Koukounari, A.; Cercamondi, C.I.; Ame, S.M.; Ali, S.M.; de Dood, C.J.; Mohammed, K.A.; Utzinger, J.; Rollinson, D.; et al. Sensitivity and specificity of a urine circulating anodic antigen test for the diagnosis of *Schistosoma haematobium* in low endemic settings. *PLoS Negl. Trop. Dis.* **2015**, *9*, e0003752. [CrossRef] [PubMed]

50. Stothard, J.R.; Kabatereine, N.B.; Tukahebwa, E.M.; Kazibwe, F.; Rollinson, D.; Mathieson, W.; Webster, J.P.; Fenwick, A. Use of circulating cathodic antigen (CCA) dipsticks for detection of intestinal and urinary schistosomiasis. *Acta Trop.* **2006**, *97*, 219–228. [CrossRef] [PubMed]

51. Colley, D.G.; Binder, S.; Campbell, C.; King, C.H.; Tchuem Tchuenté, LA.; N'Goran, E.K. A Five-Country Evaluation of a Point-of-Care Circulating Cathodic Antigen Urine Assay for the Prevalence of *Schistosoma mansoni*. *Am. J. Trop. Med. Hyg.* **2013**, *88*, 426–432. [CrossRef] [PubMed]

52. Tchuem Tchuenté, L.A.; Kueté Fouodo, C.J.; Kamwa Ngassam, R.I.; Sumo, L.; Dongmo Noumedem, C.; Mérimé Kenfack, C.; Gipwe, N.F.; Dankoni Nana, E.; Stothard, J.R.; Rollinson, D. Evaluation of Circulating Cathodic Antigen (CCA) Urine-Tests for Diagnosis of *Schistosoma mansoni* Infection in Cameroon. *PLoS Negl. Trop. Dis.* **2012**, *6*, e1758. [CrossRef] [PubMed]

53. Ratard, R.C.; Kouemeni, L.E.; Ekani Bessala, M.M.; Ndamkou, K.N.; Greer, G.J.; Spilsbury, J.; Cline, B.L. Human schistosomiasis in Cameroon. I. Distribution of schistosomiasis. *Am. J. Trop. Med. Hyg.* **1990**, *42*, 561–572. [CrossRef] [PubMed]

54. WHO. *Prevention and Control of Schistosomiasis and Soil-Transmitted Helminthiasis*; World Health Organisation: Geneva, Switzerland, 2002.

55. Garba, A.; Campagne, G.; Tassie, J.M.; Barkire, A.; Vera, C.; Sellin, B.; Chippaux, J.P. Evaluation à long terme d'un traitement de masse par praziquantel sur la morbidité due à *Schistosoma haematobium* dans deux villages hyper-endémiques du Nige. *Bull. Soc. Pathol. Exot.* **2004**, *97*, 7–11. [PubMed]

56. Nsowah-Nuamah, N.N.; Aryeetey, M.E.; Jolayemi, E.T.; Yagatsuma, Y.; Mensah, G.; Dontwi, I.K.; Nkrumah, F.K.; Kojima, S. Predicting the timing of second praziquantel treatment and its effect on reduction of egg counts in southern Ghana. *Acta Trop.* **2004**, *90*, 263–720. [CrossRef] [PubMed]

57. Frenzel, K.; Grigull, L.; Odongo-Aginya, E.; Ndugwa, C.M.; Loroni-Lakwo, T.; Schweigmann, U.; Vester, U.; Spannbrucker, N.; Doehring, E. Evidence for a long-term effect of a single dose of praziquantel on *Schistosoma mansoni*–induced hepatosplenic lesions in Northern Uganda. *Am. J. Trop. Med. Hyg.* **1999**, *60*, 927–931. [CrossRef] [PubMed]

58. Keizer, J.; Utzinger, J. Efficacity of current drugs against Soil Transmitted Helminthiasis infections: Systematic review and meta-analysis. *JAMA* **2008**, *299*, 1937–1948.

59. Albonico, M.; Bickle, Q.; Ramsan, M.; Montresor, A.; Savioli, L.; Taylor, M. Efficacy of mebendazole and levamisole alone or in combination against intestinal nematode infections after repeated targeted mebendazole treatment in Zanzibar. *Bull. World Health Organ.* **2003**, *81*, 343–352. [PubMed]

4

Phylogeography of *Bulinus truncatus* (Audouin, 1827) (Gastropoda: Planorbidae) in Selected African Countries

Eniola M. Abe [1,*], Yun-Hai Guo [1], Haimo Shen [1], Masceline J. Mutsaka-Makuvaza [2],
Mohamed R. Habib [3], Jing-Bo Xue [1], Nicholas Midzi [2], Jing Xu [1], Shi-Zhu Li [1]
and Xiao-Nong Zhou [1,*]

[1] National Institute of Parasitic Diseases (NIPD), Chinese Centre for Disease Control and Prevention, Shanghai 200025, China; guoyunhaigy@163.com (Y.G.); shenhm@nipd.chinacdc.cn (H.S.); xuejb@nipd.chinacdc.cn (J.-B.X.); xujing@nipd.chinacdc.cn (J.X.); lisz@chinacdc.cn (S.-Z.L.)

[2] Department of Medical Microbiology, College of Health Sciences, University of Zimbabwe, Harare 00263, Zimbabwe; mascelinejeni@gmail.com (M.M.-M.); midzinicholas@gmail.com (N.M.)

[3] Medical Malacology Laboratory, Theodor Bilharz Research Institute, Giza 12411, Egypt; m_ramadanhabib@yahoo.com

* Correspondence: abeeniola11@126.com (E.M.A.); zhouxn1@chinacdc.cn (X.-N.Z.);

Abstract: The transmission of some schistosome parasites is dependent on the planorbid snail hosts. *Bulinus truncatus* is important in urinary schistosomiasis epidemiology in Africa. Hence, there is a need to define the snails' phylogeography. This study assessed the population genetic structure of *B. truncatus* from Giza and Sharkia (Egypt), Barakat (Sudan) and Madziwa, Shamva District (Zimbabwe) using mitochondrial cytochrome oxidase subunit 1 gene (COI) and internal transcribed spacer 1 (ITS 1) markers. COI was sequenced from 94 *B. truncatus* samples including 38 (Egypt), 36 (Sudan) and 20 (Zimbabwe). However, only 51 ITS 1 sequences were identified from Egypt (28) and Sudan (23) (because of failure in either amplification or sequencing). The unique COI haplotypes of *B. truncatus* sequences observed were 6, 11, and 6 for Egypt, Sudan, and Zimbabwe, respectively. Also, 3 and 2 unique ITS 1 haplotypes were observed in sequences from Egypt and Sudan respectively. Mitochondrial DNA sequences from Sudan and Zimbabwe indicated high haplotype diversity with 0.768 and 0.784, respectively, while relatively low haplotype diversity was also observed for sequences from Egypt (0.334). The location of populations from Egypt and Sudan on the *B. truncatus* clade agrees with the location of both countries geographically. The clustering of the Zimbabwe sequences on different locations on the clade can be attributed to individuals with different genotypes within the population. No significant variation was observed within *B. truncatus* populations from Egypt and Sudan as indicated by the ITS 1 tree. This study investigated the genetic diversity of *B. truncatus* from Giza and Sharkia (Egypt), Barakat area (Sudan), and Madziwa (Zimbabwe), which is necessary for snail host surveillance in the study areas and also provided genomic data of this important snail species from the sampled countries.

Keywords: phylogeography; *Bulinus truncatus*; planorbidae; Africa

1. Background

The snail intermediate hosts of the genus *Bulinus* play active roles in the epidemiology of urinary schistosomiasis. The schistosome parasites depend on these snails for the development of the asexual phase of their life cycle before the cercariae are released into the water bodies to look for unsuspecting human hosts for penetration, where they continue the sexual phase of their development [1–4].

Members of the genus *Bulinus* are hermaphroditic planorbid snails, and this genus includes 37 recognized species distributed in the tropic and sub-tropic regions of the world including Africa, Mediterranean countries, and parts of the Middle East [5]. They differ in their interaction with schistosome parasites and some are involved in the transmission of human and animal schistosomiasis [6].

These important snail species inhabit various types of freshwater bodies such as streams, ponds, rivers, and irrigation canals [7]. The genetic structure of snail hosts is mostly determined by their habitat distribution, which is largely influenced by the spatial and temporal fluctuations in water availability [8,9] leading to population bottlenecks [5].

Snails belonging to the *Bulinus* group have a great capacity to rapidly increase their population size through cross- or self-fertilization, but *B. truncatus* has a preference for self-fertilization [10]. Selfing and population bottlenecks increase genetic differentiation among snail population but reduce the amount of genetic diversity within a population [11].

Whilst morphological identification of snails helps with identifying snails at group or genus level, it cannot give further insights about their interaction with the parasites [12].

Assessment of snail hosts population structure using molecular markers and other genetic tools creates a robust system for species identification and differentiation [8,12–17]. This provides useful information about their genetic diversity and detailed elucidation of the host–parasite relationship [4], which can be applied to target effective integrated schistosomiasis control strategies in most endemic areas [18].

The use of different markers such as COI, microsatellites and ITS 1, has helped to achieve identification of *B. truncatus* sampled from few African countries including Senegal, Niger, Tanzania, Burkina Faso, and Cameroon [11,12]. Studies have also observed strong population subdivision and low diversity for hermaphroditic freshwater snails including *B. truncatus* [11,19–23].

It is, therefore, imperative to provide information on the diversity of important snail hosts including *B. truncatus* through assessing their phylogenic status in most countries endemic for schistosomiasis across Africa, to further improve our understanding about their phylogenetic relationships as well as the disease epidemiology.

This study provided information on the phylogeography of *B. truncatus* populations from Giza and Sharkia (Egypt), Barakat area (Sudan), and Madziwa, Shamva District (Zimbabwe), using partial mitochondrial DNA cytochrome oxidase subunit I (COI) and internal transcribed spacer 1 (ITS 1) to determine their phylogenetic relationship, which is important for epidemiological investigation and snail hosts surveillance.

2. Materials and Methods

2.1. Sample Collection

Bulinus snails were collected from different locations in freshwater bodies at Giza and Sharkia governorates (Egypt), Barakat area (Sudan) and Madziwa area, Shamva District (Zimbabwe). Snail sampling was done at selected sites along water bodies; these included water contact sites where people swim, carry out fishing activities, collect water for domestic purposes, bathing, and washing clothes and utensils. Sites with no apparent human water contact activities were also visited for snail collection. A total of 134 *Bulinus* snails was assessed from different locations across the three countries.

The snails were identified phenotypically using shell morphology [24]. Snails were then preserved in absolute ethanol. Information that includes snail collection and geographic coordinates of the study areas are shown in Table 1. A map of study areas is shown in Figure 1.

Table 1. Geographic coordinates of the study areas.

Country	Location	No. of Samples Collected	Time of Collection	Type of Water Body	Latitude	Longitude
Egypt	Giza (El-Nile river, Gezerite El-Warrak)	25	October, 2016	River	30.102	31.243
	Sharkia (El-Salam canal, El-Hesenia district)	30	November, 2016	Canal	31.258	32.270
Sudan	Barakat area, Wad Madani	14	July, 2016	Canal	14.33673	33.52736
	Barakat area, Wad Madani	22	August, 2016	Canal	14.31780	33.53167
	Barakat area, Wad Madani	5	August, 2016	Canal	14.29210	33.55261
	Barakat area, Wad Madani	8	August, 2016	Canal	14.25122	33.59070
Zimbabwe	Madziwa, Shamva District	11	March, 2016	River	16.93642	31.44603
	Madziwa	6	March, 2016	River	16.91498	31.42868
	Madziwa	10	June, 2016	River	16.85695	31.49413
	Madziwa	3	June, 2016	River	16.88070	31.49083

Figure 1. Map of Africa showing countries where snail samples were collected.

2.2. Sample Preparation and DNA Extraction

The specimens were recounted, identified by morphological characters, and re-spirited (absolute ethanol) upon arrival at the National Institute of Parasitic Diseases, Shanghai, schistosomiasis laboratory [25]. Specimens were placed in TE buffer (10 mM Tris, 0.1 mM EDTA) pH 7.4 for 1 h to remove the remaining alcohol from within the tissue, which might interfere with subsequent extraction techniques. Total genomic DNA was isolated from head-foot snail tissue using the DNeasy Blood and Tissue kit (Qiagen, Crawley, UK) according to the manufacturer's instructions. DNA was eluted into 200 μL AE buffer. The snails' genomic DNA concentration was quantified using the Nanodrop

ND-1000 Spectrophotometer (Nanodrop Technologies Inc., Thermo Fisher Scientific, Wilmington, DE, USA).

2.3. Polymerase Chain Reaction (PCR) Amplification of COI and ITS 1 Fragments

IllustraPuRe Taq Ready-To-Go PCR beads (GE Healthcare) were used for the amplification of the COI and ITS 1 fragments using the methods outlined in Kane et al. [12] with 0.4 µM each of Bulcox 5 (5'CCT TTA AGA GGN CCT ATT GC 3') (forward primer) and Bulcox 14 (5'GGA AAT CAG TAM AYA AAA CCA GC 3') (reverse primer) while ETTS10 (5' GCA TAC TGC TTT GAA CAT CG 3') (forward primer) and ETTS1(5'GC TTA AGT TCA GCG GGT 3') (reverse primer) were used for *B. truncatus* amplification. A DNA template of 1 µL was added to each tube that contained 22 µL double distilled water, 1 µL each of forward and reverse primers. The total reaction volume was 25 µL. Double distilled water was used as the negative control. PCR amplification of snail genomic DNA was done using Applied Biosystems GeneAmp Thermal Cycler 2700 version 2.08. Cycling conditions for COI and ITS 1 reactions are as follows: one cycle of 95 °C for 5 min, 45 cycles of 95 °C for 30 s, 54.3 °C for 30 s, 72 °C for 45 s and 72 °C for 10 min and one cycle of 95 °C for 5 min, 45 cycles of 95 °C for 30 s, 42 °C for 30 s, 72 °C for 45 s and 72 °C for 10 min respectively. PCR fragments were separated on 1% agarose gel and visualization was performed using a gel documentation and analysis system (UVP, EpiChem II darkroom). Sequencing was performed on an Applied Biosystems 3730XL analyser (Life Technologies, Northumberland, UK).

2.4. Phylogenetic Analysis of Sequence Data

Nucleotide sequences were visually edited using Bioedit software v 7.0. [26]. BLAST searches via the National Centre for Biotechnology Information (http://www.ncbi.nlm.nih.gov/) were performed for the obtained sequences against Genbank database to ensure that contaminant sequences had not been obtained by error [27] and aligned with the reference materials [12] using the Clustal W algorithm [28]. We performed the maximum-likelihood analyses for the COI and ITS 1 sequences using the program RAxML [29]. The maximum-likelihood estimates were bootstrapped for 1000 replicates based on the GTRGAMMA substitution model. Downloaded *B. truncatus* sequences deposited in Genbank from Niger (AM286316.2), Senegal (AM921807.1 and AM921806.1) Portugal (AM286314), Italy (AM286312.3), Burkina Faso (AM286315.2), and Tanzania (AM286313.2) [12] were used as reference isolates for COI sequences, while *B. truncatus* isolates from Tanzania (AM921983), Niger (AM921965) [16], and Cameroon (KJ157504.1, KJ157503.1, KJ157500.1, KJ157501.1, KJ157502.1) [13] were used as reference isolates for ITS 1 sequences. Sequence data from other *Bulinus* species on Genbank (detailed information on accession number and origin provided as Supplementary Data) were also included in constructing the maximum likelihood phylogenetic trees. Additionally, *Bulinus forskalii* (AM286306.2) was used as an outgroup for *Bulinus truncatus* group assessed with COI marker. *Bulinus forskalii* (AM921961.1) was used as the outgroup for the *Bulinus truncatus* group assessed with ITS 1 marker.

We also estimated the phylogenetic relationships of the COI and ITS 1 *B. truncatus* dataset using Bayesian inference in MrBayes version 3.2.0 programs [30] (Figures S1 and S2). Prior to Bayesian inference, the best fit nucleotide substitution models (HKY for COI and TrN for ITS 1) were determined using a hierarchical likelihood ratio test in jMODELTEST version 0.1.1 [31]. The posterior probabilities were calculated via 1,000,000 generations using Markov chain Monte Carlo (MCMC) simulations, and the chains were sampled every 1000 generations. At the end of this run, the average standard deviation of split frequencies was below 0.01, and the potential scale reduction factor was reasonably close to 1.0 for all parameters. A consensus tree was summarized and visualized in FigTree version 1.4.3 [32].

B. truncatus sequences from the three populations, reference isolates, and other *Bulinus* species sequences used for constructing ML trees were repeated for the construction of the Bayes ML trees Clade comprising *B. forskalii* (AM286308, AM286293.2, and AM286306.2) was used as the outgroup for COI *B. truncatus* sequences while *B. forskalii* (AM921961.1) was used the outgroup for ITS 1 *B. truncatus* sequences.

The minimum spanning tree was built using NETWORK 5.0.0.0 [33] (Figure S3). We built the network to support the COI ML tree and it showed the torso of the genetic structure.

DNA sequences have been submitted to the National Centre for Biotechnology Information Archive with accession numbers MG759386–MG759479 (*B. truncatus* group assessed with COI marker) and MG757840-757890 (*B. truncatus* group assessed with ITS 1 marker).

2.5. Determination of Haplotype and Nucleotide Diversity

The level of sequence diversity, which includes number of haplotype (h), haplotype diversity (hd), nucleotide diversity (π), Tajima's D (D), and theta per site statistics, were calculated for *B. truncatus* populations assessed with both COI and ITS 1 markers in Arlequin software version 3.5 [34]. In addition, we compared Fst of *B. truncatus* studied populations using Arlequin software version 3.5 [34].

3. Results

3.1. Phylogeny

Altogether, 94 individual snail samples including 38 (Giza and Sharkia; Egypt), 36 (Barakat area; Sudan), and 20 (Madziwa, Shamva District; Zimbabwe) were successfully sequenced at the COI region (Table 2), and 51 including 28 (Egypt) and 23 (Sudan) were sequenced at the ITS 1 locus (Table 2), because of failure in either amplification or sequencing. Following the sequencing alignment and trimming of all the sequences, the final fragments of 737 bp (COI) and 580 bp (ITS 1) were obtained. Among these, 6, 11, and 6 unique COI haplotypes of *B. truncatus* sequences were observed from Giza and Sharkia (Egypt), Barakat area (Sudan) and Madziwa, Shamva district (Zimbabwe), respectively (Table 2). In Egypt and Sudan, respectively, 3 and 2 unique ITS 1 haplotypes of *B. truncatus* sequences were observed (Table 2). No information on *B. truncatus* ITS 1 sequences from Zimbabwe was recorded in this study due to failure in either amplification or sequencing.

Table 2. Estimation of nucleotide diversity and summary statistics of *Bulinus truncatus* identified using COI I and ITS 1 markers.

		N	H	Hd	π	S.D.π	Θs	s.d.S	Tajima's D	p-Value
	Egypt	38	6	0.334	0.00205	0.001445	0.002916	0.001299	−0.85621	0.24
COI	Sudan	36	11	0.768	0.009359	0.005067	0.009602	0.003341	−0.08761	0.538
	Zimbabwe	20	6	0.784	0.014701	0.007859	0.011655	0.004442	1.01745	0.898
ITS 1	Egypt	28	3	0.14	0.005589	0.003362	0.020107	0.006909	−2.69592	0
	Sudan	23	2	0.443	0.00169	0.001367	0.001034	0.000769	1.41416	0.923

Number of sequences (N), number of haplotypes (h), haplotype diversity (Hd), nucleotide diversity (pi), theta per site (Θs), standard deviation (s.d.).

Phylogenetic analyses indicated some measures of variation in the genetic population structure of *B. truncatus* population from Giza and Sharkia (Egypt), Barakat area (Sudan), and Madziwa (Zimbabwe). A large quantity of COI sequence data from Giza and Sharkia (Egypt) and Barakat area (Sudan) cluster together on the *B. truncatus* clade but the COI sequence data of Madziwa (Zimbabwe) *B. truncatus* population cluster at different locations on the tree (Figure 2 and Figure S1). No significant variation was observed between *B. truncatus* populations from Giza and Sharkia (Egypt) and Barakat area (Sudan) (Figure 3 and Figure S2). The minimum spanning tree indicated the torso of *B. truncatus* populations genetic structure (Figure S3). The tree showed five haplotypes for *B. truncatus* obtained from Zimbabwe, while five and two haplotypes were indicated for Sudan and Egypt *B. truncatus* populations respectively. Cryptic lineages or other known species of *B. truncatus* were not detected.

Figure 2. A rooted maximum likelihood tree of *Bulinus truncatus* for CO1 sequences. Maximum likelihood tree of a 737 bp fragment of the cytochrome oxidase subunit 1 (CO1) gene for *B. truncatus* in this study with an additional 51 published Genbank sequences including *B. truncatus* reference isolates. Values on the branches are bootstrap support based on 1000 replications. *B. forskalii* (AM286306.2) was defined as outgroup. * UGD-Uganda, TZ-Tanzania, SAF-South Africa, KY-Kenya, ZB-Zanzibar, SG-Senegal, BFS, Burkina Faso, Nig-Niger, Agl-Angola, Mlw-Malawi.

Figure 3. A rooted maximum likelihood tree of *Bulinus truncatus* for ITS 1 sequences. Maximum likelihood tree of a 580 bp fragment of the internal transcribed spacer 1 (ITS 1) for *B. truncatus* in this study with an additional 33 published Genbank sequences including *B. truncatus* reference isolates. Values on the branches are bootstrap support based on 1000 replications. *B. forslkalii* (AM921961.1) was defined as outgroup. * UGD-Uganda, TZ-Tanzania, SF-South Africa, KY-Kenya, SE-Senegal, BFS, Burkina Faso, Nig-Niger, AG-Angola, MA-Mauritius, OM-Oman.

3.2. Haplotype and Nucleotide Diversity

Nucleotide polymorphism obtained for all *B. truncatus* sequences assessed in this study is shown in Table 2. Haplotype diversity observed of sequences from the three populations assessed with COI includes 0.334 (Giza and Sharkia, Egypt), 0.768 (Barakat area, Sudan), and 0.784 (Madziwa, Zimbabwe) while their nucleotide diversity includes 0.00205 (s.d. = 0.001445), 0.009359 (s.d. = 0.005067), and 0.014701 (s.d. = 0.007859) for Egypt, Sudan, and Zimbabwe, respectively (Table 2). Haplotype diversity for the two populations assessed with ITS 1 is 0.14 and 0.443 while nucleotide diversity includes 0.005589 (s.d. π 0.003362) and 0.00169 (s.d. π 0.001367) for (Giza and Sharkia, Egypt) and (Barakat area, Sudan), respectively. F_{ST} values in the pairwise population comparisons are shown in Table 3.

Table 3. Population pairwise Φst.

	Egypt	Sudan
Sudan	0.34860 *	
Zimbabwe	0.59653 *	0.36160 *

* Significant p value < 0.05.

4. Discussion

Urinary schistosomiasis burden is widely reported in Africa and this is a consequence of the unabated distribution of the important snail intermediate hosts of the genus *Bulinus* that serves as host to the schistosome parasite [4]. The *Bulinus* group is made up of about 37 recognized species and has been divided into four different groups for convenience [5].

This study assessed the genetic diversity of *B. truncatus* populations, the snail host implicated in the transmission of *S. haematobium* in Africa using mitochondrial cytochrome oxidase 1 (COI) gene and internal transcribed spacer (ITS 1).

Snail host identification using morphological characters is unreliable and sometimes ambiguous but the development and application of molecular techniques have been helpful, providing good species discrimination [4,5].

We observed that mitochondrial DNA sequences from Barakat area (Sudan) and Madziwa, Shamva (Zimbabwe) indicated high haplotype diversity including 0.768 and 0.784, respectively, a similar observation was earlier reported by Zein-Eddine et al. [14]. The level of haplotype diversity observed from the two populations in our study is less than the values reported by Zein-Eddine et al. [14]. However, relatively low haplotype diversity was also observed for sequences from Giza and Sharkia (Egypt), with 0.334. Nevertheless, the low levels of haplotype diversity observed for *B. truncatus* in this study were similar to findings by Zein-Eddine et al. [11] and those observed by Goodall-Copestake et al. [19,35], with low diversity species.

Our findings indicated some degree of variation in the *Bulinus* species population structure across Africa. *Bulinus* species populations on both COI and ITS 1 trees (Figures 2 and 3, Figures S1 and S2) separated into populations that correspond to *Bulinus* species groups [12,36]. However, we observed that *B. globosus* from West Africa clusters separately from the East African species as indicated by the COI sequence data.

Kane et al. [12] reported the division between *B. globosus* from the two regions in Africa and that *Bulinus africanus* has a close affinity with West African *B. globosus* species. This is also evident from the information provided by our COI sequence data (Figure 2).

Some levels of segregation were observed within the COI *B. truncatus* populations. The location of populations from Giza and Sharkia (Egypt) and Barakat area (Sudan) on the *B. truncatus* clade agrees with the location of both countries geographically (Figure 2). The clustering of the Madziwa, Shamva (Zimbabwe) sequences in different locations on the *B. truncatus* clade can be attributed to individuals with different genotypes within the population (Figure 2).

Findings from this study using COI identified two reciprocally monophyletic *B. truncatus* sister subclades and this corresponds to *B. truncatus* and *B. tropicus* respectively [12,36]. Nalugwa et al. [36] also obtained similar results from findings on the *B. truncatus/tropicus* complex collected from Albertine Rift freshwater bodies in Uganda. Brown and Shaw [37] have shown that *B. truncatus* is a tetraploid and *B. tropicus* is diploid; however, it is difficult to distinguish *B. truncatus* and *B. tropicus* morphologically.

The minimum spanning network was constructed to support the ML tree and this informed our decision to include some outgroup sequences. The network did not indicate a substantial difference from the information on the tree (Figure S3).

Although *Bulinus* species populations separated distinctly into groups as earlier indicated [12], no significant variation was observed within *B. truncatus* populations from Giza and Sharkia (Egypt) and Barakat area (Sudan) as indicated by the ITS 1 tree (Figure 3). Kane et al. [12] stated that

Bulinus wrighti has a characteristic COI sequence that positions the species and other members of the *Bulinus reticulatus* group close to the *Bulinus truncatus* complex. This was also observed from our ITS 1 result (Figure 3).

This study is not unique; however, it has investigated the genetic diversity of *B. truncatus* from Giza and Sharkia (Egypt), Barakat area (Sudan), and Madziwa (Zimbabwe), which is necessary for snail host surveillance in the study areas and it has also provided genomic data of this important snail species from the sampled countries.

Although no infection was detected from the snails when screened for patent and prepatent infection, the presence and distribution of *B. truncatus* in the studied areas poses a threat to the inhabitants of these areas should an infected person visit the water bodies and urinate inside or near enough for the schistosome eggs released with the urine to have contact with the water bodies, especially water contact sites such as the Nile River and El-Salam Canal (Egypt), where inhabitants engage in a lot of fishing activities, and the river at Madziwa (Zimbabwe) that people visit frequently to carry out their domestic chores as well as engage in activities such as swimming.

Previous studies implicated *B. truncatus* as the only *Bulinus* species that transmits *S. haematobium* in Egypt and other parts of northern Africa, while *Bulinus globosus* is implicated for schistosomiasis transmission in Zimbabwe [4]. The presence of *B. truncatus* in the southern African country can be attributed to the favorable environmental factors and migration of snail population; however, human activities have also increased the number of snail hosts of *S. haematobium*. This is a cause for concern and there is a need to improve measures for effective snail control strategies.

Differentiating snail host populations to assess their diversity should be prioritized in Africa, where host snails' genome data is scarce for most schistosomiasis endemic countries [18]. Efforts should be made to initiate a continent-wide snail host genome project to help develop a more comprehensive and robust snail host genome database for the African continent.

5. Conclusions

This study identified *B. truncatus*, the snail host of *S. haematobium* obtained from Giza and Sharkia (Egypt), Barakat area (Sudan), and Madziwa, Shamva District (Zimbabwe) using COI and ITS 1 markers, as well as provided information on their genetic diversity.

With the increasing global call that effective schistosomiasis control programmes should target snail control, there is a need to prioritize snail studies for effective mapping of schistosomiasis transmission [38], as well as to strengthen surveillance strategies.

Supplementary Materials:

S1A–S1J, data were used to prepare Table 2, S1A: Egypt B. truncatus COI.out, S1B: Egypt B. truncatus COI Tajima D.out, S1C: Egypt B. truncatus Fu_Li Test.out, S1D: Egypt_SUD_ZWE B. truncatus COI final.out, S1E: Fu_Li Egypt_SUD_ZWE B. truncatus COI.out, S1F: Sudan B. truncatus COI.out, S1G: Sudan B. truncatus COI Tajima D.out, S1H: Sudan B. truncatus Fu_Li test.out, S1I: Zimbabwe B. truncatus.out, S1J: Zimbabwe B. truncatus COI Tajima D.out, S2A–S2F data were used to prepare Table 3, S2A: Egypt B. truncatus ITS Fu_Li test.out, S2B: Egypt B. truncatus ITS Tajima D.out, S2C: Egypt B. truncatus ITS.out, S2D: Sudan B. truncatus ITS.out, S2E: Sudan B. truncatus ITS Fu_Li test.out, S2F: Sudan B. truncatus ITS Tajima D.out, S3A–S3M were used to prepare Figure 2A,B, S3A: Egypt Bulinus truncatus GENBANK PROTEIN SEQ NEW.fas, S3B: Egypt Bulinus truncatus GENBANK SEQ NEW.d.txt, S3C: Egypt B. truncatus GENBANK SEQ NEW.fas, S3D: SUDAN B. truncatus COI Protein SEQ1.fas, S3E: SUDAN B. truncatus COI genbankSEQ.fas, S3F: SUDAN B. truncatus Genbank SEQ COI.txt, S3G: Zimbabwe B.truncatus COI protein SEQ for genbank submission.fas, S3H: Zimbabwe B. truncatus COI SEQ for genbank submission.fas, S3I: Zimbabwe B. truncatus COI SEQ for genbank submission.txt, S3J: ZWE_SUDAN_EGYPT_BT_REF_COI_OUTGROUP.txt, S3K.ZWE_SUDAN_EGYPT_BT_REF_COI_OUTGROUP2-v2NEW.fas, S3L: Summary of the STRUCTURE analysis for B. truncatus COI.docx, S3M: Table 1. Information on B. truncatus sequences submitted to genbank, S4A–S4H were used to prepare Figure 3A,B, S4A: Information B. truncatus ITS 1 sequences submitted to genbank.xls, S4B: Egypt B. truncatus ITS.fas, S4C: Egypt B. truncatus ITS.txt, S4D: Egypt_Sudan_REF B. truncatus ITS.fas, S4E: Egypt_Sudan_REF_Outgroup B. truncatus ITS.txt, S4F: SUDAN B. truncatus ITS.fas, S4G: SUDAN B. truncatus ITS.txt, S4H: Summary of STRUCTURE analysis for B truncatus.docx.

Author Contributions: E.M.A. and X.N.Z. conceived the study; E.M.A., M.J.M. and Y.H.G. carried out laboratory analysis; H.S., X.J.B. and E.M.A. carried out data analysis; M.M., M.H. and N.M. conducted fieldwork; J.X. and S.Z.L. contributed reagents, materials, and analysis tools; E.M.A., S.Z.L. and X.N.Z. wrote the paper.

Acknowledgments: E.M.A. acknowledges the funding and support received from the National Institute of Parasitic Diseases, WHO Collaborating Centre for Tropical Diseases, and the China CDC for the postdoctoral fellowship.

References

1. WHO. *Country Profile: Preventive Chemotherapy and Transmission Control*; World Health Organization: Geneva, Switzerland, 2010; Available online: http://www.who.int/neglected_diseases/preventive_chemotherapy/databank/CP (accessed on 10 February 2018).

2. Hanington, P.C.; Forys, M.A.; Loker, E.S. A somatically diversified defense factor, FREP3, is a determinant of snail resistance to schistosome infection. *PLoS Negl. Trop. Dis.* **2012**. [CrossRef] [PubMed]

3. Gordy, M.A.; Kish, L.; Tarrabain, M.; Hanington, P.C. A comprehensive survey of larval digenean trematodes and their snail hosts in central Alberta, Canada. *Parasitol. Res.* **2016**. [CrossRef] [PubMed]

4. Rollinson, D.; Stothard, J.R.; Southgate, V.R. Interactions between intermediate snail hosts of the genus *Bulinus* and schistosomes of the *Schistosoma haematobium* group. *Parasitology* **2001**, *123*, S245–S260. [CrossRef] [PubMed]

5. Brown, D.S. *Fresh Water Snails of Africa and Their Medical Importance*, 2nd ed.; Taylor and Francis: London, UK, 1994; p. 609.

6. Akinwale, O.P.; Kane, R.A.; Rollinson, D.; Stothard, J.R.; Ajayi, M.B.; Akande, D.O.; Ogungbemi, M.O.; Duker, C.; Gyang, P.V.; Adeleke, M.A. Molecular approaches to the identification of *Bulinus* species in south-west Nigeria and observations on natural snail infections with schistosomes. *J. Helminthol.* **2010**, *85*, 283–293. [CrossRef] [PubMed]

7. Jarne, P. Mating system, bottlenecks and genetic-polymorphism in hermaphroditic animals. *Genet. Res.* **1995**, *65*, 193–207. [CrossRef]

8. Djuikwo-Teukenga, F.F.; Da Silva, A.; Njiokou, F.; Kamgang, B.; Same Ekobo, A.; Dreyfuss, G. Significant population genetic structure of the Cameroonian freshwater snail, *Bulinus globosus*, (Gastropoda: Planorbidae) revealed by nuclear microsatellite loci analysis. *Acta Trop.* **2014**, *137*, 111–117. [CrossRef] [PubMed]

9. Brown, D.S. *Freshwater Snails of Africa and Their Medical Importance*; Taylor and Francis: London, UK, 1980; p. 487.

10. Jarne, P.; Charlesworth, D. The evolution of the selfing rate in functionally hermaphrodite plants and animals. *Annu. Rev. Ecol. Syst.* **1993**, *24*, 441–466. [CrossRef]

11. Zein-Eddine, R.; Djuikwo-Teukeng, F.F.; Dar, Y.; Dreyfuss, G.; Van den Broeck, F. Population genetics of the *Schistosoma* snail host *Bulinus truncatus* in Egypt. *Acta Trop.* **2017**, *172*, 36–43. [CrossRef]

12. Kane, R.A.; Stothard, J.R.; Emery, A.M.; Rollinson, D. Molecular characterization of freshwater snails in the genus *Bulinus*: A role for bar codes? *Parasites Vectors* **2008**, *1*, 15. [CrossRef]

13. Standley, C.J.; Goodacre, S.L.; Wade, C.M.; Stothard, J.R. The population genetic structure of *Biomphalaria choanomphala* in Lake Victoria, East Africa: Implications for schistosomiasis transmission. *Parasites Vectors* **2014**, *7*, 524. [CrossRef]

14. Zein-Eddine, R.; Djuikwo-Teukeng, F.F.; Al-Jawhari, M.; Senghor, B.; Huyse, T.; Dreyfuss, G. Phylogeny of seven *Bulinus* species originating from endemic areas in three African countries, in relation to the human blood fluke *Schistosoma haematobium*. *BMC Evol. Biol.* **2014**, *14*, 271. [CrossRef] [PubMed]

15. Mohamed, A.H.; Sharaf El-Din, A.T.; Mohamed, A.M.; Habib, M.R. The relationship between genetic variability and the susceptibility of *Biomphalaria alexandrina* snails to *Schistosoma mansoni* infection. *Mem. Inst. Oswaldo Cruz* **2012**, *107*, 326–337. [CrossRef] [PubMed]

16. Abdel-Hamid, Z.A.; Rawi, S.M.; Arafa, A.F. Identification of a genetic marker associated with the resistance to *Schistosoma mansoni* infection using random amplified polymorphic DNA analysis. *Mem. Inst. Oswaldo Cruz* **2006**, *101*, 863–868. [CrossRef] [PubMed]

17. Emery, A.M.; Loxton, N.J.; Stothard, J.R.; Jones, C.S.; Spinks, J.; Llewellyn-Hughes, J.; Noble, L.R.; Rollinson, D. Microsatellites in the freshwater snail *Bulinus globosus* (Gastropoda: Planorbidae) from Zanzibar. *Mol. Ecol. Notes* **2003**, *3*, 108–110. [CrossRef]

18. Abe, E.M.; Guan, W.; Guo, Y.H.; Kassegne, K.; Qin, Z.Q.; Xu, J.; Chen, J.H.; Ekpo, U.F.; Li, S.Z.; Zhou, X.N. Differentiating snail intermediate hosts of *Schistosoma* spp. using molecular approaches: Fundamental to successful integrated control mechanism in Africa. *Infect. Dis. Poverty* **2018**. [CrossRef] [PubMed]

19. Djuikwo-Teukeng, F.F.; Njiokou, F.; Nkengazong, L.; De Meeus, T.; SameEkobo, A.; Dreyfuss, G. Strong genetic structure in Cameroonian populations of *Bulinus truncatus* (Gastropoda: Planorbidae), intermediate host of *Schistosoma haematobium*. *Infect. Genet. Evol.* **2001**, *11*, 17–22. [CrossRef] [PubMed]

20. Viard, F.; Bremond, P.; Labbo, R.; Justy, F.; Delay, B.; Jarne, P. Microsatellites and the genetics of highly selfing populations in the freshwater snail *Bulinus truncatus*. *Genetics* **1996**, *142*, 1237–1247.

21. Viard, F.; Justy, F.; Jarne, P. Population dynamics inferred from temporal variation at microsatellite loci in the selfing snail *Bulinus truncatus*. *Genetics* **1997**, *146*, 973–982.

22. Chlyeh, G.; Henry, P.Y.; Jarne, P. Spatial and temporal variation of life-history traits documented using capture-mark-recapture methods in the vector snail *Bulinus truncatus*. *Parasitology* **2003**, *127*, 243–251. [CrossRef]

23. Jarne, P.; Viard, F.; Delay, B.; Cuny, G. Variable microsatellites in the highly selfing snail *Bulinus truncatus* (Basommatophora: Planorbidae). *Mol. Ecol.* **1994**, *3*, 527–528. [CrossRef]

24. Brown, D.S.; Kristensen, T.K. *A Fish Guide to Fresh Water Snails*; Danish Bilharziasis Laboratory: DK-2920 Charlottenlund, Denmark, 1993.

25. Emery, A.M.; Allan, F.E.; Rabone, M.E.; Rollinson, D. Schistosomiasis collection at NHM (SCAN). *Parasit Vectors* **2012**, *5*, 185. [CrossRef] [PubMed]

26. Hall, T.A. BioEdit: A user-friendly biological sequence alignment editor and analysis program for Windows 95/98/NT. In *Nucleic Acids Symposium Series*; Information Retrieval Ltd.: London, UK, 1999; pp. 95–98.

27. Altschul, S.F.; Gish, W.; Miller, W.; Myers, E.W.; Lipman, D.J. Basic local alignment search tool. *J. Mol. Biol.* **1990**, *215*, 403–410. [CrossRef]

28. Thompson, J.D.; Higgins, D.G.; Gibson, T.J. CLUSTALW: Improving the sensitivity of progressive multiple sequence alignment through sequence weighting, position-specific gap penalties and weight matrix choice. *Nucleic Acids Res.* **1994**, *22*, 4673–4680. [CrossRef] [PubMed]

29. Stamatakis, A. RAxML version 8: A tool for phylogenetic analysis and post-analysis of large phylogenies. *Bioinformatics* **2014**, *30*, 1312–1313. [CrossRef] [PubMed]

30. Ronquist, F.; Teslenko, M.; van der Mark, P.; Avres, D.L.; Darling, A.; Hohna, S.; Larget, B.; Liu, L.; Suchard, M.A.; Huelsenbeck, J.P. MrBayes 3.2: Efficient Bayesian phylogenetic inference and model choice across a large model space. *Syst. Biol.* **2012**, *61*, 539–542. [CrossRef] [PubMed]

31. Posada, D. jModelTest: Phylogenetic model averaging. *Mol. Biol. Evol.* **2008**, *25*, 1253–1256. [CrossRef] [PubMed]

32. Rambaut, A. Evolution and phylogenetics software. FigTree version 1.4.3. Available online: http://tree.bio.ed.ac.uk/software/figtree/ (accessed on 8 December 2018).

33. Polzin, T.; Daneshmand, S.V. On Steiner trees and minimum spanning trees in hypergraphs. *Oper. Res. Lett.* **2003**, *31*, 12–20. [CrossRef]

34. Excoffier, L.; Laval, G.; Schneider, S. Arlequin ver.3.1: An integrated software package for population genetics data analysis. *Evol. Bioinform.* **2005**, *1*, 47–50. [CrossRef]

35. Goodall-Copestake, W.P.; Tarling, G.A.; Murphy, E.J. On the comparison of population-level estimates of haplotype and nucleotide diversity: A case study using the gene *cox1* in animals. *Heredity* **2012**, *109*, 50–56. [CrossRef]

36. Nalugwa, A.; Jørgensen, A.; Nyakaana, S.; Kristensen, TK. Molecular phylogeny of *Bulinus* (Gastropoda: Planorbidae) reveals the presence of three species complexes in the Albertine Rift freshwater bodies. *Int. J. Genet. Mol. Biol.* **2010**, *2*, 130–139.

37. Brown, D.S.; Shaw, K.M. Freshwater snails of thee *Bulinus truncatus/tropicus* complex in Kenya: Tetraploid species. *J. Mollus. Stud.* **1989**, *55*, 509–532. [CrossRef]

38. Allan, F.; Sousa-Figueiredo, J.C.; Emery, A.M.; Paulo, R.; Mirante, C.; Sebastião, A.; Brito, M.; Rollinson, D. Mapping freshwater snails in north-western Angola: Distribution, identity and molecular diversity of medically important taxa. *Parasites Vectors* **2017**, *10*, 460. [CrossRef] [PubMed]

5

Artemether and Praziquantel: Origin, Mode of Action, Impact and Suggested Application for Effective Control of Human Schistosomiasis

Robert Bergquist [1] and Hala Elmorshedy [2,3,*]

[1]   Ingerod, SE-454 94 Brastad, Sweden; robert.bergquist@outlook.com
[2]   College of Medicine, Princess Nourah bint Abdulrahman University, Riyadh 11671, Saudi Arabia
[3]   Department of Tropical Health, High Institute of Public Health, Alexandria University, Alexandria 21561, Egypt
*   Correspondence: elmorshedyh@hotmail.com

Abstract: The stumbling block for the continued, single-drug use of praziquantel (PZQ) against schistosomiasis is less justified by the risk of drug resistance than by the fact that this drug is inactive against juvenile parasites, which will mature and start egg production after chemotherapy. Artemisinin derivatives, currently used against malaria in the form of artemisinin-based combination therapy (ACT), provide an opportunity as these drugs are not only active against malaria plasmodia, but surprisingly also against juvenile schistosomes. An artemisinin/PZQ combination would be complementary, and potentially additive, as it would kill two schistosome life cycle stages and thus confer a transmission-blocking modality to current chemotherapy. We focus here on single versus combined regimens in endemic settings. Although the risk of artemisinin resistance, already emerging with respect to malaria therapy in Southeast Asia, prevents use in countries where ACT is needed for malaria care, an artemisinin-enforced praziquantel treatment (APT) should be acceptable in regions of North Africa (including Egypt), the Middle East, China, and Brazil that are not endemic for malaria. Thanks to recent progress with respect to high-resolution diagnostics, based on circulating schistosome antigens in humans and molecular approaches for snail surveys, it should be possible to keep areas scheduled for schistosomiasis elimination under surveillance, bringing rapid response to bear on problems arising. The next steps would be to investigate where and for how long APT should be applied to make a lasting impact. A large-scale field trial in an area with modest transmission should tell how apt this approach is.

Keywords: schistosomiasis; elimination; praziquantel; artemether; combination therapy

1. Background

The World Health Organization (WHO) includes schistosomiasis among the neglected tropical diseases (NTDs) and has selected it for elimination [1]; this may be premature as there is still a large discrepancy between the number of people requiring preventive chemotherapy (PCT) and those presently receiving it [2]. The disease is caused by trematode parasites with a predilection for abdominal capillary veins in the mammalian definitive host. Various freshwater snails act as intermediate hosts for the six different species capable of infecting humans. Out of these, *Schistosoma mansoni*, *S. haematobium*, and *S. japonicum* together cause almost all cases of schistosomiasis, which amounts to about 240 million infected and 700 million at risk worldwide [3]. The prevalence is often focal with high transmission in some spots and none in others and the lesions caused, intestinal or urogenital depending on the species of the parasite, tend to be chronic rather than acute. The attributes of infection include poor sanitation, proximity to water bodies, type and extent of water contact, snail population density, as well as age and gender of the human population in the endemic areas. For example, the prevalence and intensity of infection are significantly higher in males and in school-age children [2,4,5]. Theoretically, successful schistosomiasis control should be possible through a multidisciplinary approach focusing on chemotherapy, snail control, provision of water, sanitation, and hygiene (WASH) as well as behavioural change [6,7]. Nevertheless, elimination will be difficult to achieve in practice, and very few endemic countries have been entirely successful in controlling the disease. Interestingly, Japan managed to eradicate the infection (in 1977), mainly thanks to snail control based on environmental management, as described by Tanaka and Tsuji [2,4,5].

The cornerstone strategy for schistosomiasis control was for a long time directed at its snail intermediate host using broad-spectrum molluscicides. However, when praziquantel (PZQ) was introduced [8] and soon afterwards used for mass drug administration (MDA), it not only replaced other drugs thanks to safety, high efficacy and easy administration [9–11] but effectively became the only approach. This modality also changed the focus from snail control and infection prevention to morbidity reduction, reflected in a declining disability-adjusted life years (DALY) metric for schistosomiasis [12,13].

In China, Chairman Mao Zedong, not only instigated the National Schistosomiasis Control Programme [14] but also took an interest in malaria. The launch of the malaria research programme (under code name 523) in 1967 focused on herbs used in traditional Chinese medicine. Working in this programme, Youyou Tu, soon identified the ingredient artemisinin (qinghaosu) in extracts from wormwood (*Artemisia annua*) as a powerful antimalarial [15,16]. Qinghaosu has been used in China for more than 2,000 years for the treatment of fevers, and the story of how it was discovered has eloquently been told by Faurant [17] and Miller [18]. Already in 1971, Chinese chemists isolated the active lactone with its peroxide grouping [19]. However, this knowledge did not reach the West until the late 1970s when it was mentioned in a Welcome News Supplement [20]. Youyou Tu's own remarks [15] at the Fourth Meeting of the WHO Scientific Working Group on the Chemotherapy of Malaria, held in Beijing 1981, provided further details of the new drug. The landmark work carried out under her direction [21] constituted a break-through for malaria therapy and led to the development of artemisinin-based combination therapy (ACT) that has since revolutionized the care of malaria patients [22] eventually leading to Youyou Tu being awarded the Nobel prize in Medicine for 2015, together with Campbell and Ōmura for ivermectin [23,24]. However, the story does not end there since, amazingly, it was found that the artemisinin do not only affect the malaria parasites, but are also active against juvenile schistosomes, which was first shown by Chen et al. [25] at the end of the golden decade of antiparasitic drug discovery in the 1970s. In fact, this discovery predates that of scholarly articles on qinghaosu's use against malaria, which remains its main application.

2. Pharmacological Aspects

Single-celled malaria plasmodia and schistosome worms are phylogenetically very distant from each other, and one might think that the damage caused by the artemisinins to both these organisms would be due to different principles. However, there are reasons to believe otherwise, considering that both parasites feed by the digestion of haemoglobin in host erythrocytes, leading to a surplus of haeme (protoporphyrin-IX with a ferric ion at its centre) or haemin (ferriprotoporphyrin-IX characterized by an extra chloride ion bound to the ferric ion), both of which produce destructive hydroxyl radicals capable of provoking the alkylation of parasite proteins [26]. Faced with this threat, both parasites detoxify these compounds by crystallizing them into the inert polymer haemozoin (ferriprotoporphyrin-IX) that is found in quantity, both in *Plasmodium* [27] and adult schistosomes [28]. It seems that haeme and haemin are implicated in the destruction of *Plasmodium* and *Schistosoma* due to interference with the formation of hemozoin. Various drugs besides artemisinins (e.g., trioxalanes [29–31], trioxaquines [32], and ozonides [33,34]) are also capable to form alkylates with free haeme and haemin and use them for further alkylation, this time between parasite proteins.

Indeed, this seems to be an example of independent parallel evolution making chemical pathways available when needed, thus appearing de novo without connection to previous genetic information.

2.1. The Artemisinins

The active principle in qinghaosu is a lactol endoperoxide, which was used to produce artemether (ART) and artesunate, two semisynthetic artemisinin derivatives which become active after being metabolised in the blood into dihydro-artemisinin [35]. The current working hypothesis is that this drug acts through haeme-dependent reduction to sequentially generate free radicals: the haeme iron first attacks and breaks the endoperoxide linkage to artemisinin, producing an oxygen-free radical, which is then rearranged to produce a carbon-free radical that causes lethal damage through the alkylation of parasite proteins [36]. Work by Xiao et al. [31,37–39] and Chaturvedi et al. [36], further developed and summarized by Xiao and Sun [26], indicates that the same pathway is followed with respect to *Schistosoma*. Antioxidant enzymes systems available in adult worms, but not common in immature ones, can prevent this effect. However, to be effective, the drug needs to be ingested by the parasite, enabling the interaction with haemin or haeme causing damage to the worm gut by generating one or many substances toxic to these worms in amounts overwhelming the pathway leading to the hemozoin. The fact that the gut suffers particularly severe damage after ART treatment supports this chain of events [37]. A disadvantage of the artemisinin derivatives is their short in vivo half-life, typically ~2 h in humans [40].

2.2. Praziquantel

In spite of being used for 40 years, and most of that time in the form of MDA, the exact molecular mechanism of PZQ remains unknown. However, the drug has no effect on the enzymes discussed above but relies on a rapid influx of Ca^{2+} into the worm (interestingly, immature forms are refractory), leading to intense muscular paralysis together with damage to the tegument [41,42]. How this disruption is linked to the original binding of the drug is still unknown, but it is thought that the exposure of parasite surface antigens leads to recognition and parasite clearance through immunological means, something which may indirectly account for the difference in sensitivity between juvenile and mature stages [43]. Although the receptor is not known, it has been shown that PZQ disrupts ion transport and recent experimental evidence indicates that transient potential (TRP) channels are targeted by the drug; this could result in the increased permeability of adult schistosome cell membranes towards calcium ions [44].

2.3. Combination Treatment

With artemisinins active against immature schistosome worms [25,45,46] and PZQ primarily targeting adults [47,48], the combination of PZQ and ART presents a chemotherapeutic perfect storm against this parasite as shown in Figure 1, where the y-axle shows the cidal effect expressed as percentage of killed parasites in the experimental animals used. Although small susceptibility variations with respect to parasite age can be seen between the species, there is also a short period coinciding with a larval age between 4 and 5 weeks when all three species are partially refractory against both ART and PZQ. However, the main difference between the two drugs is that the former is predominantly active against juvenile stages and the latter against adult stages. In addition, although PZQ shows a similar activity against *S. haematobium* and *S. japonicum* worms, there is quite a different picture when given to *S. mansoni*, as it obviously also has some activity against juvenile stages.

S. mansoni reactions to ART according to experiments by Xiao et al. [46] and to PZQ by Gönnert and Andrews [48], were confirmed by Sabah et al. [47]; *S. japonicum* to ART by Xiao et al. [39] and to PZQ by Xiao et al. [49], were confirmed by Wu et al. [50]; and *S. haematobium* to PZQ by Botros et al. [51]. Note that *S. haematobium* reactions to ART represent indirect information on parasite susceptibility based on tegumental damage [52,53] and cannot therefore be directly compared with other measurements presented in this figure.

Figure 1. Activity of artemether and praziquantel in relation to different stages of maturity in all three main schistosome species. (**A**) *S. mansoni*; (**B**) *S. japonicum*; (**C**) *S. haematobium*.

3. Drug Resistance

3.1. Artemether

Resistance to artemisinins in malaria parasites, defined as a slower rate of parasite clearance in patients under treatment, has emerged in Southeast Asia's Mekong region [54]. The parasites are thought to mount a defensive stress response, and recent evidence suggests that this response in certain mutants is enhanced, thus promoting parasite survival leading to drug resistance [55]. These authors have shown that the enhanced cellular defence response that underlies resistance development enables very early ring stages to withstand drug exposure for longer. However, in this case, the intrinsic sensitivity to artemisinin is retained [55], which is an encouraging sign that might also play a role in schistosomiasis therapy in due course, although there is as of yet no knowledge about this. On the other hand, drug resistance may still appear in the longer perspective, and might well do so if the drug were to be incorporated in widespread control schemes. It should also be said that the determination of whether or not resistance has developed is not straightforward when the drugs are used against schistosomiasis as the parasites are localized in abdominal veins, that is, in areas where they cannot be directly observed.

A major problem preventing the use of ART for schistosomiasis control is the increased risk for the spread of drug resistance against malaria. This is very clearly a big risk, and the use of the drug against schistosomiasis should be restricted to areas outside those where there is any trace of malaria transmission. As can be seen in Figure 2, there are such areas—in China, Brazil, Mediterranean Africa including Egypt, and the Middle East—where a combination treatment would be particularly useful at the elimination stage.

= Areas endemic for malaria
= Areas endemic for schistosomiasis but non-endemic for malaria

Figure 2.   Areas where artemisinin derivates can be used for transmission interruption of schistosomiasis.

3.2. Praziquantel

Drug resistance, to be expected after long-term use of repeated, extensive application, is a clear risk, but evidence with respect to PZQ remains scant. However, if it were to emerge, current efforts to eliminate schistosomiasis would be severely challenged requiring alternative and/or complementary drugs [56,57]. Ominously, drug resistance against PZQ has been generated in the laboratory following treatments of *S. mansoni* strains with subcurative drug doses [58–61], proving that it cannot be ruled out. Furthermore, resistant *S. mansoni* isolates have been reported from various African sites (Egypt and Kenya in particular [62–64]), while several cases of failed parasite clearance following a standard treatment for *S. haematobium* infections in Africa have also been shown [65–67]. In China, the emergence of drug resistance has also been experimentally produced [68,69], including reports of resistant *S. japonicum* isolates [70]. Based on the evidence referred to above, it can be concluded that drug resistance in the field is a clear possibility and it is just a question of how fast it will spread once established.

Even if the influx of calcium ions into the worm after exposure to PZQ is regularly observed, the molecular mechanism of PZQ's mode of action is not fully unravelled. The lack of widespread resistance after long-term use may be due to the presence of multiple pharmacologically relevant targets, and Thomas and Timson [71] suggest that PZQ may act, at least in part, on a protein–protein interaction and that altered drug metabolism or enhanced drug efflux are the most likely ways resistance may arise. Additionally, laboratory tests to identify resistance to PZQ have demonstrated a specific region in the parasite genome which might be responsible for reduced drug susceptibility [72].

4. Trials and Community-based Studies

Although annual or biennial MDA with PZQ controls schistosomiasis morbidity well, even in high-transmission areas, it does not generally achieve any significant reduction in transmission [73]. ART, on the other hand, has been shown to do so in several randomized control studies [74–78], at least during the limited time covered by the studies. With regard to single-drug trials using artemether, Utzinger et al. [79] investigated the use of ART for prevention of *S. mansoni* infection using a randomized, double-blind, placebo-controlled trial in Côte d'Ivoire, demonstrating that ART resulted in a significantly lower incidence of infection (24% versus 48.6%, relative risk: 0.50 [95% CI 0.35–0.71], $p = 0.00006$), translating into a 50% risk reduction. A follow-up study on the application of ART against *S. haematobium* in the same country found similar results, although the protective efficacy was considerably lower [78]. A few studies more similar to interventions have been carried out. In Nigeria, for example, PZQ combined with artesunate was used for the treatment of urinary schistosomiasis in 312 randomly selected schoolchildren, reaching a cure rate of 89%, something statistically significant. Two groups, given either monotherapy with PZQ and artesunate to compare, showed a 73% and 71% cure, respectively, demonstrating that the use of combination treatment is both safe and more effective than treatment with either drug alone [76].

Results of a systematic reviews and meta-analysis of a large number of clinical trials have demonstrated the superior performance of the combined drug regimens versus single-drug application, as shown by Wu et al. [45], Liu et al. [35] and Perez del Villar et al. [80]. The first two reviews concerned *S. japonicum* infections only, out of which the former reports ten randomized controlled trials with participants ranging from 318 to 5098; four were multi-centre studies, and six were carried out at single centres. Artemisinin compounds (artesunate or ART) had few side effects and were found to be effective at 7-day and 15-day intervals (preferentially when used at 15-day intervals) for preventing infection during short-term exposures, such as during flooding relief work [45]. Liu et al. [35] state that protection was considerably higher when using combination therapy (84–97%), while it was only 52% with monotherapy (PZQ at 40 mg/Kg), while increasing the dosage to 60 or 100 mg/Kg resulted in a protection rate up to 91%. Interestingly, the protection rate of artemisinin derivates alone exceeded that of PZQ alone with protection rates reaching 97%, the highest rates achieved when the number of doses (3–8) were increased and the interval between them shortened from 1 month to 1 week. Confirming these results, not only for *S. japonicum* but also for *S. haematobium* and *S. mansoni*, Perez del Villar et al. [80] also reported better results with combination therapy than that achieved using either drug alone. In addition, the reviews convey the impression that ART, rather than artesunate, is the preferable choice when combined with PZQ.

In Egypt, good PZQ coverage has resulted in a substantial drop of infection intensities in most endemic settings [81–83]. However, despite a regular distribution of PZQ since almost 20 years, transmission continues at an appreciable and unacceptable level in many foci, especially in the Nile Delta. The experience in Kafer El-Sheikh Governorate, located close to the end of the Rosetta branch of the Nile River in the northern part of the Delta, is one of the hotspot areas with regard to transmission that clearly reflects the failure of controlling schistosomiasis with PZQ alone. As shown by Barakat et al. [81,82] and Haggag et al. [84], the prevalence and intensity of infection in children newly enrolled in primary schools remain almost unaffected [75]. In addition, premature interruption of MDA programmes due to the insensitivity of routinely used diagnostic tests often result in the re-emergence of infection in the span of a few years with concern that the prevalence and intensity of infection might again bounce back to higher levels.

Our own field experience in Kafer El-Sheikh Governorate have clearly demonstrated the remarkably positive effect of giving ART and PZQ in combination [74]. We conducted a double-blind, randomized controlled trial with 913 children, in which two groups (experimental and controls) received 40 mg/kg body weight of PZQ twice, four weeks apart at baseline. Afterwards, the experimental group received 6 mg/kg body weight of ART every 3 weeks in 5 cycles during the transmission season, and the control group received a placebo. At the end of the study, prevalence of infection in the group receiving ART was approximately half that of the placebo group: 6.7% versus 11.6%, and incidence of new infection for the ART group was 2.7% versus 6.5% for the placebo group, i.e., a clearly significant risk reduction. What was unique about this study is that we treated the patent infection with two doses of PZQ 4 weeks apart, 40 mg/Kg each to maximize the cure rate, thereby achieving the aim to evaluate the prophylactic effect of ART alone. It should be added that five annual rounds of PZQ treatment with a coverage rate above 90% in the same area was shown to have reduced the incidence from 29% to 12 %, while the incidence dropped from approximately 19% in 2000 to 12% in 2001 [85]. Another study including 2382 individuals of both sexes and all ages in five high-risk Nile Delta villages in Kafer El-Sheikh showed an overall prevalence of schistosomiasis of 29% with a generally low intensity of infection. Although this result was deemed positive compared to the situation before MDA using PZQ was implemented, the outcome was tempered by the insight that transmission remained largely uninterrupted after long-term uninterrupted control activities [75]. To ensure better cure rates in this area, prevent rapid re-infection, and avoid the potential development of drug resistance, the use of ART/PZQ combinations should be instituted.

5. Discussion

Treatment failure can be due to drug resistance against PZQ, but it can also be due to a lack of therapeutic efficacy of the drug with respect to juvenile trematode flukes as shown by Doenhoff et al. [86]. In this connection, it should also be considered that PZQ, though it has a strong curative effect, never reaches 100% efficacy. These facts together reveal that this drug is not transmission-blocking, making the goal of elimination of schistosomiasis illusory if not combined with other drugs or tools, such as snail control, health education, water, sanitation, and hygiene (WASH). Overall, complementing PZQ with ART would not only target all stages of the parasite, from its penetration into the host (when PZQ has an ultra-short activity to the organism covering only a few hours) over its first weeks of growth to the adult stage. Importantly, by targeting the stages before egg production has started, the artemisinin derivates are truly a transmission-blocking drugs. In addition, its already high efficacy can be raised to almost 100% by using several doses provided on a weekly basis [46]; however, this approach would not be realistic in practise. This is of course only acceptable for short periods, when prevention is needed for which it has successfully been applied in flooding interventions in China [35,45]. Prolonged treatment periods have not been tried.

The successful outcome of 40 years of schistosomiasis chemotherapy using PZQ, most of this time in the form of MDA is of a magnitude relieving morbidity and suffering of millions of people. This accomplishment has led to thoughts of worldwide elimination of the disease in the next decade, though others feel that it might take longer [87]. The stumbling block is that PZQ does not block transmission. This can, however, be achieved by conferring a transmission-blocking modality to current chemotherapy through the addition of artemisinin derivatives that act before the infection results in adult worms capable of producing eggs. However, due to the risk of drug resistance, which is already emerging in Southeast Asia, APT cannot be recommended in areas where ACT is needed for malaria care. On the other hand, China, Mediterranean Africa, and also large areas elsewhere where schistosomiasis and malaria do not overlap are also locations where the elimination of schistosomiasis would have the best chance of rapid success. As side effects of an ART treatment are mild or non-existent, we propose a precision treatment approach, involving repeated ART treatments (monthly or bimonthly) backed up with PZQ biannually until elimination has been achieved. However, the elimination of schistosomiasis from sub-Saharan Africa cannot depend on artemisinin derivates, due to the need to reserve these drugs for malaria treatment; it will therefore require more complicated, long-term schemes, preferably including a vaccine. It is encouraging that, thanks to high-resolution diagnostics, both for humans [88] and snails [89], it should be possible to keep areas scheduled for elimination under surveillance so that rapid response can be raised whenever needed [90].

Thanks to donors supporting purchase and distribution of PZQ (e.g., the Schistosomiasis Control Initiative working in Africa (http://www.imperial.ac.uk/schistosomiasis-control-initiative), the drug been made available free of charge in all large endemic areas. However, as pointed above, there is still a shortfall with respect to PZQ [2]. The addition of ART would raise the cost further but before requesting the extra funds, more convincing data is required. Although the field trials mentioned here support combination therapy, testing in conjunction with more sensitive and quantitative diagnostic tools will be needed to take us closer to the goal of applying ART/PZQ therapy for schistosomiasis elimination in non-malarious areas. Indeed, such diagnostic assays [91–93] have already shown that the extent of schistosome infection has been greatly underestimated, due to the diagnostic deficit of stool examination and urine filtration which are still commonly used in the endemic areas [94].

6. Conclusions

The obvious problem with PZQ is that it does not block transmission. Snail control has been tried with questionable results since the snails hosts of *S. mansoni* and *S. haematobium* are non-amphibious and can survive long dry periods. The outcome in China has been better, although not completely successful there either, since the intermediate snail host of *S. japonicum* is amphibious and therefore slightly easier to control. Other underlying factors favouring transmission are ecological conditions, poor sanitation, and the high intensity of unprotected water contact. Under such circumstances, additional control measures need to be adopted. One of these measures would be to change the current MDA strategy to include a combination of PZQ and ART in certain areas based on the rationale that it would confer a transmission-blocking modality to current chemotherapy. thereby ensuring higher cure rates, reducing (possibly even preventing) transmission and rapid re-infection, and avoiding a potential development of resistance to either drug.

The spatiotemporal risk for reinfection dominates in endemic areas, which in principle would require keeping people on constant chemotherapy, at least for a period of time. Although this is not a realistic approach, a strategy consisting of PZQ provided at 6-month intervals together with a monthly ART treatment might be the recipe for not only achieving elimination, but in fact also making local eradication possible. It remains to be investigated how long APT regimens should last and how realistic this approach would be.

Author Contributions: Both authors produced the main body of text together. R.B. conceived the draft, focusing on drug origin and mode of action studies. H.M. contributed field use of combined treatment and clinical trials.

References

1. WHO. Accelerating Work to Overcome the Global Impact of Neglected Tropical Diseases. Available online: http://www.who.int/neglected_diseases/NTD_RoadMap_2012_Fullversion.pdf (accessed on 3 December 2018).
2. WHO. Schistosomiasis Fact Sheet of 20 February 2018. Available online: http://www.who.int/news-room/fact-sheets/detail/schistosomiasis (accessed on 20 August 2018).
3. Hotez, P.J.; Asojo, O.A.; Adesina, A.M. Nigeria: "Ground Zero" for the high prevalence neglected tropical diseases. *PLoS Negl. Trop. Dis.* **2012**, *6*, e1600. [CrossRef]
4. Barakat, R.; El Morshedy, H. Efficacy of two praziquantel treatments among primary school children in an area of high *Schistosoma mansoni* endemicity, Nile Delta, Egypt. *Parasitology* **2011**, *138*, 440–446. [CrossRef]
5. El-Khoby, T.; Galal, N.; Fenwick, A.; Barakat, R.; El-Hawey, A.; Nooman, Z.; Habib, M.; Abdel-Wahab, F.; Gabr, N.S.; Hammam, H.M.; et al. The epidemiology of schistosomiasis in Egypt: Summary findings in nine governorates. *Am. J. Trop. Med. Hyg.* **2000**, *62*, 88–99. [CrossRef]
6. Gryseels, B. Schistosomiasis. *Infect. Dis. Clin. N. Am.* **2012**, *26*, 383–397. [CrossRef]
7. Sow, S.; de Vlas, S.J.; Stelma, F.; Vereecken, K.; Gryseels, B.; Polman, K. The contribution of water contact behavior to the high *Schistosoma mansoni* Infection rates observed in the Senegal River Basin. *BMC Infect. Dis.* **2011**, *11*, 198. [CrossRef]
8. Davis, A.; Wegner, D.H. Multicentre trials of praziquantel in human schistosomiasis: Design and techniques. *Bull. World Health Organ.* **1979**, *57*, 767–771.
9. Colley, D.G.; Bustinduy, A.L.; Secor, W.E.; King, C.H. Human schistosomiasis. *Lancet* **2014**, *383*, 2253–2264. [CrossRef]
10. Zhou, X.N.; Bergquist, R.; Leonardo, L.; Yang, G.J.; Yang, K.; Sudomo, M.; Olveda, R. Schistosomiasis japonica control and research needs. *Adv. Parasitol.* **2010**, *72*, 145–178. [CrossRef]
11. King, C.H. Parasites and poverty: The case of schistosomiasis. *Acta Trop.* **2010**, *113*, 95–104. [CrossRef]
12. Hay, S.I.; Abajobir, A.A.; Abate, K.H.; Abbafati, C.; Abbas, K.M.; Abd-Allah, F.; Abdulkader, R.S.; Abdulle, A.M.; Abebo, T.A.; Abera, S.F.; et al. Global, regional, and national disability-adjusted life-years (DALYs) for 333 diseases and injuries and healthy life expectancy (HALE) for 195 countries and territories, 1990–2016: A systematic analysis for the Global Burden of Disease Study 2016. *Lancet* **2017**, *390*, 1260–1344. [CrossRef]
13. Murray, C.J.; Vos, T.; Lozano, R.; Naghavi, M.; Flaxman, A.D.; Michaud, C.; Ezzati, M.; Shibuya, K.; Salomon, J.A.; Abdalla, S.; et al. Disability-adjusted life years (DALYs) for 291 diseases and injuries in 21 regions, 1990–2010: A systematic analysis for the Global Burden of Disease Study 2010. *Lancet* **2012**, *380*, 2197–2223. [CrossRef]
14. Chen, J.; Xu, J.; Bergquist, R.; Li, S.Z.; Zhou, X.N. "Farewell to the God of Plague": The Importance of Political Commitment Towards the Elimination of Schistosomiasis. *Trop. Med. Infect. Dis.* **2018**, *3*, 108. [CrossRef]
15. Tu, Y. The discovery of artemisinin (qinghaosu) and gifts from Chinese medicine. *Nat. Med.* **2011**, *17*, 1217–1220. [CrossRef]
16. Tu, Y. The development of the antimalarial drugs with new type of chemical structure—qinghaosu and dihydroqinghaosu. *Southeast Asian J. Trop. Med. Publ. Health* **2004**, *35*, 250–251.
17. Faurant, C. From bark to weed: The history of artemisinin. *Parasite* **2011**, *18*, 215–218. [CrossRef]
18. Miller, L.H.; Su, X. Artemisinin: Discovery from the Chinese herbal garden. *Cell* **2011**, *146*, 855–858. [CrossRef]
19. Klayman, D.L. Qinghaosu (artemisinin): An antimalarial drug from China. *Science* **1985**, *228*, 1049–1055. [CrossRef]
20. Gardner, B. A present from Chairman Mao. Welcome News Supplement 6: Research Directions in Malaria. *Wellcome Trust* **2002**, *25* Suppl. 6.
21. Li, Y.; Wu, Y.L. How Chinese scientists discovered qinghaosu (artemisinin) and developed its derivatives? What are the future perspectives? *Med. Trop. Rev. Corps Sante Colonial* **1998**, *58*, 9–12.
22. Ansari, M.T.; Saify, Z.S.; Sultana, N.; Ahmad, I.; Saeed-Ul-Hassan, S.; Tariq, I.; Khanum, M. Malaria and artemisinin derivatives: An updated review. *Mini Rev. Med. Chem.* **2013**, *13*, 1879–1902. [CrossRef]
23. Tu, Y. Artemisinin-A Gift from Traditional Chinese Medicine to the World (Nobel Lecture). *Angew. Chem.* **2016**, *55*, 10210–10226. [CrossRef] [PubMed]

24. Tambo, E.; Khater, E.I.; Chen, J.H.; Bergquist, R.; Zhou, X.N. Nobel prize for the artemisinin and ivermectin discoveries: A great boost towards elimination of the global infectious diseases of poverty. *Infec. Dis. Poverty* **2015**, *4*, 58. [CrossRef] [PubMed]

25. Chen, D.J.; Fu, L.F.; Shao, P.P.; Wu, F.Z.; Fan, C.Z.; Shu, H.; Ren, C.X.; Sheng, X.L. Experimental studies on antischistosomal activity of qinghaosu. *Chin. Med. J.* **1980**, *60*, 422–425.

26. Xiao, S.H.; Sun, J. *Schistosoma* hemozoin and its possible roles. *Int. J. Parasitol.* **2017**, *47*, 171–183. [CrossRef] [PubMed]

27. Pagola, S.; Stephens, P.W.; Bohle, D.S.; Kosar, A.D.; Madsen, S.K. The structure of malaria pigment beta-haematin. *Nature* **2000**, *404*, 307–310. [CrossRef] [PubMed]

28. Homewood, C.A.; Jewsbury, J.M. Comparison of malarial and schistosome pigment. *Trans. R. Soc. Trop. Med. Hyg.* **1972**, *66*, 1–2. [CrossRef]

29. Meunier, B.; Robert, A. Heme as trigger and target for trioxane-containing antimalarial drugs. *Acc. Chem. Res.* **2010**, *43*, 1444–1451. [CrossRef] [PubMed]

30. Creek, D.J.; Charman, W.N.; Chiu, F.C.; Prankerd, R.J.; Dong, Y.; Vennerstrom, J.L.; Charman, S.A. Relationship between antimalarial activity and heme alkylation for spiro- and dispiro-1,2,4-trioxolane antimalarials. *Antimicrob. Agents Chemother.* **2008**, *52*, 1291–1296. [CrossRef]

31. Xiao, S.H.; Keiser, J.; Chollet, J.; Utzinger, J.; Dong, Y.; Endriss, Y.; Vennerstrom, J.L.; Tanner, M. In vitro and in vivo activities of synthetic trioxolanes against major human schistosome species. *Antimicrob. Agents Chemother.* **2007**, *51*, 1440–1445. [CrossRef]

32. Pradines, V.; Portela, J.; Boissier, J.; Cosledan, F.; Meunier, B.; Robert, A. Trioxaquine PA1259 alkylates heme in the blood-feeding parasite *Schistosoma mansoni*. *Antimicrob. Agents Chemother.* **2011**, *55*, 2403–2405. [CrossRef]

33. Dong, Y.; Wang, X.; Kamaraj, S.; Bulbule, V.J.; Chiu, F.C.; Chollet, J.; Dhanasekaran, M.; Hein, C.D.; Papastogiannidis, P.; Morizzi, J.; et al. Structure-Activity Relationship of the Antimalarial Ozonide Artefenomel (OZ439). *J. Med. Chem.* **2017**, *60*, 2654–2668. [CrossRef] [PubMed]

34. Xue, J.; Wang, X.; Dong, Y.; Vennerstrom, J.L.; Xiao, S.H. Effect of ozonide OZ418 against *Schistosoma japonicum* harbored in mice. *Parasitol. Res.* **2014**, *113*, 3259–3266. [CrossRef]

35. Liu, R.; Dong, H.F.; Guo, Y.; Zhao, Q.P.; Jiang, M.S. Efficacy of praziquantel and artemisinin derivatives for the treatment and prevention of human schistosomiasis: A systematic review and meta-analysis. *Parasites Vectors* **2011**, *4*, 201. [CrossRef] [PubMed]

36. Chaturvedi, D.; Goswami, A.; Saikia, P.P.; Barua, N.C.; Rao, P.G. Artemisinin and its derivatives: A novel class of anti-malarial and anti-cancer agents. *Chem. Soc. Rev.* **2010**, *39*, 435–454. [CrossRef] [PubMed]

37. Xiao, S.H.; Mei, J.Y.; Jiao, P.Y. *Schistosoma japonicum*-infected hamsters (Mesocricetus auratus) used as a model in experimental chemotherapy with praziquantel, artemether, and OZ compounds. *Parasitol. Res.* **2011**, *108*, 431–437. [CrossRef] [PubMed]

38. Xiao, S.; Chollet, J.; Utzinger, J.; Matile, H.; Mei, J.; Tanner, M. Artemether administered together with haemin damages schistosomes in vitro. *Trans. R. Soc. Trop. Med. Hyg.* **2001**, *95*, 67–71. [PubMed]

39. Xiao, S.H.; You, J.Q.; Yang, Y.Q.; Wang, C.Z. Experimental studies on early treatment of schistosomal infection with artemether. *Southeast Asian J. Trop. Med. Publ. Health* **1995**, *26*, 306–318.

40. Djimde, A.; Lefevre, G. Understanding the pharmacokinetics of Coartem. *Malar. J.* **2009**, *8* (Suppl. 1), S4. [CrossRef]

41. Chan, J.D.; Zarowiecki, M.; Marchant, J.S. Ca^{2+} channels and praziquantel: A view from the free world. *Parasitol. Int.* **2013**, *62*, 619–628. [CrossRef] [PubMed]

42. Xiao, S.; Binggui, S.; Chollet, J.; Tanner, M. Tegumental changes in 21-day-old *Schistosoma mansoni* harboured in mice treated with artemether. *Acta Trop.* **2000**, *75*, 341–348. [CrossRef]

43. Cupit, P.M.; Cunningham, C. What is the mechanism of action of praziquantel and how might resistance strike? *Future Med. Chem.* **2015**, *7*, 701–705. [CrossRef] [PubMed]

44. Bais, S.; Greenberg, R.M. TRP channels as potential targets for antischistosomals. *Int. J. Parasitol. Drugs Drug Resist.* **2018**, *8*, 511–517. [CrossRef] [PubMed]

45. Wu, T.X.; Liu, G.J.; Zhang, M.M.; Wang, Q.; Ni, J.; Wei, J.F.; Zhou, L.K.; Duan, X.; Chen, X.Y.; Zheng, J.; et al. Systematic review of benefits and harms of artemisinin-type compounds for preventing schistosomiasis. *Zhonghua Yi Xue Za Zhi* **2003**, *83*, 1219–1224. [PubMed]

46. Shuhua, X.; Chollet, J.; Weiss, N.A.; Bergquist, R.N.; Tanner, M. Preventive effect of artemether in experimental animals infected with *Schistosoma mansoni*. *Parasitol. Int.* **2000**, *49*, 19–24. [CrossRef]

47. Sabah, A.A.; Fletcher, C.; Webbe, G.; Doenhoff, M.J. *Schistosoma mansoni*: Chemotherapy of infections of different ages. *Exp. Parasitol.* **1986**, *61*, 294–303. [CrossRef]

48. Gonnert, R.; Andrews, P. Praziquantel, a new board-spectrum antischistosomal agent. *Zeitschrift fur Parasitenkunde* **1977**, *52*, 129–150. [CrossRef] [PubMed]

49. Xiao, S.H.; Yue, W.J.; Yang, Y.Q.; You, J.Q. Susceptibility of *Schistosoma japonicum* to different developmental stages to praziquantel. *Chin. Med. J.* **1987**, *100*, 759–768.

50. Wu, W.; Wang, W.; Huang, Y.X. New insight into praziquantel against various developmental stages of schistosomes. *Parasitol. Res.* **2011**, *109*, 1501–1507. [CrossRef]

51. Botros, S.; Pica-Mattoccia, L.; William, S.; El-Lakkani, N.; Cioli, D. Effect of praziquantel on the immature stages of *Schistosoma haematobium*. *Int. J. Parasitol.* **2005**, *35*, 1453–1457. [CrossRef]

52. Xiao, S.U.; Utzinger, J.; Shen, B.G.; Tanner, M.; Chollet, J. Ultrastructural alterations of adult *Schistosoma haematobium* harbored in mice following artemether administration. *Zhongguo Ji Sheng Chong Xue Yu Ji Sheng Chong Bing Za Zhi* **2006**, *24*, 321–328.

53. Shu-Hua, X.; Utzinger, J.; Chollet, J.; Tanner, M. Effect of artemether administered alone or in combination with praziquantel to mice infected with Plasmodium berghei or *Schistosoma mansoni* or both. *Int. J. Parasitol.* **2006**, *36*, 957–964. [CrossRef] [PubMed]

54. WHO. Q&A on artemisinin resistance. 2018. Available online: https://www.who.int/malaria/media/artemisinin_resistance_qa/en/ (accessed on 11 November 2018).

55. Tilley, L.; Straimer, J.; Gnadig, N.F.; Ralph, S.A.; Fidock, D.A. Artemisinin Action and Resistance in *Plasmodium falciparum*. *Trends Parasitol.* **2016**, *32*, 682–696. [CrossRef] [PubMed]

56. Bergquist, R.; Utzinger, J.; Keiser, J. Controlling schistosomiasis with praziquantel: How much longer without a viable alternative? *Infect. Dis. Poverty* **2017**, *6*, 74. [CrossRef] [PubMed]

57. Cioli, D.; Valle, C.; Angelucci, F.; Miele, A.E. Will new antischistosomal drugs finally emerge? *Trends Parasitol.* **2008**, *24*, 379–382. [CrossRef] [PubMed]

58. Lotfy, W.M.; Hishmat, M.G.; El Nashar, A.S.; Abu El Einin, H.M. Evaluation of a method for induction of praziquantel resistance in *Schistosoma mansoni*. *Pharm. Biol.* **2015**, *53*, 1214–1219. [CrossRef] [PubMed]

59. Couto, F.F.; Coelho, P.M.; Araujo, N.; Kusel, J.R.; Katz, N.; Jannotti-Passos, L.K.; Mattos, A.C. *Schistosoma mansoni*: A method for inducing resistance to praziquantel using infected Biomphalaria glabrata snails. *Mem. Inst. Oswaldo Cruz* **2011**, *106*, 153–157. [CrossRef] [PubMed]

60. Ismail, M.; Metwally, A.; Farghaly, A.; Bruce, J.; Tao, L.F.; Bennett, J.L. Characterization of isolates of *Schistosoma mansoni* from Egyptian villagers that tolerate high doses of praziquantel. *Am. J. Trop. Med. Hyg.* **1996**, *55*, 214–218. [CrossRef] [PubMed]

61. Fallon, P.G.; Doenhoff, M.J. Drug-resistant schistosomiasis: Resistance to praziquantel and oxamniquine induced in *Schistosoma mansoni* in mice is drug specific. *Am. J. Trop. Med. Hyg.* **1994**, *51*, 83–88. [CrossRef]

62. Mwangi, I.N.; Sanchez, M.C.; Mkoji, G.M.; Agola, L.E.; Runo, S.M.; Cupit, P.M.; Cunningham, C. Praziquantel sensitivity of Kenyan *Schistosoma mansoni* isolates and the generation of a laboratory strain with reduced susceptibility to the drug. *Int. J. Parasitol. Drugs Drug Resist.* **2014**, *4*, 296–300. [CrossRef]

63. Melman, S.D.; Steinauer, M.L.; Cunningham, C.; Kubatko, L.S.; Mwangi, I.N.; Wynn, N.B.; Mutuku, M.W.; Karanja, D.M.; Colley, D.G.; Black, C.L.; et al. Reduced susceptibility to praziquantel among naturally occurring Kenyan isolates of *Schistosoma mansoni*. *PLoS Negl. Trop. Dis.* **2009**, *3*, e504. [CrossRef]

64. Ismail, M.; Botros, S.; Metwally, A.; William, S.; Farghally, A.; Tao, L.F.; Day, T.A.; Bennett, J.L. Resistance to praziquantel: Direct evidence from *Schistosoma mansoni* isolated from Egyptian villagers. *Am. J. Trop. Med. Hyg.* **1999**, *60*, 932–935. [CrossRef]

65. Alonso, D.; Munoz, J.; Gascon, J.; Valls, M.E.; Corachan, M. Failure of standard treatment with praziquantel in two returned travelers with *Schistosoma haematobium* infection. *Am. J. Trop. Med. Hyg.* **2006**, *74*, 342–344. [CrossRef] [PubMed]

66. Silva, I.M.; Thiengo, R.; Conceicao, M.J.; Rey, L.; Lenzi, H.L.; Pereira Filho, E.; Ribeiro, P.C. Therapeutic failure of praziquantel in the treatment of *Schistosoma haematobium* infection in Brazilians returning from Africa. *Mem. Inst. Oswaldo Cruz* **2005**, *100*, 445–449. [CrossRef] [PubMed]

67. Silva, I.M.; Pereira Filho, E.; Thiengo, R.; Ribeiro, P.C.; Conceicao, M.J.; Panasco, M.; Lenzi, H.L. Schistosomiasis haematobia: Histopathological course determined by cystoscopy in a patient in whom praziquantel treatment failed. *Rev. Inst. Med. Trop. São Paulo* **2008**, *50*, 343–346. [CrossRef] [PubMed]

68. Liang, Y.S.; Li, H.J.; Dai, J.R.; Wang, W.; Qu, G.L.; Tao, Y.H.; Xing, Y.T.; Li, Y.Z.; Qian, K.; Wei, J.Y. Studies on resistance of *Schistosoma* to praziquantel XIII resistance of *Schistosoma japonicum* to praziquantel is experimentally induced in laboratory. *Chin. J. Schistosomiasis Control* **2011**, *23*, 605–610.

69. Li, H.J.; Liang, Y.S.; Dai, J.R.; Wang, W.; Qu, G.L.; Li, Y.Z.; Xing, Y.T.; Tao, Y.H.; Qian, K.; Jia, Y.; et al. Studies on resistance of Schistosoma to praziquantel XIV experimental comparison of susceptibility to praziquantel between PZQ-resistant isolates and PZQ-susceptible isolates of *Schistosoma japonicum* in stages of adult worms, miracidia and cercariae. *Chin. J. Schistosomiasis Control* **2011**, *23*, 611–619.

70. Ke, Q.; You-Sheng, L.; Wei, W.; Guo-Li, Q.; Hong-Jun, L.; Zhen-Kun, Y.; Zheng-Yang, Z.; Yuntian, X.; Jian-Rong, D. Studies on resistance of *Schistosoma* to praziquantel XVII Biological characteristics of praziquantel-resistant isolates of Schistosoma japonicum in mice. *Chin. J. Schistosomiasis Control* **2017**, *29*, 683–688. [CrossRef]

71. Thomas, C.M.; Timson, D.J. The mechanism of action of praziquantel: Six hypotheses. *Curr. Top. Med. Chem.* **2018**. [CrossRef]

72. World Health Organization. Seventh Meeting of the Working Group on Monitoring of Neglected Tropical Diseases Drug Effi Cacy. Geneva, 26–27 February 2018. Available online: http://apps.who.int/iris/bitstream/handle/10665/273620/WHO-CDS-NTD-PCT-2018.06-eng.pdf?ua=1 (accessed on 3 November 2018).

73. King, C.H. The evolving schistosomiasis agenda 2007-2017-Why we are moving beyond morbidity control toward elimination of transmission. *PLoS Negl. Trop. Dis.* **2017**, *11*, e0005517. [CrossRef]

74. Elmorshedy, H.; Tanner, M.; Bergquist, R.N.; Sharaf, S.; Barakat, R. Prophylactic effect of artemether on human schistosomiasis mansoni among Egyptian children: A randomized controlled trial. *Acta Trop.* **2016**, *158*, 52–58. [CrossRef]

75. Elmorshedy, H.; Bergquist, R.; El-Ela, N.E.; Eassa, S.M.; Elsakka, E.E.; Barakat, R. Can human schistosomiasis mansoni control be sustained in high-risk transmission foci in Egypt? *Parasites Vectors* **2015**, *8*, 372. [CrossRef] [PubMed]

76. Inyang-Etoh, P.C.; Ejezie, G.C.; Useh, M.F.; Inyang-Etoh, E.C. Efficacy of a combination of praziquantel and artesunate in the treatment of urinary schistosomiasis in Nigeria. *Trans. R. Soc. Trop. Med. Hyg.* **2009**, *103*, 38–44. [CrossRef] [PubMed]

77. Hou, X.Y.; McManus, D.P.; Gray, D.J.; Balen, J.; Luo, X.S.; He, Y.K.; Ellis, M.; Williams, G.M.; Li, Y.S. A randomized, double-blind, placebo-controlled trial of safety and efficacy of combined praziquantel and artemether treatment for acute schistosomiasis japonica in China. *Bull. World Health Organ.* **2008**, *86*, 788–795. [CrossRef] [PubMed]

78. N'Goran, E.K.; Utzinger, J.; Gnaka, H.N.; Yapi, A.; N'Guessan, N.A.; Kigbafori, S.D.; Lengeler, C.; Chollet, J.; Shuhua, X.; Tanner, M. Randomized, double-blind, placebo-controlled trial of oral artemether for the prevention of patent *Schistosoma haematobium* infections. *Am. J. Trop. Med. Hyg.* **2003**, *68*, 24–32. [CrossRef] [PubMed]

79. Utzinger, J.; N'Goran, E.K.; N'Dri, A.; Lengeler, C.; Xiao, S.; Tanner, M. Oral artemether for prevention of *Schistosoma mansoni* infection: Randomised controlled trial. *Lancet* **2000**, *355*, 1320–1325. [CrossRef]

80. Perez del Villar, L.; Burguillo, F.J.; Lopez-Aban, J.; Muro, A. Systematic review and meta-analysis of artemisinin based therapies for the treatment and prevention of schistosomiasis. *PLoS ONE* **2012**, *7*, e45867. [CrossRef] [PubMed]

81. Barakat, R.; El Morshedy, H.; Farghaly, A. *Neglected Tropical Diseases—Middle East and North Africa*; McDowell, M.A., Rafati, S., Eds.; Springer: New York, NY, USA, 2014.

82. Barakat, R.M. Epidemiology of Schistosomiasis in Egypt: Travel through Time: Review. *J. Adv. Res.* **2013**, *4*, 425–432. [CrossRef]

83. Barakat, R.; Farghaly, A.; El Morshedy, H.; Hassan, M.; Miller de, W. Impact of National Schistosomiasis Control Program in Kafr El-Sheikh governorate, Nile Delta, Egypt: An independent evaluation. *J. Egypt. Public Health Assoc.* **1998**, *73*, 737–753.

84. Haggag, A.A.; Rabiee, A.; Abd Elaziz, K.M.; Gabrielli, A.F.; Abdel Hay, R.; Ramzy, R.M.R. Mapping of *Schistosoma mansoni* in the Nile Delta, Egypt: Assessment of the prevalence by the circulating cathodic antigen urine assay. *Acta Trop.* **2017**, *167*, 9–17. [CrossRef]

85. Barakat, R.; Elmorshedy, H. Annual report of the project entitled: "Establishment and monitoring of cohort school children in Kafer El-Sheikh Governorate, Egypt, in preparation for schistosomiasis vaccine candidate testing when appropriate". Vaccine Development Project (SVDP); Funded by USAID& Egyptian Ministry of Health and Population (EMHP), 1996-2001. Unpublished work.

86. Doenhoff, M.J.; Cioli, D.; Utzinger, J. Praziquantel: Mechanisms of action, resistance and new derivatives for schistosomiasis. *Curr. Opin. Infect. Dis.* **2008**, *21*, 659–667. [CrossRef]

87. Fenwick, A.; Jourdan, P. Schistosomiasis elimination by 2020 or 2030? *Int. J. Parasitol.* **2016**, *46*, 385–388. [CrossRef] [PubMed]

88. Coulibaly, J.T.; N'Gbesso, Y.K.; Knopp, S.; N'Guessan, N.A.; Silue, K.D.; van Dam, G.J.; N'Goran, E.K.; Utzinger, J. Accuracy of urine circulating cathodic antigen test for the diagnosis of *Schistosoma mansoni* in preschool-aged children before and after treatment. *PLoS Negl. Trop. Dis.* **2013**, *7*, e2109. [CrossRef]

89. Qin, Z.Q.; Jing, X.; Feng, T.; Lv, S.; Qian, Y.; Zhang, L.; Li, Y.L.; Chao, L.V.; Bergquist, R.; Li, S.Z.; Zhou, X.N. Field evaluation of a loop-mediated isothermal amplification (LAMP) platform for the detection of *Schistosoma japonicum* infection in Oncomelania hupensis snails. *Trop. Med. Infect. Dis.* **2018**. [CrossRef]

90. Bergquist, R.; Yang, G.J.; Knopp, S.; Utzinger, J.; Tanner, M. Surveillance and response: Tools and approaches for the elimination stage of neglected tropical diseases. *Acta Trop.* **2015**, *141*, 229–234. [CrossRef] [PubMed]

91. Ogongo, P.; Kariuki, T.M.; Wilson, R.A. Diagnosis of schistosomiasis mansoni: An evaluation of existing methods and research towards single worm pair detection. *Parasitology* **2018**, *145*, 1355–1366. [CrossRef] [PubMed]

92. Corstjens, P.L.; De Dood, C.J.; Kornelis, D.; Fat, E.M.; Wilson, R.A.; Kariuki, T.M.; Nyakundi, R.K.; Loverde, P.T.; Abrams, W.R.; Tanke, H.J.; et al. Tools for diagnosis, monitoring and screening of *Schistosoma* infections utilizing lateral-flow based assays and upconverting phosphor labels. *Parasitology* **2014**, *141*, 1841–1855. [CrossRef]

93. Bergquist, R. Good things are worth waiting for. *Am. J. Trop. Med. Hyg.* **2013**, *88*, 409–410. [CrossRef] [PubMed]

94. Colley, D.G.; Andros, T.S.; Campbell, C.H., Jr. Schistosomiasis is more prevalent than previously thought: What does it mean for public health goals, policies, strategies, guidelines and intervention programs? *Infect. Dis. Poverty* **2017**, *6*, 63. [CrossRef] [PubMed]

6

Elimination of Schistosomiasis Mekongi from Endemic Areas in Cambodia and the Lao People's Democratic Republic: Current Status and Plans

Virak Khieu [1,*], Somphou Sayasone [2], Sinuon Muth [1], Masashi Kirinoki [3],
Sakhone Laymanivong [4], Hiroshi Ohmae [3], Rekol Huy [1], Thipphavanh Chanthapaseuth [5],
Aya Yajima [6], Rattanaxay Phetsouvanh [7], Robert Bergquist [8] and Peter Odermatt [8,9]

[1] National Center for Parasitology, Entomology and Malaria Control, Ministry of Health, Phnom Penh 12100, Cambodia; sinuonm@gmail.com (S.M.); kolhuy@gmail.com (R.H.)
[2] Lao Tropical and Public Health Institute, Vientiane 01030, Laos; somphou.sayasone@yahoo.com
[3] School of Medicine, Dokkyo Medical University, Mibu, Shimotsuga, Tochigi 321-0293, Japan; kirinoki@dokkyomed.ac.jp (M.K.); rsa40370@nifty.com (H.O.)
[4] Centre for Malariology, Parasitology and Entomology, Vientiane 01000, Laos; sakhone07@gmail.com
[5] World Health Organization, Vientiane Office, Vientiane 01160, Laos; chanthapaseutht@who.int
[6] World Health Organization, Western Pacific Regional Office, Manila 1000, Philippines; yajimaa@who.int
[7] Department of Communicable Disease Control, Ministry of Health, Vientiane 01130, Laos; rattanaxay@gmail.com
[8] Department of Epidemiology and Public Health, Swiss Tropical and Public Health Institute, P.O. Box 4002 Basel, Switzerland; robert.bergquist@yahoo.se (R.B.); peter.odermatt@swisstph.ch (P.O.)
[9] University of Basel, P.O. Box 4001 Basel, Switzerland
* Correspondence: virak.khieu@gmail.com

Abstract: The areas endemic for schistosomiasis in the Lao People's Democratic Republic and in Cambodia were first reported 50 and 60 years ago, respectively. However, the causative parasite *Schistosoma mekongi* was not recognized as a separate species until 1978. The infection is distributed along a limited part of the Mekong River, regulated by the focal distribution of the intermediate snail host *Neotricula aperta*. Although more sensitive diagnostics imply a higher figure, the current use of stool examinations suggests that only about 1500 people are presently infected. This well-characterized setting should offer an exemplary potential for the elimination of the disease from its endemic areas; yet, the local topography, reservoir animals, and a dearth of safe water sources make transmission control a challenge. Control activities based on mass drug administration resulted in strong advances, and prevalence was reduced to less than 5% according to stool microscopy. Even so, transmission continues unabated, and the true number of infected people could be as much as 10 times higher than reported. On-going control activities are discussed together with plans for the future.

Keywords: *Schistosoma mekongi*; *Neotricula aperta*; snail; Cambodia; Lao PDR; elimination

1. Historical Background

The parasitic, trematode genus *Schistosoma* puts more than 800 million people in the world's tropical areas at risk, infecting a third of them [1,2]. Six different species of *Schistosoma* can infect humans, each depending on a specific snail species acting as intermediate host. The various endemic areas for the three main schistosome species have long been well-known, with basically *S. mansoni* in Africa and Latin America, *S. haematobium* in Africa, and *S. japonicum* in China and The Philippines (formerly also in Japan).

The adult schistosomes are miniscule worms with a preference for abdominal capillaries of the definitive human host, where they release a large number of eggs. These are excreted with either urine or feces (which route depends on the schistosome species) and infect the intermediate snail host, which releases many cercariae—a later developmental stage—into the water. The parasite's life cycle is completed when the definitive human host comes into contact with water containing schistosome cercariae that can penetrate the human skin. However, large numbers of parasite eggs fail to be excreted and, instead, cause microscopic lesions due to the host immune reactions in various organs, most often the liver. Generally, this leads to a chronic disease with comparatively low direct mortality. Schistosomiasis as a whole constitutes one of the neglected tropical diseases (NTDs) selected for elimination by the World Health Organization (WHO). Owing to the limited geographical distribution of *Schistosoma mekongi* to endemic areas in Cambodia and the Lao People's Democratic Republic (Lao PDR), strategies aiming at its elimination and eventual eradication can be implemented more effectively than for other, more widespread species.

Before effective chemotherapy became available in the late 1970s, the cornerstone for schistosomiasis control was broad-spectrum molluscicides directed at the intermediate snail host. However, when the drug praziquantel was introduced [3] and started to be used (at 40 mg/kg) for mass drug administration (MDA), it soon replaced most other control activities thanks to safety, high efficacy against the adult parasite worm, and easy administration [1,4]. Praziquantel changed the focus from infection prevention to morbidity reduction, reflected in a decline of the disability-adjusted life years (DALYs) metric for schistosomiasis [5,6]. This decline has, however, been contended since minor, so-called subtle morbidities are not considered by the DALY [5,6].

After schistosomiasis had been discovered in the Mekong River Basin (MRB), first in Lao PDR in 1957 [7] and 10 years later (1968) in Cambodia [8], biological research conducted in the 1970s demonstrated that the eggs from the MRB schistosomes were morphologically different from *S. japonicum* [8]. Furthermore, the former species had a different intermediate snail host [9,10] that could not infect water buffaloes [8] but was found in dogs [11]. By 1978, it became clear that the parasite was sufficiently different from *S. japonicum* to be named a separate species, *S. mekongi* [12]. Schistosomiasis mekongi is only found in specific areas along the MRB as it transverses Lao PDR and Cambodia. Due to the specific environmental variables required by its intermediate host snail, *Neotricula aperta* [9,10,13], transmission of *S. mekongi* is highly focal [14,15]. Compared to other schistosome species, the endemic areas for this kind of schistosomiasis are very limited, and the population at risk is unusually small, comprising only an estimated 150,000 people [14]. However, infection and re-infection sustain the disease, particularly in children, due to their high level of water contact [16,17]. Reservoir hosts, also play a role in maintaining the infection in the environment, although their diversity is not as broad as that seen with *S. japonicum*.

This paper reviews the work carried out after the rediscovery of the *S. mekongi* foci in the early 1990s in Lao PDR and Cambodia. We start with the historical background and continue by summarizing early control activities in each country. Subsequently, we list the achievements and elaborate on the organizational set-up, highlighting most relevant operational research activities. This review also features the more recent switch from morbidity control to elimination, followed by a discussion of the steps to achieve and the challenges involved.

1.1. Lao PDR

The first schistosomiasis mekongi case was diagnosed in Saint Joseph Hospital in Paris in 1957 [7], where an 18-year old Laotian patient was hospitalized, following an episode of severe hematemesis. The patient had advanced hepatosplenic pathology, and the infection was eventually traced back to his first years of life spent on Khong Island, Champasack Province, Lao PDR. Later on, a scientific paper reported on several other schistosomiasis patients originating from the same area [18]. In 1967, a WHO mission was sent to Champasack confirming the infection risk and identifying a transmission focus [19]. High village prevalence rates of schistosomiasis (up to 60%) were observed in certain districts, such as Khong and Mounlapamok in Champasack Province. Severe hepato-biliary morbidity associated with *S. mekongi* infection was frequently seen at the local health facilities. However, further follow-up studies could not be done at this point in time due to war and civil unrest in the 1970s and 1980s. In 1989, the Ministry of Health (MoH) initiated its first chemotherapy-based intervention with support from WHO in all of the endemic communities in Khong and Mounlapamok [14]. It was found that one third of all children tested were positive for *S. mekongi*, leading to the recommendation to implement health information, education, and communication (IEC) in addition to chemotherapy. This type of intervention was performed annually until 1995 and subsequently continued up to 1999 with support from the German Pharma Health Fund. After several annual MDA rounds with praziquantel, the prevalence of schistosomiasis in sentinel villages was as low as 2% [20].

1.2. Cambodia

In the late 1960s, schistosomiasis patients also started to be diagnosed at Phnom Penh's Calmette Hospital in Cambodia [21,22]. All those patients originated from Kratié Province where the presence of a transmission focus was confirmed in primary surveys [23,24]. An extended survey, including the examination of 3, 767 primary school-children in villages along the Mekong River from Strung Treng, towards the Vietnamese border, discovered variable rates of infection with the highest infection (~34%) in Kratié Province, notably lower rates in Stung Treng Province (4%) and no infections in the provinces further downstream [19]. However, intradermal sensitivity tests against *S. japonicum* antigen were positive in some children (<10%) from some downstream villages, and some exposure to the parasite was documented [19].

Early observations on Khong Island in Lao PDR confirmed severe clinical manifestations of the infection [25], such as portal hypertension with dilated superficial abdominal veins or advanced ascites and/or hepatomegaly and/or splenomegaly. Adolescents and young adults were the most heavily affected. Infection rates of 60% and higher were diagnosed with co-infections with *Opisthorchis viverrini* (64%) and hookworm (44%) being very common. However, no mortality was reported [25,26]. In Cambodia, the dramatic, historical events (Cambodian Civil War) that gained momentum in the late 1960s, deterred further studies. Schistosomiasis was only brought back into the national health agenda in 1992, when the non-governmental organization (NGO) 'Action Internationale Contre la Faim' diagnosed marked hepato-splenomegaly in 50% of 120 schoolchildren from Ampil Tuk, a village in Kratié Province [16].

When large-scale monitoring in 1994 resulted in the diagnosis of many severe cases in 20 villages in Kratié Province, the enormity of the schistosomiasis problem in the country became fully recognized [17]. A pilot schistosomiasis control program, mainly based on MDA and IEC, was started in 1995 in Kratié Province [15]. Two years later, the program was scaled up to include all endemic districts in the two hardest hit provinces, Kratié and Stung Treng, bringing the total number of villages to 114 (56 in Kratié and 58 in Stung Treng) with an estimate of 80,000 people at risk [20]. During 1994–1995, several surveys in accessible villages along the Mekong River in Kratié Province showed infection rates between 1% and 68% [17]. Based on the initial epidemiological observations, the Cambodian MoH and the health authorities in Kratié Province, in collaboration with "Médecins sans Frontières", initiated a rehabilitation program at Kratié provincial hospital and the district hospital of Sambo, with integrated community-based and hospital-based schistosomiasis control [15]. In 1996, Hatz et al. [20,27] conducted the first ultrasound profiling of *S. mekongi* infection in the Stung Treng Province in Cambodia, detecting pathological changes in 84% of the 299 participants with periportal thickening in 16% and parenchymal changes in 9% of those investigated.

2. From Morbidity Control to Elimination

2.1. Lao PDR

The first National Policy and Strategy for Control of Helminth Infections was developed and endorsed by the MoH in 2009 [28]. It served as a backbone for the helminth control program, targeting four groups of helminth diseases with public health significance, i.e., lymphatic filariasis (LF), soil-transmitted helminthiasis (STH), food-borne trematodiasis, and schistosomiasis.

2.1.1. Policy, Commitment, and Interdisciplinarity

In 2015, the National Policy and Strategy for Control of Helminth Infections was revised and extended to cover all NTDs with public health significance in Lao PDR, such as leprosy. Following the Policy and Strategy directives, the National Committee for NTD control was established. It included members from the MoH, such as the Department of Communicable Disease Control (CDC), the Lao Tropical and Public Health Institute (Lao TPHI), the National Centre of Malariology, Parasitology and Entomology (CMPE), National Centre for Environmental Health and Water Supply as well as representatives from other administrative authorities, such as the Ministry of Education and Sports, the Ministry of Agriculture and Forestry and the Ministry of Transport and Construction. Chaired by the Deputy Minister of Health, this committee guides, monitors, advocates, and authorizes all NTD control activities in Lao PDR including the MoH budget. It also comprises all activities regarding schistosomiasis control. Its status was updated and its list of members renewed in 2018.

A specific national schistosomiasis elimination action plan for the period 2016–2020 has been developed as a guidance for the National Control Program. This plan is supported by a Technical Taskforce at the central, provincial and district levels, and the taskforce members are experts from the ministries, which are already involved by the National Committee for NTD Control.

2.1.2. Activities after the Millennium Shift

With MDA and IEC discontinued after 1999 due to waning financial support, *S. mekongi* infection prevalence started—unsurprisingly—to rapidly increase. In 2003, a survey was conducted by the MoH, with support from WHO, using the Kato-Katz technique based on a single stool sample. It revealed an overall infection prevalence of 11.0% across the 64 endemic communities in Khong District, varying from 0% to 47.2%. The average infection prevalence in Mounlapamok District was 0.7%, only reaching higher levels (3.5%) in the most highly infected village, and with a majority of villages still completely negative (Figure 1). This re-emergence was later confirmed by a joint Lao–Swiss research project conducted by the Lao TPHI in the period 2005–2006. It showed a *S. mekongi* infection prevalence of 68% and 4% in Khong and Mounlapamok, respectively [29]. These rebounding prevalence rates in the two endemic districts brought infection rates up to the levels common before control was initiated in 1989.

In 2007, the Lao MoH, in collaboration with WHO and other partners, re-established a second chemotherapy-based intervention scheme with the aim to eliminate schistosomiasis as a public health problem by bringing infection intensities below 1% in all areas, using seven specifically defined sentinel villages to monitor the intervention success (MoH, Technical Report on schistosomiasis control program, unpublished). To achieve this goal, WHO recommended maintaining the annual MDA with praziquantel covering at least 75% of each community treated. The high-risk population, namely school-aged children and adults, i.e., people of ages from 5 to 60 years old, were targeted. They conducted ten rounds of MDA, with an average coverage of >80%, which brought the prevalence down to less than 10% in 2016 at all the sentinel sites, with no cases of high-intensity infection (>400 eggs per gram) detected (Figure 2) [30]. In 2017, the infection prevalence was less than 3%, with only 0.1% of them being high-intensity infections. In 2018, less than 6% of villagers at most sentinel sites were infected, with an overall prevalence of 3.2%. No patient with high-intensity infection was diagnosed (Figure 3). In addition, spot-checks were conducted in 20 randomly selected villages with a total of 3, 533 study participants. In 2017, and thus far in 2018, the average infection prevalence reached only 0.7%. No high-intensity infection was diagnosed [31], but continued MDA in the future is planned.

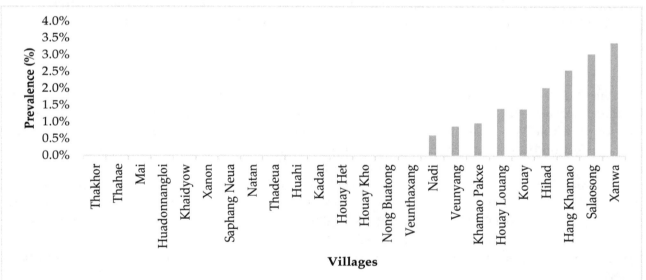

Figure 1. Prevalence of schistosomiasis in Khong (top) and Mounlapamok (bottom), detected by an approach based on a single Kato-Katz smear within the MoH and World Health Organization (WHO) survey in 2003.

With regard to investigating if transmission involving reservoir hosts could become a problem for elimination of schistosomiasis mekongi, Strandgaard et al. [32] conducted a survey focused on domestic pigs in the Khong District. Working with a total number of 98 pigs, detection of *S. mekongi* eggs in the liver, intestines, and stools of 12 (12.2%) of them confirmed this animal as a possible definitive host.

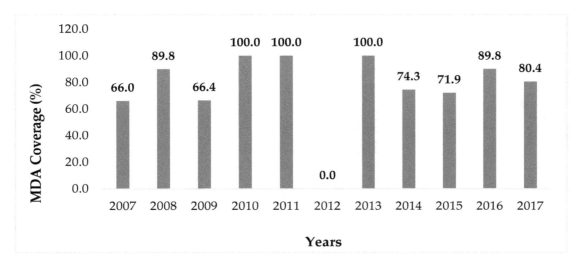

Figure 2. Mass drug administration (MDA) coverage at the *S. mekongi* endemic communities in Lao PDR in the period 2006–2017.

Figure 3. *Schistosoma mekongi* infection prevalence at the seven sentinel sites in the districts Khong and Mounlapamok in the period 2016–2018.

2.2. Cambodia

In collaboration with the MoH National Center for Parasitology, Entomology and Malaria Control (CNM) in Phnom Penh, researchers from Dokkyo Medical University, Mibu, Tochigi, Japan have been conducting epidemiological surveys in Cambodia since 1997. The aim was to elucidate the status of schistosomiasis due to *S. mekongi* [14]. Figure 4 shows the results of a seroepidemiological survey conducted in 1997 and 1998, using the enzyme-linked immunosorbent assay (ELISA) with *S. japonicum* soluble egg antigen (SEA) according to Matsuda et al. [33]. The results were consistent with the stool examinations with regard to the distribution of the infection among the endemic villages [14]. However, egg-positive rates exceeding 50% and ELISA-positive rates higher than 90% were recorded in some villages in the northern part of Kratié Province, while ELISA-positive rates of less than 30% were recorded in some villages in the southern part of the area [14]. None of these parts of Kratié Province had been targeted by surveillance prior to 1997; consequently, no stool examinations had been performed there in the period 1994–1995.

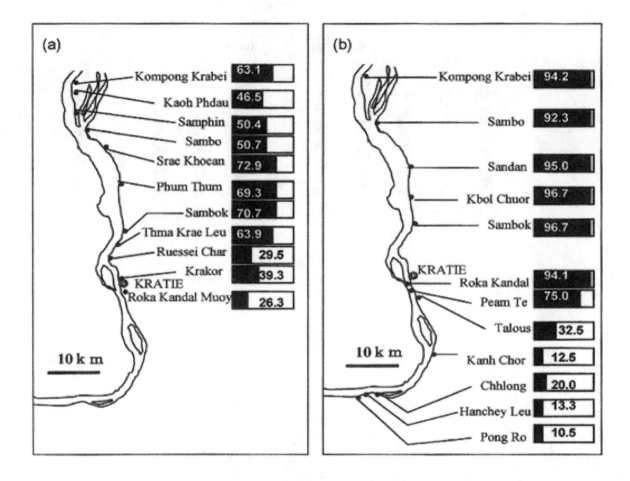

Figure 4. Comparison of results of stool examination and ELISA conducted in villages along the Mekong River in the Kratié Province [14]. Positive ratios (%) are represented by the numbers in the bar charts. (**a**) Prevalence of schistosomiasis mekongi, as determined by stool examination during 1994–1995 [17], and (**b**) prevalence of schistosomiasis mekongi, as determined by ELISA using *S. japonicum* soluble egg antigen (SEA) in the period 1997–1998 [14].

Serology surveys were part of the diagnostic approach, owing to their usefulness for the detection of schistosomiasis risk by village, particularly in low-endemic foci. Since 2003, ELISAs specific for *S. mekongi* were applied, relying on a technique using sodium metaperiodate (SMP) to reduce non-specific cross-reactions via oxidization of polysaccharide residues in the antigen molecules [34]. Ultrasound, a technique showing severe pathological changes in the liver that are often irreversible, was carried out using portable devices. However, this kind of examination can only be used for personal examination as well as for regional risk monitoring and historical evaluation [35]. Such examinations were conducted in 2003 to compare morbidity due to *S. mekongi* infection in villages in Kratié Province characterized by high and low endemicity [36].

Stool examinations were carried out using the Kato-Katz technique [37]. The SMP–ELISA technique was used for surveys in sentinel villages designated by the National Schistosomiasis Control Program (in Achen, Char Thnaol, Srae Kheun and Sambok in Kratié Province as well as several additional spot-check sites). As shown in Figure 5, ELISA-positive rates in sentinel villages and at two additional sites (Roka Kandal and Sambour) dramatically decreased to below 20%, while ELISA-positive rates remained high (>50%) at two spot-check sites (Kampong Krabei and Kbal Chuor).

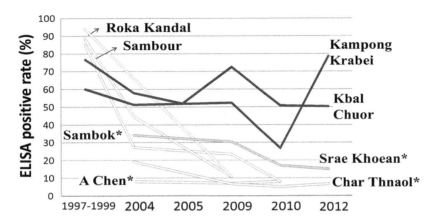

Figure 5. Changes in specific antibody rates in villages in the Kratié Province, Cambodia, during the period 1997–2012. Legend: *Sentinel villages for monitoring, as designated by the National Center for Parasitology, Entomology and Malaria Control (CNM). Black line: high-risk villages (≥50%); grey line: Moderate-risk villages (≥10% and <50%); white line: low-risk village (<10%) SMP–ELISA using *S. mekongi* SEA.

Applying ultrasound examination, dilatation of the portal vein was detected in 139 of 366 participants (38%) in a high-endemic village group and in 10 of the 117 participants (1.2%) in low-endemic villages. The characteristic ultrasound pattern of septum formation in the liver parenchyma producing the fish scale pattern noted in *S. japonicum* infection, was not observed in *S. mekongi* infections. However, in the 1990s, splenomegaly due to *S. mekongi* infection was reported to be more severe than that due to *S. japonicum* infection [38,39].

Various animals have been suspected to act as reservoir infection sources. While pigs have been experimentally shown to be possible natural reservoirs of *S. mekongi* in Lao PDR [32], this finding could only be confirmed for dogs in Cambodia. Natural schistosome infection in dogs in Cambodia was first reported by Matsumoto et al. in 2002 [40]. Schistosome eggs were detected in 1 of the 28 canine stool samples (3.6%) collected from Kbal Chuor village in Kratié Province in 2000 [40]. During a more recent survey in 2010, 15 and 17 canine stool samples were collected from two villages, Kbal Chuor and Kampong Krabei, in Kratié Province; *S. mekongi* eggs were detected in 2 (13.3%) and 1 (5.9%) of the samples from these villages, respectively.

Hisakane et al. [41] constructed a mathematical model for *S. mekongi* transmission in Cambodia, according to which dogs were considered definitive hosts in addition to humans. The simulations indicated that biannual universal and/or targeted treatment could reduce the prevalence to below 5%, within 8 years, based on 85% coverage of the residents [41]. Natural *S. mekongi* infections were not detected in cats, pigs, cows, water buffalos, horses or rats in Cambodia [40]. Rodents have been shown to be susceptible to *S. mekongi* by experimental infection; however, no natural infections have been detected to date. In 2016, ten *S. mekongi* infected *N. aperta* were found in 4840 corrected mollusks (0.2%).

A national task force for the control of STH, schistosomiasis and LF was set up in 2003. The members of the committee were representatives of different departments, ministries, and NGOs. Each department, institution and ministry involved has the responsibility to contribute to specific control/elimination activities. While CNM is responsible for developing the control/elimination strategies of NTDs, including *S. mekongi*, the Department of School Health of the Ministry of Education, Youth and Sports manages health education and support of water, sanitation and hygiene (WASH) approach in schools, the Department of Rural Health of the Ministry of Rural Development (MRD) is in charge of WASH in the communities, and WHO and the United Nations Children's Fund (UNICEF) offer technical and financial support. In 2004, the first National Policy and Guidelines for Helminth Control in Cambodia was established and adopted by the National Task Force for the Control of STH, schistosomiasis and LF [39].

3. Achievements

3.1. Lao PDR

The move from control to elimination is a challenge and recent experience suggests that interruption of MDA without adequate sanitary improvements, would within a few years lead to the parasite reclaiming its previous high endemicity. With this in mind, the MoH has started community-led initiatives to eliminate schistosomiasis by combining MDA with schistosomiasis-adapted Water, Sanitation and Hygiene (WASH) interventions (CL-SWASH) in two pilot villages in 2015, with technical support from WHO and other partners [31,42–44]. CL-SWASH integrates various ongoing MoH components of parasitic infection control with the aim to expand development of Water Safety Plans –a multi-risk management approach ranging from community participation to nationwide activities. Communities will be empowered to self-assess their environmental health risk situation, particularly in relation to schistosomiasis transmission, for instance, by interrupting transmission by eliminating open defecation. CL-SWASH continues to expand and had completed activities in 24 villages by the end of 2018, as well as outlined a plan to cover all 202 endemic villages by 2025. In addition, the MoH national action plan for elimination of schistosomiasis reflects the recommendation by the 'Expert Consultation to Accelerate Elimination of Asian Schistosomiasis' conducted in Shanghai, China under the auspices of the WHO Regional Office for the Western Pacific (WPRO) in May 2017 [45]. The main conclusion was to shift activities from the current chemotherapy-only intervention to an integrated One-Health strategy, aiming to interrupt transmission by 2025 and to achieve certified elimination by 2030 [46].

3.2. Cambodia

Since 1995, the MDA together with the IEC campaigns have been conducted annually in the two provinces endemic for *S. mekongi*. In Kratié Province, four sentinel villages were followed-up annually. Figure 6 shows the rapid decrease in the prevalence of *S. mekongi* infection from 1995 to 2018. The *S. mekongi* prevalence at four sentinel surveillance sites in Kratié Province dropped dramatically from 70% in 1995 to less than 1% in 2018. According to the CNM annual reports no new patients with *S. mekongi* infection were diagnosed in these villages over the last few years, demonstrating the positive impact of the intervention.

Figure 6. *S. mekongi* prevalence distribution in four sentinel site villages of Kratié, Cambodia 1995–2018.

In 2016, an external evaluation of schistosomiasis control in Cambodia was led by WHO and based on the formalin-detergent diagnostic method [47] proven to have higher sensitivity than the standard Kato-Katz method [37]. The evaluation demonstrated absence of high-intensity infections, both at the sentinel sites and the two additional spot-check sites [48]. Based on this finding, it was concluded that annual rounds of MDA, targeting the entire at-risk population above 5 years of age would be sufficient to achieve elimination of schistosomiasis as a public health problem defined as <1% prevalence of high-intensity infection. This success encouraged the MoH to shift gear from disease control to elimination in alignment with the recommendation of the 2017 WHO Expert Consultation [45]. In 2018, the National Strategic Plan for Elimination of Schistosomiasis (2019–2023) was developed after holding a national consultation workshop with all relevant stakeholders at the national and provincial levels, with input from MoH, MRD, Ministry of Agriculture, Forestry and Fishery, and the Ministry of Education, Youth and Sports. The aim is to interrupt transmission of schistosomiasis by 2025 and validate elimination of schistosomiasis by 2030. Three main elimination strategies were adopted:

1. Universal access to the One-Health intervention package consisting of preventive chemotherapy, CL-SWASH, and treatment of the animal reservoirs;
2. Strengthening community members' health literacy to prevent reinfection and interrupt transmission through a sustained change of sanitation and hygiene behaviour empowering people to act as drivers of schistosomiasis elimination; and
3. Adoption of effective and sustained active and passive surveillance of schistosomiasis in human and reservoirs hosts.

4. Next Steps and Challenges

The prevalence information in Lao PDR and Cambodia discussed here, is based on stool examination by the Kato-Katz technique [49], often based on a single stool sample, which implies that the real prevalence could be considerably higher than that presented. While the use of the Kato-Katz technique is acceptable in areas characterized by high-intensity of infection, the recent reduction of *S. mekongi* intensity of infection, following regular MDA with praziquantel, requires a rapid switch to more sensitive diagnostic techniques [49].

The polymerase chain reaction (PCR) and the loop-mediated isothermal amplification (LAMP) are highly sensitive and specific diagnostic assays that have been validated for schistosomiasis diagnosis [50,51]. The LAMP technique holds the advantage of being applicable in field laboratories, where it has been used to detect *Schistosoma* in the snail host [52,53], an application that should be useful for monitoring transmission. Detecting circulating schistosome antigens (cathodic circulating antigen, CCA or anodic circulating antigen, CAA) in sera from infected humans [54] represents a different approach. An added benefit is that these antigens pass from the blood circulation into the urine, allowing the testing of urine samples rather than blood [54], which should make people more receptive to the recurrent testing that will be needed in the future. A commercial point-of-care (POC-CCA) test for *S. mansoni* has delivered excellent results in Africa [55,56], identifying three to four times more infected individuals compared to the Kato-Katz technique [56]. When POC-CCA and a CAA test were compared with the Kato-Katz stool examination in Lao PDR and Cambodia, the two former assays showed 3- and 6-times better sensitivity, respectively [57]. However, cross-reactivity with other intestinal trematode infections, such as *O. viverrini*, cannot be ruled out, necessitating extended evaluations. Thus, before these tests can become standard assays in control programs, more experience with them are needed. Efforts in this direction are on-going.

The national helminth control programs in Cambodia and Lao PDR implement schistosomiasis control activities independently; however, the two teams regularly visit each other to gain insights into the operational activities and implementation of each program. This is important for sustaining the goals set, and needs now to be complemented by a database encompassing the entire area endemic for *S. mekongi*, distributed to these two countries. The preliminary database, established in Lao PDR to keep track of ongoing control activities and impact measures implemented, has proven useful by contributing to the adoption of standardized measures of infection and morbidity. An online database accessible by all stakeholders would be instrumental for exchange of surveillance data and rapid response action when needed, substantially facilitating the work towards elimination of *S. mekongi* infections. Once a *S. mekongi* database has been established, the information can be leveraged by bundling the data together with cartographic records and remotely sensed data from earth-observing satellites, displaying the information in a geographical information system (GIS) [58,59]. Thanks to the growing accessibility to the Internet and global positioning systems, relevant data can be collected from satellite sensors and analyzed in field settings, or other resource-poor environments, by laptop computers, and even mobile phones.

The multi-sectoral control approach, initiated in pilot villages in both countries, has thus far demonstrated both feasibility and suitability. Nonetheless, scaling up this kind of intervention is a challenge that will require substantial efforts when enlarging activities to cover communities and higher levels. Each endemic village initially requires six provincial-level officials from the different administrative sectors, involved to spend three working days initiating the activities needed. Later all enrolled villages receive follow-up visits to consolidate the various activities started. However, the resources needed, particularly with reference to trained personnel, to implement multi-sectoral activities in all villages endemic for schistosomiasis (114 in Cambodia and 202 in Lao PDR) are currently not available. This notwithstanding, the local health services must become more adapted to surveillance-and-response systems [60]. Today, these services do not have a defined role, neither with respect to diagnosis nor to treatment delivery. Strengthening of the health system has been recognized to be essential for the long-term success of control. Consequently, defining the role of curative and preventive health services in the surveillance and response, and diagnoses and treatment of *S. mekongi* and improving these services accordingly will be indispensable for successful control and future elimination.

In the absence of a schistosomiasis vaccine or alternative drugs, praziquantel has now been used as the mainstay for control, wherever possible complemented by WASH or CL-SWASH. Today, praziquantel treatment through annual MDA is assured as the MoHs in Cambodia and Lao PDR both make substantial efforts to maintain the annual treatment rounds. However, the move towards elimination planned will require transmission control, something which is more difficult in areas endemic for *S. mekongi* than anywhere else. Even if sufficiently sensitive snail diagnostics exist, the collection of specimens for testing is a challenge as the average shell length of *N. aperta* is less than 3 mm [60]. Further, the snails are restricted to shallow areas with water moving fast over wood or stone surfaces. As such conditions only exist during the dry season, the snails mostly originate from eggs laid the previous year [61]. Thus, every year provides new snail populations and they can only be found during a few months in the first half of the year. Transmission control should also involve reservoir host such as dogs and other domestic animals found susceptible for *S. mekongi* infection. The most expedient way of checking these would be serology, even if antibody titers will be less significant than direct tests of circulating or excreted schistosome antigens.

5. Conclusions

Despite the geographically fragmented environment along the Mekong River in Cambodia and Lao PDR, it should be feasible to achieve elimination of *S. mekongi* owing to the confinement of this parasite to extremely restricted areas. In fact, *S. mekongi* has the smallest distribution of any of the schistosome species. However, elimination has proved more difficult than initially thought. Despite strong progress in a large part of the endemic area, thanks to the MDA with praziquantel and the initiation of the multi-sectoral control approach, elimination remains a distant goal. What is needed for improved control are (i) scaling-up of the multi-sectoral control approach; (ii) application of a common database; and (iii), in the longer perspective, local health services to a surveillance-and-response system. A more thorough study of which animals can act as definitive hosts, would also be useful.

These moves, however, will only be bear fruit if a reliable representation of *S. mekongi* prevalence and intensity of infection can be ensured, something that is clearly attainable through the implementation of more sensitive diagnostics, supported by remotely sensed data and GIS technology.

Acknowledgments: We thank Jasmina Saric for her efficient English editing.

References

1. Colley, D.G.; Bustinduy, A.L.; Secor, W.E.; King, C.H. Human schistosomiasis. *Lancet* **2014**, *383*, 2253–2264. [CrossRef]
2. Steinmann, P.; Keiser, J.; Bos, R.; Tanner, M.; Utzinger, J. Schistosomiasis and water resources development: Systematic review, meta-analysis, and estimates of people at risk. *Lancet Infect Dis.* **2006**, *6*, 411–425. [CrossRef]
3. Davis, A.; Wegner, D.H. Multicentre trials of praziquantel in human schistosomiasis: Design and techniques. *Bull. World Health Organ.* **1979**, *57*, 767–771. [PubMed]
4. King, C.H. Parasites and poverty: The case of schistosomiasis. *Acta Trop.* **2010**, *113*, 95–104. [CrossRef] [PubMed]
5. Dalys, G.B.D.; Collaborators, H. Global, regional, and national disability-adjusted life-years (DALYs) for 333 diseases and injuries and healthy life expectancy (HALE) for 195 countries and territories, 1990–2016: A systematic analysis for the Global Burden of Disease Study 2016. *Lancet* **2017**, *390*, 1260–1344. [CrossRef]
6. Murray, C.J.; Vos, T.; Lozano, R.; Naghavi, M.; Flaxman, A.D.; Michaud, C.; Ezzati, M.; Shibuya, K.; Salomon, J.A.; Abdalla, S.; et al. Disability-adjusted life years (DALYs) for 291 diseases and injuries in 21 regions, 1990–2010: A systematic analysis for the Global Burden of Disease Study 2010. *Lancet* **2012**, *380*, 2197–2223. [CrossRef]
7. Vic-Dupont, B.C.; Soubrane, J.; Halle, B.; Richir, C. Bilharziose à *Schistosoma japonicum* à forme hépato-spléenique révélée par une grande hématemese. *Bull. Mem. Soc. Med. Hop. Paris* **1957**, *73*, 933–941.
8. Schneider, C.R.; Kitikoon, V.; Sornmani, S.; Thirachantra, S. Mekong schistosomiasis. III: A parasitological survey of domestic water buffalo (*Bubalus bubalis*) on Khong Island, Laos. *Ann. Trop. Med. Parasitol.* **1975**, *69*, 227–232. [CrossRef] [PubMed]
9. Davis, G.M.; Kitikoon, V.; Temcharoen, P. Monograph on "Lithoglyphopsis" aperta, the snail host of Mekong River schistosomiasis. *Malacologia* **1976**, *15*, 241–287. [PubMed]
10. Kitikoon, V.; Schneider, C.R. Notes on the aquatic ecology of Lithoglyphopsis aperta. *Southeast Asian J. Trop. Med. Public Health* **1976**, *7*, 238–243. [PubMed]
11. Sornmani, S.; Kitikoon, V.; Schneider, C.R.; Harinasuta, C.; Pathammavong, O. Mekong schistosomiasis. 1. Life cycle of *Schistosoma japonicum*, Mekong strain in the laboratory. *Southeast Asian J. Trop. Med. Public Health* **1973**, *4*, 218–225. [PubMed]
12. Voge, M.; Price, Z.; Bruckner, D.A. Changes in tegumental surface of *Schistosoma mekongi* Voge, Bruckner, and Bruce 1978, in the mammalian host. *J. Parasitol.* **1978**, *64*, 944–947. [CrossRef] [PubMed]
13. Attwood, S.W.; Fatih, F.A.; Campbell, I.; Upatham, E.S. The distribution of Mekong schistosomiasis, past and future: Preliminary indications from an analysis of genetic variation in the intermediate host. *Parasitol. Int.* **2008**, *57*, 256–270. [CrossRef] [PubMed]
14. Ohmae, H.; Sinuon, M.; Kirinoki, M.; Matsumoto, J.; Chigusa, Y.; Socheat, D.; Matsuda, H. *Schistosomiasis mekongi*: From discovery to control. *Parasitol. Int.* **2004**, *53*, 135–142. [CrossRef] [PubMed]
15. Sinuon, M.; Tsuyuoka, R.; Socheat, D.; Odermatt, P.; Ohmae, H.; Matsuda, H.; Montresor, A.; Palmer, K. Control of *Schistosoma mekongi* in Cambodia: Results of eight years of control activities in the two endemic provinces. *Trans. R. Soc. Trop. Med. Hyg.* **2007**, *101*, 34–39. [CrossRef] [PubMed]
16. Biays, S.; Stich, A.H.; Odermatt, P.; Long, C.; Yersin, C.; Men, C.; Saem, C.; Lormand, J.D. A foci of *Schistosomiasis mekongi* rediscovered in Northeast Cambodia: Cultural perception of the illness; description and clinical observation of 20 severe cases. *Trop. Med. Int. Health* **1999**, *4*, 662–673. [CrossRef] [PubMed]

17. Stich, A.H.; Biays, S.; Odermatt, P.; Men, C.; Saem, C.; Sokha, K.; Ly, C.S.; Legros, P.; Philips, M.; Lormand, J.D.; et al. Foci of *Schistosomiasis mekongi*, Northern Cambodia: II. Distribution of infection and morbidity. *Trop. Med. Int. Health* **1999**, *4*, 674–685. [CrossRef] [PubMed]

18. Barbier, M. Determination of aocus of arteriovenous bilharziosiin southern Laos (Sithadone Province). *Bull. Soc. Pathol. Exot. Filiales* **1966**, *59*, 4–83. [PubMed]

19. Iijima, T.; Garcia, R.G. *Rapport D'affectation (Enquête Préliminaire sur la Bilharziose au Laos Méridional)*; OMS, Bureau Rég. Pacif. Occid. Doc. WPRO-80, 23 Mai 1967 (11 Pages, 3 Cartes); WPRO: Manila, Philippines, 1967.

20. Urbani, C.; Sinoun, M.; Socheat, D.; Pholsena, K.; Strandgaard, H.; Odermatt, P.; Hatz, C. Epidemiology and control of mekongi schistosomiasis. *Acta Trop.* **2002**, *82*, 157–168. [CrossRef]

21. Audebaud, G.; Tournier-Lasserve, C.; Brumpt, V.; Jolly, M.; Mazaud, R.; Imbert, X.; Bazillio, R. 1st case of human schistosomiasis observed in Cambodia (Kratié area). *Bull. Soc. Pathol. Exot. Filiales* **1968**, *61*, 778–784. [PubMed]

22. Tournier-Lasserve, C.; Audebaud, G.; Brumpt, V.; Jolly, M.; Calvez, F.; Mazaud, R.; Imbert, X.; Bazillio, R. Existence of a focus of human bilharziosis, in Cambodia in the Kratié area. I. Study of the 1st three clinical cases. *Med. Trop. (Mars)* **1970**, *30*, 451–461. [PubMed]

23. Jolly, M.; Bazillio, R.; Audebaud, G.; Brumpt, V.; Sophinn, B. Existence of a focus of human bilharziosis, in Cambodia in Kratié area. II. Epidemiologic survey. Preliminary results. *Med. Trop. (Mars)* **1970**, *30*, 462–471. [PubMed]

24. Jolly, M.; Bazillio, R.; Audebaud, G.; Brumpt, V.; Sophinn, B. First epidemiologic studies on a focus of human biharziasis in Cambodia, in the region of Kratié. *Bull. Soc. Pathol. Exot. Filiales* **1970**, *63*, 476–483. [PubMed]

25. Sornmani, S.; Vivatanasesth, P.; Thirachantra, S. Clinical study of Mekong schistosomiasis at Khong Island, Southern Laos. *Southeast Asian J. Trop. Med. Public Health* **1976**, *7*, 270–281. [PubMed]

26. Sornmani, S. Current status of schistosomiasis in Laos, Thailand and Malaysia. *Southeast Asian J. Trop. Med. Public Health* **1976**, *7*, 149–154. [PubMed]

27. Hatz, C.; Odermatt, P.; Urbani, C. *Preliminary Data on Morbidity Due to Schistosomiasis mekongi Infections among the Population of Sdau Village, Northestern Cambodia*; Médecins Sans Frontières Suisse: Phnom Penh, Cambodia, 1997.

28. MOH. *National Policy and Strategy for Parasite Control 2009, Ministry of Health, Lao People Democratic Republic, Vientiane Lao PDR*; MOH: Long Beach, CA, USA, 2009.

29. Sayasone, S.; Mak, T.K.; Vanmany, M.; Rasphone, O.; Vounatsou, P.; Utzinger, J.; Akkhavong, K.; Odermatt, P. Helminth and intestinal protozoa infections, multiparasitism and risk factors in Champasack province, Lao People's Democratic Republic. *PLoS Negl. Trop. Dis.* **2011**, *5*, e1037. [CrossRef] [PubMed]

30. WHO. Report on Mass Drug Administration to Control of Schistosomiasis in Lao People's Democratic Republic 2018. Available online: https://www.who.int/neglected_diseases/preventive_chemotherapy/sch/en/ (accessed on 19 January 2019).

31. WHO. *Report on Schistosoma mekongi Paratological Surveillance from Village Sentinel Sites (2016–2018)*; WHO: Geneva, Switzerland, 2018.

32. Strandgaard, H.; Johansen, M.V.; Pholsena, K.; Teixayavong, K.; Christensen, N.O. The pig as a host for *Schistosoma mekongi* in Laos. *J. Parasitol.* **2001**, *87*, 708–709. [CrossRef]

33. Matsuda, H.; Tanaka, H.; Blas, B.L.; Nosenas, J.S.; Tokawa, T.; Ohsawa, S. Evaluation of ELISA with ABTS, 2-2′-azino-di-(3-ethylbenzthiazoline sulfonic acid), as the substrate of peroxidase and its application to the diagnosis of schistosomiasis. *Jpn. J. Exp. Med.* **1984**, *54*, 131–138. [PubMed]

34. Kirinoki, M.; Chigusa, Y.; Ohmae, H.; Sinoun, M.; Socheat, D.; Matsumoto, J.; Kitikoon, V.; Matsuda, H. Efficacy of sodium metaperiodate (SMP)-ELISA for the serodiagnosis of schistosomiasis mekongi. *Southeast Asian J. Trop. Med. Public Health* **2011**, *42*, 25–33. [PubMed]

35. Hatz, C.F. The use of ultrasound in schistosomiasis. *Adv. Parasitol.* **2001**, *48*, 225–284. [PubMed]

36. Keang, H.; Odermatt, P.; Odermatt-Biays, S.; Cheam, S.; Degremont, A.; Hatz, C. Liver morbidity due to *Schistosoma mekongi* in Cambodia after seven rounds of mass drug administration. *Trans. R. Soc. Trop. Med. Hyg.* **2007**, *101*, 759–765. [CrossRef] [PubMed]

37. Katz, N.; Chaves, A.; Pellegrino, J. A simple device for quantitative stool thick-smear technique in schistosomiasis mansoni. *Rev. Inst. Med. Trop. São Paulo* **1972**, *14*, 397–400. [PubMed]

38. Chigusa, Y.; Otake, H.; Kirinoki, M.; Ohmae, H.; Socheat, D.; Sinuon, M. Splenomegaly of *Schistosoma mekongi* infection in Kratie province Cambodia. *Clin. Parasitol.* **2001**, *12*, 63–65.

39. CNM. *National Policy and Guideline for Helminth Control in Cambodia by the National Task Force for the Control of Soil-Transmitted Helminthiasis, Schistosomiasis, and for the Elimination of Lymphatic Filariasis*; CNM: Albuquerque, NM, USA, 2004.

40. Matsumoto, J.; Muth, S.; Socheat, D.; Matsuda, H. The first reported cases of canine schistosomiasis mekongi in Cambodia. *Southeast Asian, J. Trop. Med. Public Health* **2002**, *33*, 458–461.

41. Hisakane, N.; Kirinoki, M.; Chigusa, Y.; Sinuon, M.; Socheat, D.; Matsuda, H.; Ishikawa, H. The evaluation of control measures against *Schistosoma mekongi* in Cambodia by a mathematical model. *Parasitol. Int.* **2008**, *57*, 379–385. [CrossRef] [PubMed]

42. WHO. *Report on National Meeting on Neglected Tropical Disease Control Program*; WHO: Geneva, Switzerland, 2018.

43. WHO. *Action Plan for Schistosomiasis Elimination 2016–2020*; WHO: Geneva, Switzerland, 2016.

44. WHO. Water Safety Planning Will Contribute to the Elimination of Schistosomiasis Worms and Improve Nutrition via a Community-Led Approach in the Province of Champassak. 2016. Available online: http:// www.wpro.who.int/laos/mediacentre/releases/2016/20160524-lao-cl-swash-water-safety/en/ (accessed on 19 January 2019).

45. WHO. *Expert Consultation to Accelerate Elimination of Asian Schistosomiasis, Shanghai, China, 22–23 May 2017, Meeting Report*; 2017 Report Series; RS/2017/GE/36(CHN); WHO: Geneva, Switzerland, 2017.

46. WHO. *Report on National Policy and Strategies on Neglected Tropical Diseases Prevention and Control, May 2018*; WHO: Geneva, Switzerland, 2018.

47. Elkins, D.B.; Sithithaworn, P.; Haswell-Elkins, M.; Kaewkes, S.; Awacharagan, P.; Wongratanacheewin, S. *Opisthorchis viverrini*: Relationships between egg counts, worms recovered and antibody levels within an endemic community in northeast Thailand. *Parasitology* **1991**, *102*, 283–288. [CrossRef] [PubMed]

48. Kirinoki, M.; Ohmae, H.; Chigusa, Y.; Muth, S.; Khieu, V. *Evaluation of the Status of Schistosomiasis Elimination as a Public Health Problem in Cambodia and Development of Monitoring Protocol and Indicators for Interruption of Transmission of Mekong Schistosomiasis*; Technical Report to WPRO; WHO: Geneva, Switzerland, 2016.

49. Bergquist, R.; Johansen, M.V.; Utzinger, J. Diagnostic dilemmas in helminthology: What tools to use and when? *Trends Parasitol.* **2009**, *25*, 151–156. [CrossRef] [PubMed]

50. Lodh, N.; Mikita, K.; Bosompem, K.M.; Anyan, W.K.; Quartey, J.K.; Otchere, J.; Shiff, C.J. Point of care diagnosis of multiple schistosome parasites: Species-specific DNA detection in urine by loop-mediated isothermal amplification (LAMP). *Acta Trop.* **2017**, *173*, 125–129. [CrossRef] [PubMed]

51. He, P.; Gordon, C.A.; Williams, G.M.; Li, Y.; Wang, Y.; Hu, J. Real-time PCR diagnosis of *Schistosoma japonicum* in low transmission areas of China. *Infect. Dis. Poverty* **2018**, *7*, 8. [CrossRef] [PubMed]

52. Hamburger, J.; Abbasi, I.; Kariuki, C.; Wanjala, A.; Mzungu, E.; Mungai, P. Evaluation of loop-mediated isothermal amplification suitable for molecular monitoring of schistosome-infected snails in field laboratories. *Am. J. Trop. Med. Hyg.* **2013**, *88*, 344–351. [CrossRef] [PubMed]

53. Qin, Z.Q.; Xu, J.; Feng, T.; Lv, S.; Qian, Y.J.; Zhang, L.J.; Li, Y.; Lv, C. Field Evaluation of a Loop-Mediated Isothermal Amplification (LAMP) Platform for the Detection of *Schistosoma japonicum* Infection in *Oncomelania hupensis* Snails. *Trop. Med. Infect. Dis.* **2018**, *3*, 124. [CrossRef] [PubMed]

54. Bergquist, R.; van Dam, G.J.; Xu, J. Diagnostic tests for schistosomiasis. In *Schistosoma: Biology, Pathology and Control*; Jamieson, B.G.M., Ed.; CRC Press: Boca Raton, FL, USA, 2016; pp. 401–439.

55. Colley, D.G.; Binder, S.; Campbell, C.; King, C.H.; Tchuem Tchuente, L.A.; N'Goran, E.K.; Erko, B.; Karanja, D.M.; Kabatereine, N.B.; van Lieshout, L.; et al. A five-country evaluation of a point-of-care circulating cathodic antigen urine assay for the prevalence of *Schistosoma mansoni*. *Am. J. Trop. Med. Hyg.* **2013**, *88*, 426–432. [CrossRef] [PubMed]

56. Kittur, N.; Castleman, J.D.; Campbell, C.H., Jr.; King, C.H.; Colley, D.G. Comparison of *Schistosoma mansoni* Prevalence and Intensity of Infection, as Determined by the Circulating Cathodic Antigen Urine Assay or by the Kato-Katz Fecal Assay: A Systematic Review. *Am. J. Trop. Med. Hyg.* **2016**, *94*, 605–610. [CrossRef] [PubMed]

57. Vonghachack, Y.; Sayasone, S.; Khieu, V.; Bergquist, R.; van Dam, G.J.; Hoekstra, P.T.; Corstjens, P.L.A.M.; Nickel, B.; Marti, H.; Utzinger, J.; et al. Comparison of novel and standard diagnostic tools for the detection of *Schistosoma mekongi* infection in Lao People's Democratic Republic and Cambodia. *Infect. Dis. Poverty* **2017**, *6*, 127. [CrossRef] [PubMed]

58.   Malone, J.; Bergquist, R.; Rinaldi, L. Geospatial Surveillance and Repsonse Systems for Schistosomiasis. In *Schistosoma: Biology, Pathology and Control*; Jamieson, B.G.M., Ed.; CRC Press: Boca Raton, FL, USA, 2016; pp. 479–497.

59.   Malone, J.B.; Bergquist, R.; Luvall, J.C. Use of Geospatial Surveillance and Response Systems for Vector-borne Diseases in the Elimination Phase. *Trop. Med. Infect. Dis.* **2019**, *18*, 4. [CrossRef] [PubMed]

60.   Bergquist, R.; Yang, G.J.; Knopp, S.; Utzinger, J.; Tanner, M. Surveillance and response: Tools and approaches for the elimination stage of neglected tropical diseases. *Acta Trop.* **2015**, *141 Pt B*, 229–234. [CrossRef]

61.   Attwood, S.W.; Upatham, E.S. Observations on *Neotricula aperta* (Gastropoda: Pomatiopsidae) population densities in Thailand and central Laos: Implications for the spread of Mekong schistosomiasis. *Parasit. Vectors* **2012**, *5*, 126. [CrossRef] [PubMed]

7

Current Status of the Sm14/GLA-SE Schistosomiasis Vaccine: Overcoming Barriers and Paradigms towards the First Anti-Parasitic Human(itarian) Vaccine

Miriam Tendler *, Marília S. Almeida, Monica M. Vilar, Patrícia M. Pinto and Gabriel Limaverde-Sousa

FIOCRUZ—Instituto Oswaldo Cruz, Laboratório de Esquistossomose Experimental, Av. Brasil, 4365, Manguinhos, Rio de Janeiro 21045-900, Brazil; sirianni@ioc.fiocruz.br (M.S.A.); mvilar@ioc.fiocruz.br (M.M.V.); pmpinto@ioc.fiocruz.br (P.M.P.); gabriel.sousa@ioc.fiocruz.br (G.L.-S.)
* Correspondence: tendlermiriam@gmail.com

Abstract: Schistosomiasis, a disease historically associated with poverty, lack of sanitation and social inequality, is a chronic, debilitating parasitic infection, affecting hundreds of millions of people in endemic countries. Although chemotherapy is capable of reducing morbidity in humans, rapid re-infection demonstrates that the impact of drug treatment on transmission control or disease elimination is marginal. In addition, despite more than two decades of well-executed control activities based on large-scale chemotherapy, the disease is expanding in many areas including Brazil. The development of the Sm14/GLA-SE schistosomiasis vaccine is an emblematic, open knowledge innovation that has successfully completed phase I and phase IIa clinical trials, with Phase II/III trials underway in the African continent, to be followed by further trials in Brazil. The discovery and experimental phases of the development of this vaccine gathered a robust collection of data that strongly supports the ongoing clinical phase. This paper reviews the development of the Sm14 vaccine, formulated with glucopyranosyl lipid A (GLA-SE), from the initial experimental developments to clinical trials including the current status of phase II studies.

Keywords: schistosomiasis; vaccine; Sm14; FABP

1. Introduction

Schistosomiasis is the second-most socioeconomically devastating parasitic disease after malaria. The disease is both chronic and debilitating with an estimated 200 million people infected, most of whom (85%) live in Africa. Of those infected, 120 million are symptomatic and 20 million present severe disease symptoms [1]. These estimates may err on the low side since meta-analysis has found the number of people at risk to be closer to 800 million [2]. Globally, the impact of schistosomiasis remains high and the estimated number of disability-adjusted life years (DALYs) has increased with the inclusion of previously under-recognized morbidities not previously included in the DALY index (for example, stunted growth and anemia associated with retarded intellectual development) in infants, toddlers and school age children, whose physical health and intellectual capacity are fundamental to nation development and sustainability [3,4]. In addition, high-definition circulating antigen tests, such as the POC-CCA assay, indicate that the current number of infections may be at least 10 times higher than that shown by egg detection [5]. In Brazil, the largest endemic country for schistosomiasis, 6 million individuals are estimated to be infected and 25 million are at risk of contracting the disease [6,7].

Mass chemotherapy has been the strategy of choice for the control schistosomiasis with the support of international health funding agencies. Estimates show that at least 206.5 million people were treated in 2016 [8]. However, the strategy of large-scale chemotherapeutic treatment, also equivocally called 'prophylactic treatment', over a period of 30 years has failed to control schistosome transmission. Approximately 300 million US dollars are being spent annually on treatments applied to the same populations year after year with no prospect of preventing reinfection or the need for repeat treatments [9]. 'Deworming' initiatives, originally applied to animal species only, were proposed as a tool for schistosomiasis control programs focused on school children in endemic countries [10,11].

In the veterinary field, under One Health policies for the control of helminth infections such as *Fasciola hepatica*, the major parasitic infection of livestock worldwide, there is a strong demand for the replacement of anti-helminthic drugs with vaccines. This would significantly reduce the amount of chemical residues in meat, milk and added-value products. Indeed, vaccines are considered to be the most environmentally- and human health-friendly method of control of fascioliasis in livestock [12].

The potential introduction of vaccines into schistosomiasis control programs brings hope to the poor living in endemic areas. The Brazilian Sm14 vaccine project was launched in the 1990s and strongly pushed in the context of a formal WHO program aimed at the development of an anti-schistosomiasis vaccine. The main outcome of this initiative was the selection of six priority antigen candidates of which only Sm14, continues to be developed (Table 1, adapted from [13]).

With strategic support from WHO, the Sm14 vaccine, which is based on a recombinant protein, is moving forward in an endemic country towards final development. It is being developed utilizing sophisticated and modern technological platforms and professionally conducted within a network of outstanding companies and collaborators. It is the result of long-term scientific developments carried under the coordination of FIOCRUZ, a public institution linked to the Brazilian Ministry of Health and is protected by strong patents, owned by FIOCRUZ, in all countries of interest worldwide.

Recently, the Consultative Expert Working Group on Research and Development: Financing and Coordination (CEWG/WHO) selected the Sm14 vaccine as one of six demonstration projects, globally, following an extensive review process. It was recognized as being fully in accordance with the principles of CEWG, such as clear mechanisms of de-linkage of costs from investments in research and development (R&D) from costs of final product, accessibility, affordability, viability and open knowledge innovation. The CEWG recognized that the Sm14 vaccine may become a key tool for the implementation of effective infection reduction and transmission control programs for schistosomiasis that would not rely only on chemotherapy [14].

Over recent years it has been possible to complete important milestones in the development of the vaccine including scaling up production process from laboratory bench to a clinical trial scale as well as the successful conclusion of two phase I human trials in healthy adults (male and female) living in a Brazilian non-endemic area (2011–2014) [15] together with a first phase II trial in 30 male adults living in highly endemic area for both *Schistosoma mansoni* and *S. haematobium* at the Senegal River Basin (2015–2017). In the latter, safety was extensively confirmed and strong and long-lasting immunogenicity was also demonstrated (manuscript in preparation). Master cell bank generation has recently been completed and production in good manufacturing practices (GMP) of a second Sm14 lot is currently ongoing, under the coordination of the Infectious Disease Research Institute (IDRI, Seattle, US). This article is an overview of the development of the Sm14 schistosomiasis vaccine development from antigen discovery to the current human studies (Figure 1). The need to overcome barriers for the establishment of a truly humanitarian vaccine—addressing the needs of the developing world—will be discussed.

Table 1. Schistosomiasis priority antigens selected by the WHO for independent testing (adapted from [13]).

Antigen	Size (kDa)	Stage Expressed	Description	Protection (%)	Place of Development
Glutathione S-transferase (P28/GST)	28	Adult/somula/egg	Enzyme	30–60	Institut Pasteur, Lille, France
Paramyosin (Sm97)	97	Adult/somula	Muscle protein	30	Case Western Reserve University/National Institute of Health/Cornell University, USA
IrV-5	62	Adult/somula/egg	Muscle protein	50–70	Johns Hopkins School of Medicine, Baltimore, USA
Triose phosphate isomerase (TPI)	28	Adult/somula/egg	Enzyme	30–60	Harvard School of Public Health, Boston, USA
Sm23	23	Adult/somula/egg	Integrated membrane protein	40–50	Johns Hopkins School of Medicine/Harvard School of Public Health, USA
Sm14	14	Adult/somula	Fatty acid-binding protein	65	Instituto Oswaldo Cruz, Rio de Janeiro, Brazil

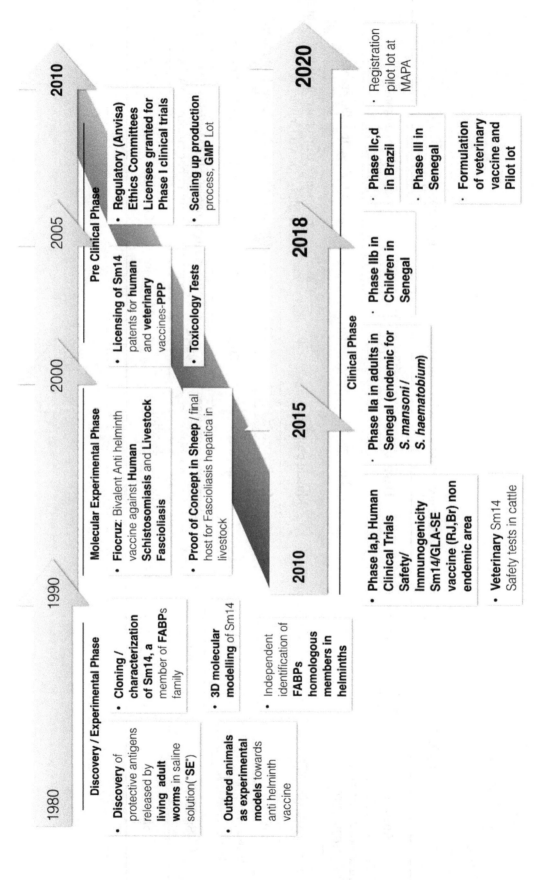

Figure 1. Timeline: Sm14/GLA-SE anti-schistosomiasis vaccine - from discovery phase to final product. MAPA: Brazilian Ministry of Agriculture.

2. Innovative Strategies Adopted for Antigen Discovery and Early Development Phases

Biotechnological advances in various areas of vaccine research have contributed to the development of safer and more effective formulations. Efforts to develop anti-helminth vaccines have been ongoing for many years and are continuing to progress in the identification of candidate antigens. These efforts have recently been boosted by the generation of a number of helminth genome sequences [16]. The development of a vaccine against schistosomiasis would represent an important step in the context of research and development in public health for poor populations infected and exposed to schistosomes. There have been initiatives to develop a vaccine against schistosomiasis from research groups in different countries. The Brazilian Sm14-based anti-schistosomiasis vaccine is the only one of these initiatives that is currently undergoing clinical trials [17].

In contrast to the current 'OMICS' strategies, in which high-throughput screening of potential target antigens are processed in parallel by automated 'discovery protocols and platforms', the Sm14 project was initiated by gathering observations from animal models of infection together with logical progression based on experimental evidence.

The first original approach was in the methodology for generating a worm extract that was subsequently used to assess protective immunity. Rather than lyophilized parasites, generally used by other research groups, a saline extract containing secreted/excreted antigens derived from living adult schistosomes was utilized for initial immunizations. The restricted number of potential protective antigens released in this saline extract allowed an accelerated identification of strong antigen candidates for molecular analysis and gene cloning [18–22]. Innovative methods were also adopted for the assessment of immunity, where the use of outbred models, in contrast to the commonly-employed inbred animals, allowed a better representation of the ultimate target population and provided a unique opportunity to develop an alternative strategy for the assessment of protective immunity. The analyses were stratified based on the measurement of frequencies of worm burdens within vaccinated animal populations as compared with non-vaccinated infected controls, as opposed to evaluation of mean values of parasite loads, as usually adopted. A solid base of pre-clinical data was generated establishing the immunization protocols that would be adopted during the following steps of the development [23–31].

As molecular biology tools evolved and gene-cloning techniques became available, several antigens released in the saline culture medium of live schistosomes, were cloned and sequenced. Serum from rabbits immunized with the 'saline extract' was used to screen an adult *S. mansoni* cDNA library and the most promising antigen was identified as a member of the fatty acid binding protein (FABP) family, termed Sm14 [32]. Molecular modeling studies from our group predicted the beta-barrel structure of the Sm14 [33] that was later experimentally confirmed by crystallography [34] and nuclear magnetic resonance [35]. These analyses allowed the engineering of a stabilizing mutation that conferred a remarkable long-term stability, while maintaining the function and immunogenicity of the antigen [36].

Sm14 was shown to be particularly important to helminths, which are not capable of synthetizing fatty acids but rely on these being provided by the host species. Lipids, apart from being constituents of membranes, have important roles in development of different lifecycle stages and the evasion of immune responses both by adult worms and larvae [37]. In addition to the publication describing the a FABP family member in *Schistosoma mansoni* [32], different groups published the identification of homologous FABP protein members from FABP family in many helminths of human and veterinary importance. Of particular importance was the identification of the *F. hepatica* FABP [38]. *F. hepatica* is the main parasite of livestock worldwide. We have managed to successfully test Sm14 vaccination against *F. hepatica* in mice, followed by two independent experiments in sheep, one of the definitive host species for fascioliasis [39]. These experiments that demonstrated that Sm14 is also protective against *F. hepatica* infection has led to Sm14 being developed in parallel as the molecular basis for a veterinary vaccine by FIOCRUZ, in collaboration with the private Brazilian company Ourofino Animal Health.

3. Clinical Studies

The licensing of the Sm14 patents for veterinary use gave birth to a public–private partnership (PPP) model of product development that rendered significant visibility to the Sm14 vaccine project. Such a gain in momentum was followed by strong support for human vaccine development by the Brazilian government project financing agency (FINEP) that allowed the use of contract research organizations (CROs) for antigen production, quality control and fill-finish in world-class academic GMP facilities based in the United States of America in collaboration with the Ludwig Institute for Cancer Research, Cornell University and the Infectious Disease Research Institute (IDRI, Seattle, USA).

In order to have a consistent, stable and defined final product for clinical human use, the Sm14 antigen was formulated with the synthetic adjuvant glucopyranosyl lipid A (GLA-SE), an adjuvant successfully tested in clinical trials with different human vaccine candidates.

In December of 2010, the Brazilian Health Regulatory Agency (ANVISA) approved a phase Ia clinical trial in 20 healthy male volunteers from a non-endemic area (Rio de Janeiro, Brazil) to evaluate the safety of the investigational product. The study was conducted by the Brazilian National Institute of Infectious Diseases (INI/FIOCRUZ). The results of this first trial demonstrated the safety of the vaccine in the studied population, showing no systemic reactogenicity. No serious adverse events were associated to the investigational product [15]. A phase Ib clinical study, to evaluate the safety and immunogenicity of the vaccine preparation in 10 healthy women volunteers, was also then successfully concluded in 2012 (manuscript in preparation).

In 2015–2016, within the scope of a CEWG Demonstration Project, a phase IIa trial was developed in 30 male adults living in a highly endemic area for both *S. mansoni* and *S. haematobium* in the Senegal River Basin. The trial was conducted by a specialized team from Espoir Pour La Santé (EPLS), linked to the Pasteur Institute of Lille (IPL, France), headed by Dr. Gilles Riveau (IPL) in conjunction with the FIOCRUZ group and the Brazilian biotechnology company Orygen Biotecnologia the license holder of Sm14 for human use (ClinicalTrials.gov Identifier: NCT03041766) [40]. The main objectives of the trial were safety and immunogenicity of the Sm14/GLA-SE vaccine. These objectives were fully achieved. The investigational product rSm14 (50 µg) formulated with GLA-SE in two dosages (2.5 µg and 5 µg/dose, denominated groups 1 and 2, respectively) and administered intramuscular (IM), was shown to be safe with no observed serious adverse events in either group. The most common reactions were local pain and heaviness of the vaccinated arm. These reactions were transitory and mild. Seroconversion of 92% of individuals after the second dose were observed, similar to the pattern observed in the phase I trials [15]. Immunogenicity based on additional cellular responses, memory cells and T cell activation markers were analyzed at IDRI in an extensive panel focusing on the identification of a vaccine-related immune response.

After the completion of the phase IIa trial and based on the observed induction of a strong and long-lasting immune response, an extension study to assess the possible persistence and profile of this response beyond the initial schedule of the trial was duly authorized by Senegalese Ministry of Health (MoH). This was carried out between August and December 2017 with the inclusion of two additional time points, 9 and 12 months, after the first vaccine injection. ELISA tests performed at Centre de Recherche Biomédicale/Espoir Pour La Santé (EPLS) showed the persistence of significant specific antibody titers up to 12 months after the first vaccination dose with Sm14/GLA-SE (manuscript in preparation).

A phase IIb trial design and protocol were defined in January 2018, based on the results of the phase IIa trial in adults. The phase IIb trial will involve 95 school children from 7–11 years of age living in the same endemic area for both *S. mansoni* and *S. hamatobium* of the Senegal River Basin region. Ethical committee approval and regulatory approval from the Senegalese MoH have been obtained. EPLS has already initiated the trial in the same region as the original phase IIa trial in adults, using the same lot of GMP Sm14 under a regimen of three IM doses of 50 µg/dose formulated with 2.5 µg of GLA-SE, 30 days apart. The phase IIa and b trials are largely funded by Orygen Biotecnologia in conjunction with FIOCRUZ and with support of CEWG-WHO platform and financial fund.

4. Sm14 +GLA-SE: A Humanitarian Anti-Schistosomiasis Vaccine

During the process of analysis by WHO member state representatives, within a regional structure, and extensive subsequent analysis by technical experts and ad hoc committees, the Sm14 schistosomiasis vaccine, was selected by the WHO Executive Board as one of the current list of six demonstration projects. A stakeholders meeting organized by WHO at its Geneva headquarters was held in June 2015 prior to the release of the first installment of funding. During the process of selection and shortlisting of the candidate demonstration projects presented projects, discussions on the scientific merits, state of the art of the project and requirement for full adherence to CEWG principles, much was learned concerning the mandatory need to assure the accessibility and affordability of this vaccine to the poor endemic countries in which it will ultimately be used [14].

From its inception, the Sm14 schistosomiasis vaccine has been designed to be both effective and low-cost. To achieve this goal, several innovations for vaccine development were implemented and a strong effort was made to choose intellectual property-free components [36]. This has led to the successful development of a very low-cost, stable product involving a large-scale production process.

De-linkage of final product price from the costs of the long R&D phases has been achieved by Sm14 being initially developed at a governmental scientific foundation (FIOCRUZ) with support from funds from public Brazilian financial institutions (FINEP and FAPERJ).

After 2005, licensing of FIOCRUZ patent rights for human use to a private Brazilian company was through contracts designed to protect the accessibility, affordability and supply strategies for the lower- and middle-income countries (LMIC) that are the target areas to receive the anti-schistosomiasis vaccine. The presently licensee company, Orygen Biotecnologia, is a startup company wholly owned by two of the largest Brazilian pharmaceutical companies. Its involvement in the final development of the Sm14 human vaccine is crucial. The company has agreed to a cost plus pricing strategy, as adopted by WHO for vaccine pricing [41].

In parallel, the veterinary anti-fasciola vaccine is being developed in keeping with current European guidelines to reduce the presence of anti-helminthic drug chemical residues in milk and meat of livestock. It is aimed at rich countries and markets and designed to contribute/support future potential large-scale delivery programs.

We are no longer at a stage when an anti-schistosomiasis vaccine is to be discussed, attacked or delayed, as it was for decades along with all anti-parasite vaccines. Our knowledge concerning vaccines has improved enormously, as have the technical resources available. Vaccines represent the intervention strategy with the best cost–benefit ratio thus far applied in public health. Moreover, transmission control of infectious/transmissible diseases has only been achieved through vaccination. Sanitation, chemotherapy and health education are not sufficient to eliminate parasitic diseases that disproportionally affect people living in poor countries. Immunization with a safe and effective vaccine can contribute to a long-term reduction of schistosome egg excretion from the host, thus truly controlling transmission. So far, there are no vaccines against the parasites that afflict countries fighting to emerge from poverty and reach better conditions of health and overall development.

The Sm14 vaccine against schistosomiasis is being developed as a humanitarian vaccine to be included in effective schistosomiasis transmission control programs that will hopefully invert the paradigm for a north-to-south route for technology generation and contribute to the broad use of the most safe, effective and environmentally and human-friendly health-promoting strategy, prophylactic vaccination.

Acknowledgments: The authors would like to thank Steven Reed, Rhea Coler, Tracey Day, Anna Marie Beckman and IDRI team for immunogenicity tests and stability tests on Sm14 GMP lot; Orygen Biotechnologia technical team; Marcia Ciol, statistician from WA University; Gilles Riveau and Anne-Marie Schacht from EPLS/IPL; Tatiane dos Santos, FIOCRUZ—Instituto Oswaldo Cruz, Laboratório de Esquistossomose Experimental, for part of immunology tests.

References

1.   Chitsulo, L.; Engels, D.; Montresor, A.; Savioli, L. The global status of schistosomiasis and its control. *Acta Trop.* **2000**, *77*, 41–51. [CrossRef]

2.   Steinmann, P.; Keiser, J.; Bos, R.; Tanner, M.; Utzinger, J. Schistosomiasis and water resources development: Systematic review, meta-analysis, and estimates of people at risk. *Lancet Infect. Dis.* **2006**, *6*, 411–425. [CrossRef]

3.   Osakunor, D.N.M.; Woolhouse, M.E.J.; Mutapi, F. Paediatric schistosomiasis: What we know and what we need to know. *PLoS Negl. Trop. Dis.* **2018**, *12*, e0006144. [CrossRef] [PubMed]

4.   Poole, H.; Terlouw, D.J.; Naunje, A.; Mzembe, K.; Stanton, M.; Betson, M.; Lalloo, D.G.; Stothard, J.R. Schistosomiasis in pre-school-age children and their mothers in Chikhwawa district, Malawi with notes on characterization of schistosomes and snails. *Parasit. Vectors* **2014**, *7*, 153. [CrossRef] [PubMed]

5.   Bergquist, R.; van Dam, G.J.; Xu, J. Diagnostic tests for schistosomiasis. In *Schistosoma: Biology, Pathology and Control*, 1st ed.; Jamieson, B.G.M., Ed.; CRC Press: Boca Raton, FL, USA, 2016; pp. 401–439.

6.   Coura, J.R.; Amaral, R.S. Epidemiological and control aspects of schistosomiasis in Brazilian endemic areas. *Mem. Inst. Oswaldo Cruz* **2004**, *99*, 13–19. [CrossRef] [PubMed]

7.   Barbosa, C.S.; Araújo, K.C.; Antunes, L.; Favre, T.; Pieri, O.S. Spatial distribution of schistosomiasis foci on Itamaracá Island, Pernambuco, Brazil. *Mem. Inst. Oswaldo Cruz* **2004**, *99*, 79–83. [CrossRef] [PubMed]

8.   Schistosomiasis. Available online: http://www.who.int/news-room/fact-sheets/detail/schistosomiasis (accessed on 14 September 2018).

9.   Ahuja, A.; Baird, S.; Hicks, J.H.; Kremer, M.; Miguel, E. Economics of Mass Deworming Programs. In *Child and Adolescent Health and Development*; Bundy, D.A.P., de Silva, N., Horton, S., Jamison, D.T., Patton, G.C., Eds.; The International Bank for Reconstruction and Development/The World Bank: Washington, DC, USA, 2017; ISBN 978-1-4648-0423-6.

10.   Guidelines for School-Based Deworming Programs. Available online: https://www.globalpartnership.org/content/guidelines-school-based-deworming-programs (accessed on 5 September 2018).

11.   WHO School Deworming at a Glance. Available online: http://www.who.int/intestinal_worms/resources/joint_statement_WHO_World_Bank/en/ (accessed on 25 September 2018).

12.   Molina-Hernández, V.; Mulcahy, G.; Pérez, J.; Martínez-Moreno, Á.; Donnelly, S.; O'Neill, S.M.; Dalton, J.P.; Cwiklinski, K. *Fasciola hepatica* vaccine: We may not be there yet but we're on the right road. *Vet. Parasitol.* **2015**, *208*, 101–111. [CrossRef] [PubMed]

13.   Bergquist, N.R.; Colley, D.G. Schistosomiasis vaccine: Research to development. *Parasitol. Today* **1998**, *14*, 99–104. [CrossRef]

14.   WHO CEWG Demonstration Projects: Background and Process. Available online: http://www.who.int/phi/implementation/cewg_background_process/en/ (accessed on 25 September 2018).

15.   Santini-Oliveira, M.; Coler, R.N.; Parra, J.; Veloso, V.; Jayashankar, L.; Pinto, P.M.; Ciol, M.A.; Bergquist, R.; Reed, S.G.; Tendler, M. Schistosomiasis vaccine candidate Sm14/GLA-SE: Phase 1 safety and immunogenicity clinical trial in healthy, male adults. *Vaccine* **2016**, *34*, 586–594. [CrossRef] [PubMed]

16.   Lustigman, S.; Geldhof, P.; Grant, W.N.; Osei-Atweneboana, M.Y.; Sripa, B.; Basáñez, M.-G. A research agenda for helminth diseases of humans: Basic research and enabling technologies to support control and elimination of helminthiases. *PLoS Negl. Trop. Dis.* **2012**, *6*, e1445. [CrossRef] [PubMed]

17.   Tendler, M.; Almeida, M.; Simpson, A. Development of the Brazilian anti-schistosomiasis vaccine based on the recombinant fatty acid binding protein Sm14 plus GLA-SE adjuvant. *Front. Immunol.* **2015**, *6*. [CrossRef] [PubMed]

18.   Scapin, M.; Tendler, M. Immunoprecipitins in human schistosomiasis detected with adult worm antigens released by 3M KCl. *J. Helminthol.* **1977**, *51*, 71–72. [CrossRef] [PubMed]

19. Tendler, M.; Scapin, M. The presence of *Schistosoma mansoni* antigens in solutions used for storing adult worms. *Rev. Inst. Med. Trop. Sao Paulo* **1979**, *21*, 293–296. [PubMed]

20. Scarpin, M.; Tendler, M.; Messineo, L.; Katz, N. Preliminary studies with a *Schistosoma mansoni* saline extract inducing protection in rabbits against the challenge infection. *Rev. Inst. Med. Trop. Sao Paulo* **1980**, *22*, 164–172. [PubMed]

21. Tendler, M.; Scapin, M.; Tendler, M.; Scapin, M. *Schistosoma mansoni* antigenic extracts obtained by different extraction procedures. *Mem. Inst. Oswaldo Cruz* **1981**, *76*, 103–109. [CrossRef] [PubMed]

22. Tendler, M.; Lima, A.O.; Pinto, R.M.; Cruz, M.Q.; Brascher, H.M.; Katz, N.; Tendler, M.; Lima, A.O.; Pinto, R.M.; Cruz, M.Q.; et al. Immunogenetic and protective activity of an extract of *Schistosoma mansoni*. *Mem. Inst. Oswaldo Cruz* **1982**, *77*, 275–283. [CrossRef] [PubMed]

23. Tendler, M.; Pinto, R.M.; Bambirra, E.A.; Cruz, M.Q.; Lima, A.O.; Tendler, M.; Pinto, R.M.; Bambirra, E.A.; Cruz, M.Q.; Lima, A.O. Acquired resistance of mice against *S. mansoni* and lung granulomatous reaction induced by BCG. *Mem. Inst. Oswaldo Cruz* **1983**, *78*, 147–151. [CrossRef] [PubMed]

24. Tendler, M.; Magalhães Pinto, R.; Côrtes, M.; Gebara, G. *Schistosoma mansoni*: Comparative evaluation of different routes of experimental infection. *Rev. Inst. Med. Trop. São Paulo* **1985**, *27*, 111–114. [CrossRef] [PubMed]

25. Tendler, M.; Pinto, R.M.; Lima, A.O.; Gebara, G.; Katz, N. *Schistosoma mansoni*: Vaccination with adult worm antigens. *Int. J. Parasitol.* **1986**, *16*, 347–352. [CrossRef]

26. Tendler, M. *Schistosoma mansoni*: Protective antigens. *Mem. Inst. Oswaldo Cruz* **1987**, *82*, 125–128. [CrossRef] [PubMed]

27. Almeida, M.S.S.; Pinto, R.M.; Noronha, D.; Tendler, M.; Katz, N.; Almeida, M.S.S.; Pinto, R.M.; Noronha, D.; Tendler, M.; Katz, N. *Schistosoma mansoni*—NZ rabbit-model: Resistance due to infection and active immunization with adult worm antigen. *Mem. Inst. Oswaldo Cruz* **1987**, *82*, 233. [CrossRef] [PubMed]

28. Almeida, M.S.; Pinto, R.M.; Noronha, D.; Katz, N.; Tendler, M. Curative and protective activity in rabbits after reinfection with *Schistosoma mansoni*: A new model of immunity? *J. Parasitol.* **1989**, *75*, 308–310. [CrossRef] [PubMed]

29. Tendler, M.; Almeida, M.S.; Pinto, R.M.; Noronha, D.; Katz, N. *Schistosoma mansoni*-New Zealand rabbit model: Resistance induced by infection followed by active immunization with protective antigens. *J. Parasitol.* **1991**, *77*, 138–141. [CrossRef] [PubMed]

30. Tendler, M.; Pinto, R.M.; de Oliveira Lima, A.; Savino, W.; Katz, N. Vaccination in murine schistosomiasis with adult worm-derived antigens: Variables influencing protection in outbred mice. *Int. J. Parasitol.* **1991**, *21*, 299–306. [CrossRef]

31. Tendler, M.; Pinto, R.M.; de Oliveira Lima, A.; Savino, W.; Katz, N. Vaccination in murine schistosomiasis with adult worm derived antigens—II. Protective and immune response in inbred mice. *Mem. Inst. Oswaldo Cruz* **1992**, *87*, 281–286. [CrossRef] [PubMed]

32. Moser, D.; Tendler, M.; Griffiths, G.; Klinkert, M.Q. A 14-kDa *Schistosoma mansoni* polypeptide is homologous to a gene family of fatty acid binding proteins. *J. Biol. Chem.* **1991**, *266*, 8447–8454. [PubMed]

33. Tendler, M.; Brito, C.A.; Vilar, M.M.; Serra-Freire, N.; Diogo, C.M.; Almeida, M.S.; Delbem, A.C.; Silva, J.F.D.; Savino, W.; Garratt, R.C.; et al. A *Schistosoma mansoni* fatty acid-binding protein, Sm14, is the potential basis of a dual-purpose anti-helminth vaccine. *Proc. Natl. Acad. Sci. USA* **1996**, *93*, 269–273. [CrossRef] [PubMed]

34. Angelucci, F.; Johnson, K.A.; Baiocco, P.; Miele, A.E.; Brunori, M.; Valle, C.; Vigorosi, F.; Troiani, A.R.; Liberti, P.; Cioli, D.; et al. *Schistosoma mansoni* fatty acid binding protein: Specificity and functional control as revealed by crystallographic structure. *Biochemistry* **2004**, *43*, 13000–13011. [CrossRef] [PubMed]

35. Pertinhez, T.A.; Sforça, M.L.; Alves, A.C.; Ramos, C.R.R.; Ho, P.L.; Tendler, M.; Zanchin, N.I.T.; Spisni, A. Letter to the Editor: 1H, 15N and 13C resonance assignments of the apo Sm14-M20(C62V) protein, a mutant of *Schistosoma mansoni* Sm14. *J. Biomol. NMR* **2004**, *29*, 553–554. [CrossRef] [PubMed]

36. Ramos, C.R.R.; Spisni, A.; Oyama, S.; Sforça, M.L.; Ramos, H.R.; Vilar, M.M.; Alves, A.C.; Figueredo, R.C.R.; Tendler, M.; Zanchin, N.I.T.; et al. Stability improvement of the fatty acid binding protein Sm14 from *S. mansoni* by Cys replacement: Structural and functional characterization of a vaccine candidate. *Biochim. Biophys. Acta BBA-Proteins Proteom.* **2009**, *1794*, 655–662. [CrossRef] [PubMed]

37. Giera, M.; Kaisar, M.M.M.; Derks, R.J.E.; Steenvoorden, E.; Kruize, Y.C.M.; Hokke, C.H.; Yazdanbakhsh, M.; Everts, B. The *Schistosoma mansoni* lipidome: Leads for immunomodulation. *Anal. Chim. Acta* **2018**, *1037*, 107–118. [CrossRef] [PubMed]

38.   Rodríguez-Pérez, J.; Rodríguez-Medina, J.R.; García-Blanco, M.A.; Hillyer, G.V. *Fasciola hepatica*: Molecular cloning, nucleotide sequence, and expression of a gene encoding a polypeptide homologous to a *Schistosoma mansoni* fatty acid-binding protein. *Exp. Parasitol.* **1992**, *74*, 400–407. [CrossRef]

39.   Almeida, M.S.; Torloni, H.; Lee-Ho, P.; Vilar, M.M.; Thaumaturgo, N.; Simpson, A.J.G.; Tendler, M. Vaccination against *Fasciola hepatica* infection using a *Schistosoma mansoni* defined recombinant antigen, Sm14. *Parasite Immunol.* **2003**, *25*, 135–137. [CrossRef] [PubMed]

40.   Study of Safety and Immune Response of the Sm14 Vaccine in Adults of Endemic Regions. Available online: https://clinicaltrials.gov/ct2/show/NCT03041766 (accessed on 17 September 2018).

41.   *WHO Guideline on Country Pharmaceutical Pricing Policies*; WHO Guidelines Approved by the Guidelines Review Committee; World Health Organization: Geneva, Switzerland, 2013.

8

DNA Diagnostics for Schistosomiasis Control

Kosala G. Weerakoon [1,2,3,*], **Catherine A. Gordon** [1] and **Donald P. McManus** [1,*]

[1]   Molecular Parasitology Laboratory, Infectious Diseases Division, QIMR Berghofer Medical Research Institute, Brisbane 4006, Australia; Catherine.Gordon@qimrberghofer.edu.au

[2]   School of Public Health, University of Queensland, Brisbane 4006, Australia

[3]   Department of Parasitology, Faculty of Medicine and Allied Sciences, Rajarata University of Sri Lanka, Saliyapura 50008, Sri Lanka

*   Correspondence: kosala.weerakoon@qimrberghofer.edu.au (K.G.W.); Don.McManus@qimrberghofer.edu.au (D.P.M.)

Abstract: Despite extensive efforts over the last few decades, the global disease burden of schistosomiasis still remains unacceptably high. This could partly be attributed to the lack of accurate diagnostic tools for detecting human and animal schistosome infections in endemic areas. In low transmission and low prevalence areas where schistosomiasis elimination is targeted, case detection requires a test that is highly sensitive. Diagnostic tests with low sensitivity will miss individuals with low infection intensity and these will continue to contribute to transmission, thereby interfering with the efficacy of the control measures operating. Of the many diagnostic approaches undertaken to date, the detection of schistosome DNA using DNA amplification techniques including polymerase chain reaction (PCR) provide valuable adjuncts to more conventional microscopic and serological methods, due their accuracy, high sensitivity, and the capacity to detect early pre-patent infections. Furthermore, DNA-based methods represent important screening tools, particularly in those endemic areas with ongoing control where infection prevalence and intensity have been reduced to very low levels. Here we review the role of DNA diagnostics in the path towards the control and elimination of schistosomiasis.

Keywords: schistosomiasis; diagnosis; control and elimination; DNA; polymerase chain reaction

1. Introduction

The public health and socioeconomic impact of schistosomiasis is such that, to date, over 230 million people have acquired the disease, including many children, mainly in the tropics and subtropics. Further, this chronic debilitating disease leads to around 11,500 deaths a year and it is responsible for the loss of over 3.5 million DALYs, the majority (more than 80%) from sub-Saharan Africa [1,2]. The major schistosome species that cause infection in humans include *S. haematobium*, the agent of urinary schistosomiasis, and *S. mansoni, S. japonicum, S. mekongi, S. intercalatum* and *S. guineensis*, which cause intestinal schistosomiasis. These blood-feeding flukes are responsible for substantial long-term clinical complications with multiple organ involvement including the liver, intestine, and urinary bladder. Infective cercariae in fresh water sources penetrate the host skin and enter the blood circulation as schistosomules and inhabit mesenteric or vesical (intestinal and urinary schistosomiasis respectively) venous plexuses after pulmonary and hepatic migrations. Mature female worms lay eggs in these sites, and eggs then penetrate the intestinal walls (in intestinal schistosomiasis) to be excreted in stool or penetrate the bladder wall (in urinary schistosomiasis) to be excreted in urine while some of the eggs migrate towards ectopic sites such as the liver and other organs, leading to chronic inflammation and fibrosis. The eggs released to the environment hatch in fresh water sources releasing miracidia that penetrate specific snail hosts within which they undergo asexual reproduction and become cercariae to continue the life cycle.

Successful disease prevention and elimination programs for schistosomiasis involve the implementation of intensive intervention and efficient monitoring measures, with different countries having their own modified approaches tailored to the sociocultural and economic situations prevailing [3–5]. For example, in China the number of human schistosomiasis cases was reduced by 90% over the decade from 2004 through human case detection and treatment, health education and snail control [6]. Additionally, China has had a strong political will for many decades to eliminate schistosomiasis, since control options were first instigated by Chairman Mao in 1956, who made its elimination a national health priority [7]. In general, accurate community diagnosis of the infection and continued surveillance is helpful in the control of transmission of schistosomiasis, while prompt treatment following early detection can minimize the associated morbidity and mortality [8,9]. With continuing multiple prevention and control efforts, the prevalence and intensity of schistosomiasis in many endemic regions have gone down, so that in many infected individuals, the disease may go undetected with commonly-used conventional diagnostic tools such as the Kato-Katz fecal smear (KK) test or urine egg filtration methods, due to their low sensitivity [10–13]. As a result, a schistosomiasis-endemic area may appear to be free of the disease infection whereas in reality transmission continues and may even spread to other communities, thereby increasing the time for control and eventual elimination. A recent World Health Organization (WHO) expert committee report [12] highlighted the significance of a One Health approach focusing on preventive chemotherapy, improvement of water, sanitation and hygiene (WASH), health promotion, snail control, and detection and treatment of animal reservoirs for the sustained control and elimination of Asian schistosomiasis [12]. This further emphasizes the importance and essential need for accurate diagnostics, if the target goals of transmission interruption by 2025 and elimination of transmission by 2030 are to be achieved.

2. A General Overview of Diagnostics for Schistosomiasis

Procedures that have been commonly applied in schistosomiasis diagnosis include conventional microscopy-based tests, different antibody-based serological assays, parasite antigen detection assays and DNA detection methods including polymerase chain reaction (PCR)-based procedures (Figure 1). As considered earlier, the KK and microscopy-based egg detection in urine have the major drawbacks of low sensitivity and can be labor intensive [14–17]. Antibody detection assays also have low diagnostic accuracy, particularly in terms of test specificity, as well as being unable to distinguish between past and current infections [16]. Recent improvements in circulating parasite antigen detection assays have resulted in relatively higher accuracy in comparison with microscopic and antibody detection methods but frequent fluctuations in assay replicates have suggested the need for multiple testing to improve diagnostic accuracy [18,19].

Furthermore, the circulating antigen (circulating anodic antigen (CAA) and circulating cathodic antigen (CCA))-based assays are not currently applicable for all schistosome species. The CCA-based assay is used as a point of care test to diagnose *S. mansoni* but does not work for *S. haematobium* [20]. CAA-based lateral flow assays combined with up-converting phosphor reporter technology, work for both *S. mansoni* and *S. haematobium*. However, they have not as yet proven as effective with other schistosome species [20–22]. As a result, DNA, especially PCR-based parasite DNA detection assays, have stimulated much interest as alternative options due to their proven diagnostic accuracy, higher sensitivity, and wider range of applicability, including the ability to detect early pre-patent infections. Here we review the different DNA detection methods that have been employed in the diagnosis of human and animal schistosomiasis, discuss their application in control programs and consider their value in surveillance leading to elimination goals.

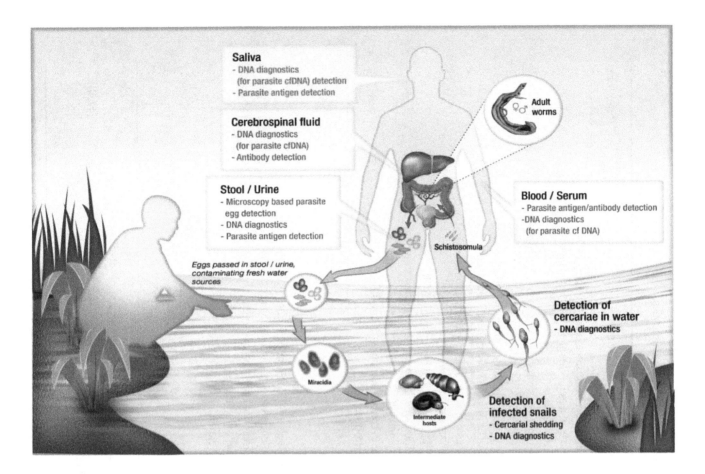

Figure 1. Applicability of diagnostic tools for the detection of different lifecycle stages of schistosomes.

3. DNA-Based Diagnostics for Schistosomiasis

Technological advances and the substantial genomic data now available for schistosomes [23–25] have opened up new avenues for the development of novel diagnostics as well as identifying new therapeutic and vaccine targets. Recent advances in DNA amplification assays include the application of real-time quantitative PCR (qPCR) and droplet digital PCR (ddPCR) for the detection of circulating cell-free parasite DNA using different clinical samples and the development of isothermal amplification assays such as loop-mediated isothermal amplification (LAMP) and recombinase polymerase amplification (RPA) techniques [26–29]. Measures of accuracy including diagnostic sensitivity and specificity of DNA detection assays vary depending on the type of the assay, target gene sequence used, as well as the type of sample tested [30]. Some of the key advantages and limitations of these different DNA detection assays along with the relative costs involved are summarized in Table 1. One of the key factors in the development of a highly sensitive DNA amplification assay is the selection of a specific amplification target sequence with numerous copies that is available in abundance within a single parasite cell; such sequences include both nuclear and mitochondrial genes [27,30–33]. In addition to being highly abundant, a target gene sequence for diagnostic DNA amplification needs to be highly specific for the targeted species so that the resulting assay is highly sensitive and specific. The *SjR2* retrotransposon [34–36] and the *nad1* mitochondrial gene [37,38] are two target sequences that have been commonly used in the diagnosis of *S. japonicum* infection. Similarly, the *SM1-7* tandem repeat sequence [39] and 18S rDNA are two targets used in the diagnosis of *S. mansoni* while mitochondrial *cox1* [40] and the *Dra1* repeat sequence [41] have been utilized for *S. haematobium* detection.

Table 1. Advantages and limitations of different DNA diagnostics.

Assay Type	Advantages	Limitations	Relative Cost*	References
cPCR	- Low cost compared to qPCR and ddPCR - Can be multiplexed when target amplicon sizes are different	- Requires post PCR processing—running PCR products in a gel—which allows high chance of contamination - More time consuming and labor intensive compared to most other PCR methods - Prone to potential laboratory contamination with the need of manual handling of PCR products	$$	[42–44]
nPCR	- Use of two sets of primers improves the specificity while the need of two rounds of cPCR provide a higher sensitivity	- Relatively time consuming and complicated initial optimization process - Need to complete two rounds of cPCR amplifications, hence more time consuming and labor intensive - Prone to contamination with amplified PCR products	$$	[45,46]
qPCR	- Higher sensitivity compared to cPCR - Higher specificity, specifically when probes are used - No post PCR processing (such as running a gel in cPCR) required for final results - No manual handling of PCR products which limits the potential laboratory contamination - Can quantify the amount of amplicons (relative quantification) - Can be multiplexed for the detection of multiple species within a single reaction - Less time consuming and less labor intensive compared to cPCR	- Relatively time consuming and complicated initial optimization process in multiplexed assays - Requires triplicate reactions to improve the accuracy of final calculations - More expensive than cPCR, LAMP, direct PCR	$$$	[13,29,38]
LAMP	- Cost effective - Less equipment required - Can visualize the end products directly without running in a gel - Faster procedures compared to other types of PCR	- Relatively time consuming and complicated initial optimization process - Prone to carryover contamination	$	[47,48]

Table 1. *Cont.*

Assay Type	Advantages	Limitations	Relative Cost *	References
RPA	- Cost effective - Less equipment required - End products can be visualized on a chip/lateral flow device - Has a great potential to be developed as a point of care diagnostic tool	- Relatively time consuming and complicated initial optimization process - Prone to contamination with the need of transferring amplified products to a detection device	$	[49–51]
ddPCR	- Higher sensitivity compared to most other types of PCR - Higher specificity, specifically when probes are used - Can quantify the amount of amplicons (absolute quantification) - No manual handling of PCR products which limits the potential laboratory contamination - Can be multiplexed for the detection of multiple species within a single reaction	- Requires specific and expensive machinery for the initial establishment - Relatively time consuming and complicated initial optimization process in multiplexed assays	$$$	[35,52,53]
Direct PCR	- Raw sample is used as the template for PCR amplification, eliminating the need of a DNA extraction step - Less time consuming and convenient	- Initial development and optimization is relatively complicated and time consuming, as it is required to overcome PCR inhibitors in raw samples.	$	[54]

* The cost of diagnostics is given as a relative scale to each other: $—low, $$—moderate, $$$—high. The individual cost of DNA diagnostics can be variable depending on factors such as the type and brand of commercial reagents used and the regional source where these reagents are purchased. Abbreviations: cPCR: conventional PCR, ddPCR: droplet digital PCR, LAMP: Loop mediated isothermal amplification, nPCR: nested PCR, RPA: Recombinase polymerase amplification.

3.1. Sample Preservation and DNA Isolation for DNA Amplification Assays

DNA extraction is a key procedure but it can be a methodological bottleneck in PCR-based diagnostic assays since the yield and quality of DNA directly affects the outcome of the amplification procedure; it is also often the most expensive part of DNA-based diagnosis, particularly when using commercially-available extraction kits [55,56]. Furthermore, sample collection and preservation techniques have a significant influence on DNA extraction and amplification outcomes. DNA extraction from fresh clinical samples is not feasible in the field and generally needs to be performed in a central laboratory. Hence appropriate measures are required to preserve samples until DNA extraction can be undertaken. These methods can vary depending on the type of clinical sample involved [56,57]. For example, common methods used in plasma sample preservation and storage include addition of K3EDTA at the time of blood sampling, and freezing [57]. K3EDTA is preferred over heparin as it stabilizes DNA and, unlike heparin, does not inhibit downstream amplification reactions [57]. Similarly, fecal samples for parasite DNA extraction can be readily preserved by immediate freezing, storage with alcohol, addition of commercial solutions such as RNA later and PAXgene, and preservation on Whatman FTA cards [58]. However, these preservation/storage reagents need to be carefully removed prior to DNA extraction since they can interfere with DNA yield as well as downstream assay procedures [58].

Major aims of DNA isolation for PCR include the removal of PCR inhibitors and nucleases, and maximizing DNA recovery and quality of DNA. In the diagnosis of schistosomiasis, stool and urine are the most commonly used clinical samples for DNA isolation; other bio-fluids (serum, saliva, and cerebrospinal fluid) are also used, particularly for cell-free DNA (cfDNA) detections assays. Conventional DNA extraction methods include precipitation techniques with phenol-chloroform and ethanol or isopropanol. However, the feasibility of applying these methods has in the past been affected by the potential for direct exposure of hazardous chemicals to operators and the significant time involved. However, the availability of commercial DNA extraction kits has markedly reduced these limitations and improved the quality and yield of isolated DNA [59,60]. The protocols involve techniques such as spin column-based purification and magnetic bead DNA separation. Furthermore, these kits have been developed for use on different clinical sample types to overcome the unique challenges related to each. Moreover, recent advances in DNA purification technology have resulted in high-throughput automated platforms minimizing the time spent, the labor involved and manual handling, making the process convenient, efficient and accurate [61–63]. However, as is common to most high-tech applications these automated techniques involve costly equipment, and are currently not suitable for field application in disease-endemic, resource-poor settings.

Most DNA amplification methods generally need to be performed in well-equipped centralized facilities that are generally located distant from the clinical specimen collection site. Therefore, under these circumstances it is important that feasible and rapid sample preservation methods are available prior to DNA extraction and amplification. Potential solutions to these issues include the preservation of clinical specimens such as fingerprick blood, urine, or stool on filter papers as dried spots for convenient transportation to a central laboratory for DNA extraction and amplification, or for direct PCR [45,64–66].

3.2. Conventional and Quantitative Real Time PCR

Of nucleic acid amplification tests, conventional PCR (cPCR) was developed first. A key advantage of the technique is the ability to observe the amplification products corresponding to appropriate base pair size that can be conveniently used in specific genomic detection through sequencing. cPCR has been applied in different surveys including the evaluation of therapeutic responses in schistosomiasis [16,67]. Another important aspect of cPCR is the feasibility to develop a multiplex assay to detect multiple infections within a single clinical sample [68]. Multiplexing in cPCR requires differing target amplicon sizes to be distinctively identified in gel electrophoresis. Specific target gene segment detection in stool or urine samples using cPCR has been widely applied in the diagnosis of schistosomiasis [42–44]. The method is highly sensitive compared with conventional microscopy methods, particularly with low intensity infections [33,43,69,70]. The accuracy of cPCR assays has been improved with the combination of other techniques, such as PCR-ELISA analysis [71] and restriction fragment length polymorphism analysis of PCR amplified fragments (PCR-RFLP) for the diagnosis of schistosome infections. The PCR-RFLP technique involves restriction endonucleases digestion of the PCR amplicon, giving rise to different electrophoretic patterns thereby providing a method for simultaneous analysis of multiple species/strains [72]. This technique has been used in characterization of snails as well as in the detection of schistosomiasis and other helminth infections [72–75].

Nested PCR (nPCR) is a more sensitive and a specific approach than cPCR, and has been successfully applied in different instances in the diagnosis of schistosomiasis [46,76]. However, the procedure includes duplication of cPCR for the initial amplification of a larger gene fragment and then another sequence within the initial fragment, which involves more labor and a higher cost.

qPCR has been widely applied in the detection of human schistosome infections of different species including large-scale epidemiological surveys and monitoring of the therapeutic response. The qPCR technique is generally more sensitive than cPCR and, importantly, can provide a measurement of infection intensity. Additionally, the procedures involved with qPCR are streamlined compared with cPCR which needs an additional electrophoresis step to detect PCR end-products [27,77,78]. Another important characteristic of qPCR is that, like cPCR, it has the ability to utilise multiplex assays to detect multiple infections within a single clinical sample using specific DNA probes. Generally, however, qPCR assays are preferred over cPCR in the development of multiplex assays, having the additional advantage of improved specificity with the use of probes and convenience in high-throughput applications. Moreover, recent studies have demonstrated the ability to detect a very high spectrum of parasites in a single sample (multi-parallel PCR) further improving multiplex qPCR assays [79–82]. Multiplexing capability has clear practical significance largely in terms of cost-effective application in epidemiological studies and for monitoring of schistosomiasis control programs, particularly in co-endemic settings, an example being the detection of *S. mansoni* and *S. haematobium* in human fecal or urine samples in areas where both species are present [27,83].

3.3. Loop-Mediated Isothermal Amplification (LAMP)

The LAMP technique is a relatively simple, cost-effective and rapid DNA detection approach compared with the commonly-used PCR-based assays and is more field-friendly. Application of the assay does not require specific equipment such as a thermocycler, electrophoresis apparatus or gel documentation units [84]; hence it is simple, and applicable in resource-poor settings once optimized. Moreover, the use of specific inner and outer primer sets makes the assay highly specific to the intended target sequence, combined with high sensitivity [85,86]. However, the initial optimization process is complicated and time consuming with the use of multiple primers. Furthermore, it is known that the LAMP technique, being highly sensitive, is highly vulnerable to carryover contamination of LAMP products from previous reactions, which can be re-amplified leading to false-positive results [87,88].

LAMP assays have demonstrated high sensitivity in the detection of *S. mansoni* and *S. haematobium* infections in co-endemic areas using urine samples, indicating the possible use of the technique as a point of care (POC) diagnostic [65]. Furthermore, a LAMP assay has been used in the sensitive detection of early pre-patent schistosome infection in an animal model [89]. In a recent field survey to detect *S. mansoni* infection in a low-transmission area, a LAMP assay was successfully applied in both snail and human stool samples and the study emphasized the potential application of this molecular approach for the identification of transmission foci and for building risk maps in support of control programs [48]. Furthermore, the LAMP method was successfully used recently in China for surveillance, including in snail surveys, indicating its usefulness, and applicability as a rapid screening and environmental risk assessment tool to identify areas suitable for targeted intervention [12].

Recent research has raised the possibility of developing multiplex LAMP assays, a concept that could be adapted for the diagnosis of multiple parasitic species, including different schistosomes, in infected individuals. Multiplex LAMP procedures incorporate an additional endpoint readout option to discriminate between amplified products, such as melting curve analysis to test for different melting temperatures or detection of distinctive gel-electrophoretic banding patterns reflecting different species characters [90,91]. The LAMP technique could provide an effective method, applicable in resource-poor endemic communities, to diagnose co-infections of *S. mansoni* and *S. haematobium*, multiple co-infections of soil-transmitted helminths (STH), or co-infections of intestinal protozoa and schistosomes, as achieved using qPCR [27,92–94].

3.4. Recombinase Polymerase Amplification (RPA)

The RPA technique is another isothermal amplification technique usually conducted under lower temperatures (around 40 °C). In RPA, DNA sequences are amplified with the use of DNA polymerase, DNA binding proteins and recombinase; primer binding to the template DNA is facilitated by nucleoprotein complexes made of recombinase proteins and oligonucleotide primers [49,95]. Similar to LAMP, the application of the RPA technique is straight forward and applicable in resource-poor settings since it does not require specific equipment such as a thermocycler, electrophoresis apparatus or gel documentations units. This novel technique has now been integrated with a chip and lateral flow devices making it a convenient portable application as a point of care diagnostic tool [95,96]. RPA has been applied in the diagnosis of both intestinal and urinary schistosomiasis, including its use in field evaluation, and has been shown to be superior to microscopy and serology in terms of convenience, detection time and diagnostic sensitivity [49–51]. However, the technique does have some practical limitations such as the need for transferring amplified products to the detection device, which can lead to potential nucleic acid contamination resulting in false positives [50,96].

3.5. Droplet Digital PCR (ddPCR)

Due to a recent advance in PCR technology, ddPCR is proving to be more sensitive and precise compared with qPCR [97–99]. ddPCR has been successfully used in the detection of cfDNA and in the diagnosis of infections and other clinical conditions, including cancer [53,97,100–104]. Moreover, it was recently applied in the diagnosis of *S. japonicum* in both an animal model and in diverse human clinical samples, and was able to quantify intensity of infection in terms of direct target gene copy number [35,53]. The technique can also be used for multiple target testing, thereby providing an effective diagnostic approach for detecting multiple parasites in an infected individual [105,106].

3.6. Direct PCR

The need for a prior DNA isolation step is a major limitation in routine PCR analysis, resulting in the requirement for additional resources and costs, delays in obtaining a result, and added complexity. Attempts have been made to overcome this constraint by optimizing PCR protocols so that clinical specimens can be added directly into the PCR reaction. However, the initial development and optimization of a 'direct PCR' assay has multiple challenges, particularly the potential negative effect of PCR inhibitors present in clinical samples. Application of modified, inhibitor-resistant polymerases and inclusion of additional reagents such as chelating agents and protease inhibitors are some strategies used to overcome these effects [107,108]. Direct application of the PCR technique has been undertaken in clinical diagnosis, including the identification of parasitic infections, with the use of conveniently preserved clinical samples such as dry blood spots [109,110]. This technique has been tested for applicability in schistosomiasis diagnosis using animal models [54], and its further improvement and evaluation would be a helpful advance for undertaking molecular diagnostics directly under field conditions rather than in a central laboratory, far from the disease-endemic community.

3.7. Parasite cfDNA Detection in Clinical Samples

Application of the PCR technique was mostly restricted to schistosome egg DNA detection until the recent development of parasite cfDNA detection methods in different clinical samples. Compared with the DNA originating from schistosome eggs in stool or urine samples, cfDNA is generally homogenously distributed in plasma and other bodily fluids, which potentially eliminates one of the major sampling problems associated with copro PCR or urine PCR, where eggs are the primary source of DNA [16,33,35,53,111,112]. Parasite cfDNA is released from schistosome stages (schistosomula, adult worms and eggs) within the mammalian host, and could possibly be the result of dead or decaying parasites within the circulation and tissues, active shedding from the parasite or from disintegrating inactive eggs [29,113,114]. Infections with all the three major human schistosomes have been diagnosed using DNA amplification-based cfDNA detection assays, and parasite cfDNA can be detected in host serum in early prepatent schistosomiasis [115–117]. In addition to serum/plasma, parasite cfDNA can be excreted in bodily fluids such as urine, saliva, and cerebrospinal fluid, and can be effectively quantified using qPCR and ddPCR assays [33,53,112,118,119].

As it is likely that the amount of parasite cfDNA in a given clinical sample will be low compared with one containing parasite eggs, a higher level of detection sensitivityis imperative. Of the different PCR-based DNA detection methods available, ddPCR and qPCR are optimal for this purpose [35,52,53]. Recent studies have demonstrated the successful amplification of the *SjR2* retrotransposon gene and *nad1* mitochondrial gene for the detection of both early pre-patent and late *S. japonicum* infection [35,53]. Furthermore, detection of cfDNA using ddPCR and qPCR has proven to be effective in individual case detection, in large scale field application and for monitoring therapeutic responses [111,118,120].

4. Applications of DNA Diagnostics for Schistosomiasis

4.1. Individual Case Detection

Early confirmation of the diagnosis of acute schistosome infection is imperative for early intervention and to achieve a good prognosis for the patient with minimum complications. Acute schistosomiasis cases include returned travelers, immigrants, and refugees [121,122], where patients present to health care facilities with early clinical manifestations such as cercarial dermatitis. These patients need to be carefully clinically evaluated and investigated but most of the commonly applied diagnostics are unable to detect these pre-patent schistosome infections. Schistosome cfDNA detection is an ideal option to diagnose these cases either using serum or non-invasive clinical samples like urine [114]. Furthermore, cfDNA detection is helpful in situations such as neuroschistosomiasis, where parasite DNA can be detected in host cerebrospinal fluid [46,120].

4.2. Diagnosis of Zoonotic Schistosomiasis in Animal Reservoirs

Accurate diagnosis of *S. japonicum*-infected mammalian reservoirs is key to achievingthe elimination of zoonotic schistosomiasis in China and the Philippines [42,123,124]. Similar to the diagnosis of human cases, insensitive conventional microscopy-based diagnostic procedures often do not detect infected animals that continue to contribute to schistosomiasis transmission. DNA amplification-based methods have now been shown to be highly effective in the diagnosis of animal reservoirs of Asian schistosomiasis. Recent surveys undertaken on carabao in the Philippines disclosed a substantially higher prevalence of schistosomiasis using qPCR on fecal samples, compared with copro-microscopic diagnosis [42,125]. Moreover, a recently-developed nPCR assay has also shown potential for field application in the sensitive diagnosis of early cases of schistosomiasis in domestic animals, using serum samples [45].

4.3. Detection of Infected Snail Hosts

Bulinus spp., *Biomphalaria* spp., and *Oncomelania* spp. act as the intermediate hosts of *S. haematobium*, *S. mansoni* and *S. japonicum* respectively. Detection of infected snail hosts—xeno-monitoring—is a pivotal indicator of an existence of schistosomiasis in a particular area, and the potential for transmission. Furthermore, xeno-monitoring is important in identifying infection risk areas to guide surveillance and necessary interventions, and represents a critical measure for achieving schistosomiasis elimination goals [126–128]. The example of Japan is one of the best to show the importance of snail control in schistosomiasis elimination, where the main control strategy was to target susceptible snail colonies using chemical molluscicides and environmental modifications [129].

Commonly used techniques in xeno-monitoring include cercarial shedding with light exposure, microscopic detection of sporocysts and cercariae in crushed snails. These traditional methods have detection limitations particularly in situations where there is a low parasite burden, or where there is aborted development of sporocysts [130]. Moreover, the labor-intensive nature of these procedures, including the collection and handling of snails and the associated costs, are both major disadvantages [131].

Molecular tools are now being widely applied in the detection of schistosome-infected snail hosts, providing promising results in support of control and elimination efforts particularly with large scale screening programs [132]. One early study described the detection of *S. haematobium* in *Bulinus truncatus* snails using cPCR targeting the *DraI* repeat sequence [128]. As well as demonstrating high sensitivity, the study highlighted the cost-effective application of the assay through the grouping and pooling of snails in the analysis. Moreover, PCR and LAMP assays were used in recent studies to detect *S. mansoni* DNA in *Biomphalaria* snails [133,134]. One of the studies showed that the LAMP assay could detect one infected snail within a pool of a thousand uninfected snails [133]. Hence this approach can provide an important low cost, rapid and highly sensitive tool for the monitoring of infected snails to provide important information required before appropriate control measures are undertaken [133]. Similar efforts have also been successful in the detection of *S. japonicum*-infected *Oncomelania* snails using LAMP-based DNA detection [135]. The application of multiplex qPCR assays have the additional advantage of identifying both snail and infecting schistosome species, another helpful consideration for successful schistosome and snail control programs [136]. Furthermore, molecular methods are of considerable help in developing transmission risk maps prior to the instigation of control efforts [48,135].

4.4. Surveillance of Environmental Sources

In addition to xeno-monitoring, the other important surveillance measure to determine the existence of environmental contamination with schistosomes is the detection of miracidia and cercariae in water sources. Evaluating the presence of cercariae is an important factor in detecting infection transmission sites. Commonly used conventional microscopic methods lack sensitivity and are highly labor-intensive [137,138]. Testing for the presence of cercariae is helpful in determining their diurnal variation, seasonal patterns, and spatial distribution. PCR-based molecular tools are now being increasingly applied to this area of surveillance [131,139,140]. qPCR has been successfully used in quantitative detection of *S. japonicum* cercariae in water samples, showing potential for the rapid and high throughput analysis of environmental samples and its application in the field [140,141].

4.5. Assessment of Progress of Control Measures

One of the key elements of sustained efforts on control and elimination measures is the frequent monitoring and surveillance of the effects/progress of the strategies already implemented. While effective control measures need to be continued with high priority, identification of less effective interventions are important in early application of appropriate modifications to improve the effect on control and elimination efforts. Application of highly sensitive and accurate diagnostics is imperative for this purpose since the ongoing control measures lead to lowered prevalence of infection and lowered infection intensity in the community [6,131,142,143]. Further, these assays also need to have the capability to perform in a short time period, with a minimum requirement of equipment and expertise and they have to be cost-effective [144]. The equipment, reagents, and setup required for conventional diagnostics, particularly parasitological methods, are relatively inexpensive, but they can be laborious especially as they need to be repeated multiple times to reach a certain diagnostic accuracy, which can also affect the costs involved. Both molecular and serological diagnostics performed in specific laboratories are more expensive, particularly with the requirements of costly equipment and reagents, specific maintenance requirements, and the need of trained personnel to carry out the tests. Field/community applicable POC immunodiagnostics are simple to use and require only a minimum amount of labor and equipment, but may involve a higher production cost [145,146]. As a result, despite being highly sensitive and accurate, DNA diagnostics cannot currently completely replace the conventional diagnostic methods for community, field, and environmental surveillance. However, the combined application of different techniques is a reasonable approach whereby, for example, an initial diagnosis is undertaken with traditional methods followed by further screening of any test-negatives with molecular tools to capture any missed infections.

5. Challenges and the Way Forward

While there has been substantial focus on mass drug administration (MDA) as a measure to control and eliminate schistosomiasis, efforts to establish accurate, field-deployable novel diagnostics, particularly in resource-poor endemic settings, have been comparatively limited. Microscopy-basedprocedures are recognized as being imprecise, making it important that more sensitive diagnostic tools are developed and deployed. Parasite DNA amplification-based molecular tools are showing encouraging promise towards reaching the level of sensitivity and specificity required to monitor the effectiveness of control programs that will lead to the elimination of schistosomiasis. These molecular assays have a wide range of applications including human case detection, detection of infection in animal reservoir hosts and snails, and in environmental surveillance, which are essential requirements to achieve elimination targets.

Despite the fact that highly sensitive and accurate, ddPCR technology is not yet at the level where it can be used routinely in the field. This is likely in the near future as it can be readily applied for the diagnosis of many other pathogens such as HIV and *Mycobacterium tuberculosis*, which are also endemic in many areas endemic for schistosomiasis. Hence the development of central laboratories that are able to undertake molecular diagnostics targeting multiple infections in these regions would be a cost-effective approach for infection control, and rather than relying on less sensitive, less accurate diagnostics which miss infected individuals, thereby hindering control efforts. Other promising advances include the diagnostic application of the LAMP and RPA techniques, which are applicable to resource-poor settings. Simplifying available DNA extraction procedures, so that they are more convenientand less expensive, and the increased use of fingerprick blood spots and urine filtrates on filter papers [65], should be advocated for field-friendly DNA detection-based molecular diagnosis. Furthermore, improvement and adaption of direct PCR approaches, without the need for DNA extraction, modifications to nucleic acid amplification procedures making them simpler, reducing equipment requirements and expertise while maintaining accuracy, would invariably favor the field use of molecular assays. Altogether these advances have the potential to provide a mechanism for the wider application of more accurate and convenient DNA detection methods that will be invaluable in future schistosomiasis control and elimination efforts.

Acknowledgments: We thank Madeleine Flynn, QIMR Berghofer Medical Research Institute, for preparing the figure.

Abbreviations

cfDNA	Cell-free DNA
CAA	Circulating anodic antigen
CCA	Circulating cathodic antigen
PCR	Polymerase chain reaction
cPCR	Conventional PCR

ddPCR	Droplet digital PCR
KK	Kato-Katz fecal smear
LAMP	Loop-mediated isothermal amplification
MDA	Mass drug administration
nPCR	Nested PCR
PCR-RFLP	Restriction fragment length polymorphism analysis of PCR products
POC	Point of care
qPCR	Real time quantitative PCR
RPA	Recombinase polymerase amplification
STH	Soil transmitted helminths
WASH	Water, sanitation and hygiene

References

1. Hotez, P.J.; Alvarado, M.; Basáñez, M.G.; Bolliger, I.; Bourne, R.; Boussinesq, M.; Brooker, S.J.; Brown, A.S.; Buckle, G.; Budke, C.M.; et al. The global burden of disease study 2010: Interpretation and implications for the neglected tropical diseases. *PLoS Negl. Trop. Dis.* **2014**, *8*, e2865. [CrossRef] [PubMed]

2. WHO. *Prevention and Control of Schistosomiasis and Soil-Transmitted Helminthiasis: WHO Technical Report Series (912)*; WHO: Geneva, Switzerland, 2002.

3. WHO. *Schistosomiasis: Progress Report 2001–2011 and Strategic Plan 2012–2020*; WHO: Geneva, Switzerland, 2013.

4. Ross, A.G.P.; Olveda, R.M.; Acosta, L.; Harn, D.A.; Chy, D.; Li, Y.; Gray, D.J.; Gordon, C.A.; McManus, D.P.; Williams, G.M. Road to the elimination of schistosomiasis from Asia: The journey is far from over. *Microbes Infect.* **2013**, *15*, 858–865. [CrossRef] [PubMed]

5. Boatin, B.A.; Basáñez, M.G.; Prichard, R.K.; Awadzi, K.; Barakat, R.M.; García, H.H.; Gazzinelli, A.; Grant, W.N.; McCarthy, J.S.; N'Goran, E.K.; et al. A research agenda for helminth diseases of humans: Towards control and elimination. *PLoS Negl. Trop. Dis.* **2012**, *6*, e1547. [CrossRef] [PubMed]

6. Sun, L.P.; Wang, W.; Hong, Q.B.; Li, S.Z.; Liang, Y.S.; Yang, H.T.; Zhou, X.N. Approaches being used in the national schistosomiasis elimination programme in China: A review. *Infect. Dis. Poverty* **2017**, *6*, 55. [CrossRef] [PubMed]

7. Fan, K.; Lai, H. Mao Zedong's fight against schistosomiasis. *Perspect. Biol. Med.* **2008**, *51*, 176–187. [PubMed]

8. WHO. *Accelerating Work to Overcome the Global Impact of Neglected Tropical Diseases: A Roadmap for Implementation*; WHO: Geneva, Switzerland, 2012.

9. WHO. *Integrating Neglected Tropical Diseases into Global Health and Development: Fourth WHO Report on Neglected Tropical Diseases*; WHO: Geneva, Switzerland, 2017.

10. Bergquist, R.; Zhou, X.N.; Rollinson, D.; Reinhard-Rupp, J.; Klohe, K. Elimination of schistosomiasis: The tools required. *Infect. Dis. Poverty* **2017**, *6*, 158. [CrossRef] [PubMed]

11. Shiff, C. Accurate diagnostics for schistosomiasis: A new role for PCR? *Rep. Parasitol.* **2015**, *4*, 23–29. [CrossRef]

12. WHO. *Expert Consultation to Accelerate Elimination of Asian Schistosomiasis*; WHO: Shanghai, China, 2017.

13. He, P.; Gordon, C.A.; Williams, G.M.; Li, Y.; Wang, Y.; Hu, J.; Gray, D.J.; Ross, A.G.; Harn, D.; McManus, D.P. Real-time PCR diagnosis of *Schistosoma japonicum* in low transmission areas of China. *Infect. Dis. Poverty* **2018**, *7*, 8. [CrossRef] [PubMed]

14. Spear, R.C.; Seto, E.Y.W.; Carlton, E.J.; Liang, S.; Remais, J.V.; Zhong, B.; Qiu, D. The challenge of effective surveillance in moving from low transmission to elimination of schistosomiasis in China. *Int. J. Parasitol.* **2011**, *41*, 1243–1247. [CrossRef] [PubMed]

15. Kongs, A.; Marks, G.; Verlé, P.; Van der Stuyft, P. The unreliability of the Kato-Katz technique limits its usefulness for evaluating *S. mansoni* infections. *Trop. Med. Int. Health* **2001**, *6*, 163–169. [CrossRef] [PubMed]

16. Weerakoon, K.G.A.D.; Gobert, G.N.; Cai, P.; McManus, D.P. Advances in the diagnosis of human schistosomiasis. *Clin. Microbiol. Rev.* **2015**, *28*, 939–967. [CrossRef] [PubMed]

17. Xu, B.; Gordon, C.A.; Hu, W.; McManus, D.P.; Chen, H.G.; Gray, D.J.; Ju, C.; Zeng, X.J.; Gobert, G.N.; Ge, J.; et al. A novel procedure for precise quantification of *Schistosoma japonicum* eggs in bovine feces. *PLoS Negl. Trop. Dis.* **2012**, *6*, e1885. [CrossRef]

18. Legesse, M.; Erko, B. Field-based evaluation of a reagent strip test for diagnosis of *Schistosoma mansoni* by detecting circulating cathodic antigen in urine before and after chemotherapy. *Trans. R. Soc. Trop. Med. Hyg.* **2007**, *101*, 668–673. [CrossRef] [PubMed]

19. Stothard, J.R.; Kabatereine, N.B.; Tukahebwa, E.M.; Kazibwe, F.; Rollinson, D.; Mathieson, W.; Webster, J.P.; Fenwick, A. Use of circulating cathodic antigen (CCA) dipsticks for detection of intestinal and urinary schistosomiasis. *Acta Trop.* **2006**, *97*, 219–228. [CrossRef] [PubMed]

20. Ochodo, E.A.; Gopalakrishna, G.; Spek, B.; Reitsma, J.B.; van Lieshout, L.; Polman, K.; Lamberton, P.; Bossuyt, P.M.M.; Leeflang, M.M.G. Circulating antigen tests and urine reagent strips for diagnosis of active schistosomiasis in endemic areas. *Cochrane Database Syst. Rev.* **2015**, *11*, CD009579. [CrossRef] [PubMed]

21. Van Grootveld, R.; van Dam, G.J.; de Dood, C.; de Vries, J.J.C.; Visser, L.G.; Corstjens, P.L.A.M.; van Lieshout, L. Improved diagnosis of active *Schistosoma* infection in travellers and migrants using the ultra-sensitive in-house lateral flow test for detection of circulating anodic antigen (CAA) in serum. *Eur. J. Clin. Microbiol. Infect. Dis.* **2018**, in press. [CrossRef] [PubMed]

22. Knopp, S.; Corstjens, P.L.A.M.; Koukounari, A.; Cercamondi, C.I.; Ame, S.M.; Ali, S.M.; de Dood, C.J.; Mohammed, K.A.; Utzinger, J.; Rollinson, D.; et al. Sensitivity and specificity of a urine circulating anodic antigen test for the diagnosis of *Schistosoma haematobium* in low endemic settings. *PLoS Negl. Trop. Dis.* **2015**, *9*, e0003752. [CrossRef] [PubMed]

23. Liu, F.; Zhou, Y.; Wang, Z.Q.; Lu, G.; Zheng, H.; Brindley, P.J.; McManus, D.P.; Blair, D.; Zhang, Q.H.; Zhong, Y.; et al. *Schistosoma japonicum* genome sequencing and functional analysis consortium the *Schistosoma japonicum* genome reveals features of host-parasite interplay. *Nature* **2009**, *460*, 345–351.

24. Young, N.D.; Jex, A.R.; Li, B.; Liu, S.; Yang, L.; Xiong, Z.; Li, Y.; Cantacessi, C.; Hall, R.S.; Xu, X.; et al. Whole-genome sequence of *Schistosoma haematobium*. *Nat. Genet.* **2012**, *44*, 221–225. [CrossRef] [PubMed]

25. Le, T.H.; Blair, D.; Agatsuma, T.; Humair, P.F.; Campbell, N.J.; Iwagami, M.; Littlewood, D.T.; Peacock, B.; Johnston, D.A.; Bartley, J.; et al. Phylogenies inferred from mitochondrial gene orders—A cautionary tale from the parasitic flatworms. *Mol. Biol. Evol.* **2000**, *17*, 1123–1125. [CrossRef] [PubMed]

26. Lier, T.; Simonsen, G.S.; Wang, T.; Lu, D.; Haukland, H.H.; Vennervald, B.J.; Hegstad, J.; Johansen, M.V. Real-time polymerase chain reaction for detection of low-intensity *Schistosoma japonicum* infections in China. *Am. J. Trop. Med. Hyg.* **2009**, *81*, 428–432. [PubMed]

27. Ten Hove, R.J.; Verweij, J.J.; Vereecken, K.; Polman, K.; Dieye, L.; van Lieshout, L. Multiplex real-time PCR for the detection and quantification of *Schistosoma mansoni* and *S. haematobium* infection in stool samples collected in northern Senegal. *Trans. R. Soc. Trop. Med. Hyg.* **2008**, *102*, 179–185. [CrossRef] [PubMed]

28. Obeng, B.B.; Aryeetey, Y.A.; Amoah, A.S.; Larbi, I.A.; Deelder, A.M.; Yazdanbakhsh, M.; Hartgers, F.C.; Boakye, D.A.; Verweij, J.J.; van Dam, G.J.; et al. Application of a circulating-cathodic-antigen (CCA) strip test and real-time PCR, in comparison with microscopy, for the detection of *Schistosoma haematobium* in urine samples from Ghana. *Ann. Trop. Med. Parasitol.* **2008**, *102*, 625–633. [CrossRef] [PubMed]

29. Cnops, L.; Soentjens, P.; Clerinx, J.; Van Esbroeck, M. A *Schistosoma haematobium*-specific real-time PCR for diagnosis of urogenital schistosomiasis in serum samples of international travelers and migrants. *PLoS Negl. Trop. Dis.* **2013**, *7*, e2413. [CrossRef] [PubMed]

30. He, P.; Song, L.G.; Xie, H.; Liang, J.Y.; Yuan, D.Y.; Wu, Z.D.; Lv, Z.Y. Nucleic acid detection in the diagnosis and prevention of schistosomiasis. *Infect. Dis. Poverty* **2016**, *5*, 25. [CrossRef] [PubMed]

31. Lier, T.; Johansen, M.V.; Hjelmevoll, S.O.; Vennervald, B.J.; Simonsen, G.S. Real-time PCR for detection of low intensity *Schistosoma japonicum* infections in a pig model. *Acta Trop.* **2008**, *105*, 74–80. [CrossRef] [PubMed]

32. Gobert, G.N.; Chai, M.; Duke, M.; McManus, D.P. Copro-PCR based detection of *Schistosoma* eggs using mitochondrial DNA markers. *Mol. Cell. Probes* **2005**, *19*, 250–254. [CrossRef] [PubMed]

33. Pontes, L.A.; Dias-Neto, E.; Rabello, A. Detection by polymerase chain reaction of *Schistosoma mansoni* DNA in human serum and feces. *Am. J. Trop. Med. Hyg.* **2002**, *66*, 157–162. [CrossRef] [PubMed]

34. Laha, T.; Brindley, P.J.; Smout, M.J.; Verity, C.K.; McManus, D.P.; Loukas, A. Reverse transcriptase activity and untranslated region sharing of a new RTE-like, non-long terminal repeat retrotransposon from the human blood fluke, *Schistosoma japonicum*. *Int. J. Parasitol.* **2002**, *32*, 1163–1174. [CrossRef]

35. Weerakoon, K.G.; Gordon, C.A.; Cai, P.; Gobert, G.N.; Duke, M.; Williams, G.M.; McManus, D.P. A novel duplex ddPCR assay for the diagnosis of schistosomiasis japonica: Proof of concept in an experimental mouse model. *Parasitology* **2017**, *144*, 1005–1015. [CrossRef] [PubMed]

36. Xu, X.; Zhang, Y.; Lin, D.; Zhang, J.; Xu, J.; Liu, Y.M.; Hu, F.; Qing, X.; Xia, C.; Pan, W. Serodiagnosis of *Schistosoma japonicum* infection: Genome-wide identification of a protein marker, and assessment of its diagnostic validity in a field study in China. *Lancet Infect. Dis.* **2014**, *14*, 489–497. [CrossRef]

37. Lier, T.; Simonsen, G.S.; Haaheim, H.; Hjelmevoll, S.O.; Vennervald, B.J.; Johansen, M.V. Novel real-time PCR for detection of *Schistosoma japonicum* in stool. *Southeast Asian J. Trop. Med. Public Health* **2006**, *37*, 257–264. [PubMed]

38. Gordon, C.; Acosta, L.P.; Gobert, G.N.; Olveda, R.M.; Ross, A.G.; Williams, G.M.; Gray, D.J.; Harn, D.; Li, Y.; McManus, D.P. Real-time PCR demonstrates high prevalence of *Schistosoma japonicum* in the Philippines: Implications for surveillance and control. *PLoS Negl. Trop. Dis.* **2015**, *9*, e0003483. [CrossRef] [PubMed]

39. Espírito-Santo, M.; Alvarado-Mora, M.; Dias-Neto, E.; Botelho-Lima, L.; Moreira, J.; Amorim, M.; Pinto, P.; Heath, A.R.; Castilho, V.; Gonçalves, E.; et al. Evaluation of real-time PCR assay to detect *Schistosoma mansoni* infections in a low endemic setting. *BMC Infect. Dis.* **2014**, *14*, 558. [CrossRef] [PubMed]

40. Umar, S.; Shinkafi, S.H.; Hudu, S.A.; Neela, V.; Suresh, K.; Nordin, S.A.; Malina, O. Prevalence and molecular characterisation of *Schistosoma haematobium* among primary school children in Kebbi State, Nigeria. *Ann. Parasitol.* **2017**, *63*, 133–139. [PubMed]

41. Lodh, N.; Naples, J.M.; Bosompem, K.M.; Quartey, J.; Shiff, C.J. Detection of parasite-specific DNA in urine sediment obtained by filtration differentiates between single and mixed infections of *Schistosoma mansoni* and *S. haematobium* from endemic areas in Ghana. *PLoS ONE* **2014**, *9*, e91144. [CrossRef] [PubMed]

42. Gordon, C.A.; Acosta, L.P.; Gray, D.J.; Olveda, R.M.; Jarilla, B.; Gobert, G.N.; Ross, A.G.; McManus, D.P. High prevalence of *Schistosoma japonicum* infection in Carabao from Samar Province, the Philippines: Implications for transmission and control. *PLoS Negl. Trop. Dis.* **2012**, *6*, e1778. [CrossRef] [PubMed]

43. Pontes, L.A.; Oliveira, M.C.; Katz, N.; Dias-Neto, E.; Rabello, A. Comparison of a polymerase chain reaction and the Kato-Katz technique for diagnosing infection with *Schistosoma mansoni*. *Am. J. Trop. Med. Hyg.* **2003**, *68*, 652–656. [PubMed]

44. Ibironke, O.A.; Phillips, A.E.; Garba, A.; Lamine, S.M.; Shiff, C. Diagnosis of *Schistosoma haematobium* by detection of specific DNA fragments from filtered urine samples. *Am. J. Trop. Med. Hyg.* **2011**, *84*, 998–1001. [CrossRef] [PubMed]

45. Zhang, X.; He, C.C.; Liu, J.M.; Li, H.; Lu, K.; Fu, Z.Q.; Zhu, C.G.; Liu, Y.P.; Tong, L.B.; Zhou, D.-B.; et al. Nested-PCR assay for detection of *Schistosoma japonicum* infection in domestic animals. *Infect. Dis. Poverty* **2017**, *6*, 86. [CrossRef] [PubMed]

46. Bruscky, I.S.; de Melo, F.L.; de Medeiros, Z.M.; Albuquerque, F.F.; Wanderley, L.B.; da Cunha-Correia, C. Nested polymerase chain reaction in cerebrospinal fluid for diagnosing spinal cord schistosomiasis: A promising method. *J. Neurol. Sci.* **2016**, *366*, 87–90. [CrossRef] [PubMed]

47. Mwangi, I.N.; Agola, E.L.; Mugambi, R.M.; Shiraho, E.A.; Mkoji, G.M. Development and evaluation of a loop-mediated isothermal amplification assay for diagnosis of *Schistosoma mansoni* infection in faecal samples. *J. Parasitol. Res.* **2018**, *2018*, 1267826. [CrossRef] [PubMed]

48. Gandasegui, J.; Fernández-Soto, P.; Muro, A.; Simões Barbosa, C.; Lopes de Melo, F.; Loyo, R.; de Souza Gomes, E.C. A field survey using LAMP assay for detection of *Schistosoma mansoni* in a low-transmission area of schistosomiasis in Umbuzeiro, Brazil: Assessment in human and snail samples. *PLoS Negl. Trop. Dis.* **2018**, *12*, e0006314. [CrossRef] [PubMed]

49. Poulton, K.; Webster, B. Development of a lateral flow recombinase polymerase assay for the diagnosis of *Schistosoma mansoni* infections. *Anal. Biochem.* **2018**, *546*, 65–71. [CrossRef] [PubMed]

50. Xing, W.; Yu, X.; Feng, J.; Sun, K.; Fu, W.; Wang, Y.; Zou, M.; Xia, W.; Luo, Z.; He, H.; et al. Field evaluation of a recombinase polymerase amplification assay for the diagnosis of *Schistosoma japonicum* infection in Hunan province of China. *BMC Infect. Dis.* **2017**, *17*, 164. [CrossRef] [PubMed]

51. Rosser, A.; Rollinson, D.; Forrest, M.; Webster, B.L. Isothermal recombinase polymerase amplification (RPA) of *Schistosoma haematobium* DNA and oligochromatographic lateral flow detection. *Parasit. Vectors* **2015**, *8*, 446. [CrossRef] [PubMed]

52. Weerakoon, K.G.; Gordon, C.A.; Gobert, G.N.; Cai, P.; McManus, D.P. Optimisation of a droplet digital PCR assay for the diagnosis of *Schistosoma japonicum* infection: A duplex approach with DNA binding dye chemistry. *J. Microbiol. Methods* **2016**, *125*, 19–27. [CrossRef] [PubMed]

53. Weerakoon, K.G.; Gordon, C.A.; Williams, G.M.; Cai, P.; Gobert, G.N.; Olveda, R.M.; Ross, A.G.; Olveda, D.U.; McManus, D.P. Droplet digital PCR diagnosis of human schistosomiasis: Parasite cell-free DNA detection in diverse clinical samples. *J. Infect. Dis.* **2017**, *216*, 1611–1622. [CrossRef] [PubMed]

54. Eraky, M.; Aly, N.M. Assessment of diagnostic performance of a commercial direct blood PCR kit for the detection of *Schistosoma mansoni* infection in mice compared with the pre-extracted PCR assay. *Parasitol. United J.* **2016**, *9*, 13. [CrossRef]

55. Silva, M.A.L.D.; Medeiros, Z.; Soares, C.R.P.; Silva, E.D.D.; Miranda-Filho, D.B.; Melo, F.L. De. A comparison of four DNA extraction protocols for the analysis of urine from patients with visceral leishmaniasis. *Rev. Soc. Bras. Med. Trop.* **2014**, *47*, 193–197. [CrossRef] [PubMed]

56. Van den Broeck, F.; Geldof, S.; Polman, K.; Volckaert, F.A.M.; Huyse, T. Optimal sample storage and extraction procotols for reliable multilocus genotyping of the human parasite *Schistosoma mansoni. Infect. Genet. Evol.* **2011**, *11*, 1413–1418. [CrossRef] [PubMed]

57. El Messaoudi, S.; Rolet, F.; Mouliere, F.; Thierry, A.R. Circulating cell free DNA: Preanalytical considerations. *Clin. Chim. Acta* **2013**, *424*, 222–230. [CrossRef] [PubMed]

58. Papaiakovou, M.; Pilotte, N.; Baumer, B.; Grant, J.; Asbjornsdottir, K.; Schaer, F.; Hu, Y.; Aroian, R.; Walson, J.; Williams, S.A. A comparative analysis of preservation techniques for the optimal molecular detection of hookworm DNA in a human fecal specimen. *PLoS Negl. Trop. Dis.* **2018**, *12*, e0006130. [CrossRef] [PubMed]

59. Gutiérrez-López, R.; Martínez-de la Puente, J.; Gangoso, L.; Soriguer, R.C.; Figuerola, J. Comparison of manual and semi-automatic DNA extraction protocols for the barcoding characterization of hematophagous louse flies (Diptera: Hippoboscidae). *J. Vector Ecol.* **2015**, *40*, 11–15. [CrossRef] [PubMed]

60. Warton, K.; Graham, L.J.; Yuwono, N.; Samimi, G. Comparison of 4 commercial kits for the extraction of circulating DNA from plasma. *Cancer Genet.* **2018**, in press. [CrossRef] [PubMed]

61. Mathay, C.; Hamot, G.; Henry, E.; Mommaerts, K.; Thorlaksdottir, A.; Trouet, J.; Betsou, F. Method validation for extraction of nucleic acids from peripheral whole blood. *Biopreserv. Biobank.* **2016**, *14*, 520–529. [CrossRef] [PubMed]

62. Kang, S.H.; Lee, E.H.; Park, G.; Jang, S.J.; Moon, D.S. Comparison of MagNA Pure 96, Chemagic MSM1, and QIAamp MinElute for hepatitis B virus nucleic acid extraction. *Ann. Clin. Lab. Sci.* **2012**, *42*, 370–374. [PubMed]

63. Lee, J.H.; Park, Y.; Choi, J.R.; Lee, E.K.; Kim, H.S. Comparisons of three automated systems for genomic DNA extraction in a clinical diagnostic laboratory. *Yonsei Med. J.* **2010**, *51*, 104–110. [CrossRef] [PubMed]

64. Schunk, M.; Kebede Mekonnen, S.; Wondafrash, B.; Mengele, C.; Fleischmann, E.; Herbinger, K.H.; Verweij, J.J.; Geldmacher, C.; Bretzel, G.; Löscher, T.; et al. Use of occult blood detection cards for real-time PCR-based diagnosis of *Schistosoma mansoni* infection. *PLoS ONE* **2015**, *10*, e0137730. [CrossRef] [PubMed]

65. Lodh, N.; Mikita, K.; Bosompem, K.M.; Anyan, W.K.; Quartey, J.K.; Otchere, J.; Shiff, C.J. Point of care diagnosis of multiple schistosome parasites: Species-specific DNA detection in urine by loop-mediated isothermal amplification (LAMP). *Acta Trop.* **2017**, *173*, 125–129. [CrossRef] [PubMed]

66. Zainabadi, K.; Adams, M.; Han, Z.Y.; Lwin, H.W.; Han, K.T.; Ouattara, A.; Thura, S.; Plowe, C.V.; Nyunt, M.M. A novel method for extracting nucleic acids from dried blood spots for ultrasensitive detection of low-density *Plasmodium falciparum* and *Plasmodium vivax* infections. *Malar. J.* **2017**, *16*, 377. [CrossRef] [PubMed]

67. Fung, M.S.; Xiao, N.; Wang, S.; Carlton, E.J. Field evaluation of a PCR test for *Schistosoma japonicum* egg detection in low-prevalence regions of China. *Am. J. Trop. Med. Hyg.* **2012**, *87*, 1053–1058. [CrossRef] [PubMed]

68. Moreira, O.C.; Verly, T.; Finamore-Araujo, P.; Gomes, S.A.O.; Lopes, C.M.; de Sousa, D.M.; Azevedo, L.R.; da Mota, F.F.; D'Avila-Levy, C.M.; Santos-Mallet, J.R.; et al. Development of conventional and real-time multiplex PCR-based assays for estimation of natural infection rates and *Trypanosoma cruzi* load in triatomine vectors. *Parasit. Vectors* **2017**, *10*, 404. [CrossRef] [PubMed]

69. Sandoval, N.; Siles-Lucas, M.; Pérez-Arellano, J.L.; Carranza, C.; Puente, S.; López-Abán, J.; Muro, A. A new PCR-based approach for the specific amplification of DNA from different *Schistosoma* species applicable to human urine samples. *Parasitology* **2006**, *133*, 581–587. [CrossRef] [PubMed]

70. Oliveira, L.M.A.; Santos, H.L.C.; Gonçalves, M.M.L.; Barreto, M.G.M.; Peralta, J.M. Evaluation of polymerase chain reaction as an additional tool for the diagnosis of low-intensity *Schistosoma mansoni* infection. *Diagn. Microbiol. Infect. Dis.* **2010**, *68*, 416–421. [CrossRef] [PubMed]

71. Gomes, L.I.; Dos Santos Marques, L.H.; Enk, M.J.; de Oliveira, M.C.; Coelho, P.M.Z.; Rabello, A. Development and evaluation of a sensitive PCR-ELISA system for detection of *Schistosoma* infection in feces. *PLoS Negl. Trop. Dis.* **2010**, *4*, e664. [CrossRef] [PubMed]

72. Sørensen, E.; Bøgh, H.O.; Johansen, M.V.; McManus, D.P. PCR-based identification of individuals of *Schistosoma japonicum* representing different subpopulations using a genetic marker in mitochondrial DNA. *Int. J. Parasitol.* **1999**, *29*, 1121–1128. [CrossRef]

73. Mikaeili, F.; Mathis, A.; Deplazes, P.; Mirhendi, H.; Barazesh, A.; Ebrahimi, S.; Kia, E.B. Differentiation of *Toxocara canis* and *Toxocara cati* based on PCR-RFLP analyses of rDNA-ITS and mitochondrial *cox1* and *nad1* regions. *Acta Parasitol.* **2017**, *62*, 549–556. [CrossRef] [PubMed]

74. González, L.M.; Montero, E.; Morakote, N.; Puente, S.; Díaz De Tuesta, J.L.; Serra, T.; López-Velez, R.; McManus, D.P.; Harrison, L.J.S.; Parkhouse, R.M.E.; et al. Differential diagnosis of *Taenia saginata* and *Taenia saginata asiatica* taeniasis through PCR. *Diagn. Microbiol. Infect. Dis.* **2004**, *49*, 183–188. [CrossRef] [PubMed]

75. Caldeira, R.L.; Teodoro, T.M.; Jannotti-Passos, L.K.; Lira-Moreira, P.M.; Goveia, C.D.O.; Carvalho, O.D.S. Characterization of South American snails of the genus *Biomphalaria* (Basommatophora: Planorbidae) and *Schistosoma mansoni* (Platyhelminthes: Trematoda) in molluscs by PCR-RFLP. *BioMed Res. Int.* **2016**, *2016*, 1045391. [CrossRef] [PubMed]

76. Gray, D.J.; Ross, A.G.; Li, Y.S.; McManus, D.P. Diagnosis and management of schistosomiasis. *BMJ* **2011**, *342*, d2651. [CrossRef] [PubMed]

77. Gomes, A.L.D.V.; Melo, F.L.; Werkhauser, R.P.; Abath, F.G.C. Development of a real time polymerase chain reaction for quantitation of *Schistosoma mansoni* DNA. *Mem. Inst. Oswaldo Cruz* **2006**, *101* (Suppl. 1), 133–136. [CrossRef] [PubMed]

78. Pillay, P.; Taylor, M.; Zulu, S.G.; Gundersen, S.G.; Verweij, J.J.; Hoekstra, P.; Brienen, E.A.T.; Kleppa, E.; Kjetland, E.F.; van Lieshout, L. Real-time polymerase chain reaction for detection of *Schistosoma* DNA in small-volume urine samples reflects focal distribution of urogenital schistosomiasis in primary school girls in KwaZulu-Natal, South Africa. *Am. J. Trop. Med. Hyg.* **2014**, *90*, 546–552. [CrossRef] [PubMed]

79. Easton, A.V.; Oliveira, R.G.; O'Connell, E.M.; Kepha, S.; Mwandawiro, C.S.; Njenga, S.M.; Kihara, J.H.; Mwatele, C.; Odiere, M.R.; Brooker, S.J.; et al. Multi-parallel qPCR provides increased sensitivity and diagnostic breadth for gastrointestinal parasites of humans: Field-based inferences on the impact of mass deworming. *Parasit. Vectors* **2016**, *9*, 38. [CrossRef] [PubMed]

80. Mejia, R.; Vicuña, Y.; Broncano, N.; Sandoval, C.; Vaca, M.; Chico, M.; Cooper, P.J.; Nutman, T.B. A novel, multi-parallel, real-time polymerase chain reaction approach for eight gastrointestinal parasites provides improved diagnostic capabilities to resource-limited at-risk populations. *Am. J. Trop. Med. Hyg.* **2013**, *88*, 1041–1047. [CrossRef] [PubMed]

81. Cimino, R.O.; Jeun, R.; Juarez, M.; Cajal, P.S.; Vargas, P.; Echazú, A.; Bryan, P.E.; Nasser, J.; Krolewiecki, A.; Mejia, R. Identification of human intestinal parasites affecting an asymptomatic peri-urban Argentinian population using multi-parallel quantitative real-time polymerase chain reaction. *Parasit. Vectors* **2015**, *8*, 380. [CrossRef] [PubMed]

82. Pilotte, N.; Papaiakovou, M.; Grant, J.R.; Bierwert, L.A.; Llewellyn, S.; McCarthy, J.S.; Williams, S.A. Improved PCR-based detection of soil transmitted helminth infections using a next-generation sequencing approach to assay design. *PLoS Negl. Trop. Dis.* **2016**, *10*, e0004578. [CrossRef] [PubMed]

83. Sady, H.; Al-Mekhlafi, H.M.; Ngui, R.; Atroosh, W.M.; Al-Delaimy, A.K.; Nasr, N.A.; Dawaki, S.; Abdulsalam, A.M.; Ithoi, I.; Lim, Y.A.L.; et al. Detection of *Schistosoma mansoni* and *Schistosoma haematobium* by real-time PCR with high resolution melting analysis. *Int. J. Mol. Sci.* **2015**, *16*, 16085–16103. [CrossRef] [PubMed]

84. Tomita, N.; Mori, Y.; Kanda, H.; Notomi, T. Loop-mediated isothermal amplification (LAMP) of gene sequences and simple visual detection of products. *Nat. Protoc.* **2012**, *3*, 877–882. [CrossRef] [PubMed]

85. Notomi, T.; Okayama, H.; Masubuchi, H.; Yonekawa, T.; Watanabe, K.; Amino, N.; Hase, T. Loop-mediated isothermal amplification of DNA. *Nucleic Acids Res.* **2000**, *28*, E63. [CrossRef] [PubMed]

86. Xu, J.; Rong, R.; Zhang, H.Q.; Shi, C.J.; Zhu, X.Q.; Xia, C.M. Sensitive and rapid detection of *Schistosoma japonicum* DNA by loop-mediated isothermal amplification (LAMP). *Int. J. Parasitol.* **2010**, *40*, 327–331. [CrossRef] [PubMed]

87. Hsieh, K.; Mage, P.L.; Csordas, A.T.; Eisenstein, M.; Soh, H.T. Simultaneous elimination of carryover contamination and detection of DNA with uracil-DNA-glycosylase-supplemented loop-mediated isothermal amplification (UDG-LAMP). *Chem. Commun. (Camb.)* **2014**, *50*, 3747–3749. [CrossRef] [PubMed]

88. Ma, C.; Wang, F.; Wang, X.; Han, L.; Jing, H.; Zhang, H.; Shi, C. A novel method to control carryover contamination in isothermal nucleic acid amplification. *Chem. Commun. (Camb.)* **2017**, *53*, 10696–10699. [CrossRef] [PubMed]

89. Fernández-Soto, P.; Gandasegui Arahuetes, J.; Sánchez Hernández, A.; López Abán, J.; Vicente Santiago, B.; Muro, A. A loop-mediated isothermal amplification (LAMP) assay for early detection of *Schistosoma mansoni* in stool samples: A diagnostic approach in a murine model. *PLoS Negl. Trop. Dis.* **2014**, *8*, e3126. [CrossRef] [PubMed]

90. Nyan, D.C.; Swinson, K.L. A novel multiplex isothermal amplification method for rapid detection and identification of viruses. *Sci. Rep.* **2015**, *5*, 17925. [CrossRef] [PubMed]

91. Liu, N.; Zou, D.; Dong, D.; Yang, Z.; Ao, D.; Liu, W.; Huang, L. Development of a multiplex loop-mediated isothermal amplification method for the simultaneous detection of *Salmonella* spp. and *Vibrio parahaemolyticus*. *Sci. Rep.* **2017**, *7*, 45601. [CrossRef] [PubMed]

92. Llewellyn, S.; Inpankaew, T.; Nery, S.V.; Gray, D.J.; Verweij, J.J.; Clements, A.C.A.; Gomes, S.J.; Traub, R.; McCarthy, J.S. Application of a multiplex quantitative PCR to assess prevalence and intensity of intestinal parasite infections in a controlled clinical trial. *PLoS Negl. Trop. Dis.* **2016**, *10*, e0004380. [CrossRef] [PubMed]

93. Gordon, C.A.; McManus, D.P.; Acosta, L.P.; Olveda, R.M.; Williams, G.M.; Ross, A.G.; Gray, D.J.; Gobert, G.N. Multiplex real-time PCR monitoring of intestinal helminths in humans reveals widespread polyparasitism in Northern Samar, the Philippines. *Int. J. Parasitol.* **2015**, *45*, 477–483. [CrossRef] [PubMed]

94. Haque, R.; Roy, S.; Siddique, A.; Mondal, U.; Rahman, S.M.M.; Mondal, D.; Houpt, E.; Petri, W.A. Multiplex real-time PCR assay for detection of *Entamoeba histolytica*, *Giardia intestinalis*, and *Cryptosporidium* spp. *Am. J. Trop. Med. Hyg.* **2007**, *76*, 713–717. [PubMed]

95. Piepenburg, O.; Williams, C.H.; Stemple, D.L.; Armes, N.A. DNA detection using recombination proteins. *PLoS Biol.* **2006**, *4*, e204. [CrossRef] [PubMed]

96. Zanoli, L.M.; Spoto, G. Isothermal amplification methods for the detection of nucleic acids in microfluidic devices. *Biosensors* **2013**, *3*, 18–43. [CrossRef] [PubMed]

97. Yang, R.; Paparini, A.; Monis, P.; Ryan, U. Comparison of next-generation droplet digital PCR (ddPCR) with quantitative PCR (qPCR) for enumeration of *Cryptosporidium* oocysts in faecal samples. *Int. J. Parasitol.* **2014**, *44*, 1105–1111. [CrossRef] [PubMed]

98. Sze, M.A.; Abbasi, M.; Hogg, J.C.; Sin, D.D. A Comparison between droplet digital and quantitative PCR in the analysis of bacterial 16S load in lung tissue samples from control and COPD GOLD 2. *PLoS ONE* **2014**, *9*, e110351. [CrossRef] [PubMed]

99. Hindson, C.M.; Chevillet, J.R.; Briggs, H.A.; Gallichotte, E.N.; Ruf, I.K.; Hindson, B.J.; Vessella, R.L.; Tewari, M. Absolute quantification by droplet digital PCR versus analog real-time PCR. *Nat. Methods* **2013**, *10*, 1003–1005. [CrossRef] [PubMed]

100. Manokhina, I.; Singh, T.K.; Peñaherrera, M.S.; Robinson, W.P. Quantification of cell-free DNA in normal and complicated pregnancies: Overcoming biological and technical issues. *PLoS ONE* **2014**, *9*, e101500. [CrossRef] [PubMed]

101. Sedlak, R.H.; Cook, L.; Cheng, A.; Magaret, A.; Jerome, K.R. Clinical utility of droplet digital PCR for human cytomegalovirus. *J. Clin. Microbiol.* **2014**, *52*, 2844–2848. [CrossRef] [PubMed]

102. Olmedillas-López, S.; García-Arranz, M.; García-Olmo, D. Current and emerging applications of droplet digital PCR in Oncology. *Mol. Diagn. Ther.* **2017**, *21*, 493–510. [CrossRef] [PubMed]

103. Hudecova, I. Digital PCR analysis of circulating nucleic acids. *Clin. Biochem.* **2015**, *48*, 948–956. [CrossRef] [PubMed]

104. Hall Sedlak, R.; Jerome, K.R. The potential advantages of digital PCR for clinical virology diagnostics. *Expert Rev. Mol. Diagn.* **2014**, *14*, 501–507. [CrossRef] [PubMed]

105. Jongthawin, J.; Intapan, P.M.; Lulitanond, V.; Sanpool, O.; Thanchomnang, T.; Sadaow, L.; Maleewong, W. Detection and quantification of *Wuchereria bancrofti* and *Brugia malayi* DNA in blood samples and mosquitoes using duplex droplet digital polymerase chain reaction. *Parasitol. Res.* **2016**, *115*, 2967–2972. [CrossRef] [PubMed]

106. Srisutham, S.; Saralamba, N.; Malleret, B.; Rénia, L.; Dondorp, A.M.; Imwong, M. Four human *Plasmodium* species quantification using droplet digital PCR. *PLoS ONE* **2017**, *12*, e0175771. [CrossRef] [PubMed]

107. Hall, D.E.; Roy, R. An evaluation of direct PCR amplification. *Croat. Med. J.* **2014**, *55*, 655–661. [CrossRef] [PubMed]

108. Chin, W.H.; Sun, Y.; Høgberg, J.; Quyen, T.L.; Engelsmann, P.; Wolff, A.; Bang, D.D. Direct PCR—A rapid method for multiplexed detection of different serotypes of *Salmonella* in enriched pork meat samples. *Mol. Cell. Probes* **2017**, *32*, 24–32. [CrossRef] [PubMed]

109. Silbermayr, K.; Eigner, B.; Duscher, G.G.; Joachim, A.; Fuehrer, H.-P. The detection of different *Dirofilaria* species using direct PCR technique. *Parasitol. Res.* **2014**, *113*, 513–516. [CrossRef] [PubMed]

110. Echeverry, D.F.; Deason, N.A.; Davidson, J.; Makuru, V.; Xiao, H.; Niedbalski, J.; Kern, M.; Russell, T.L.; Burkot, T.R.; Collins, F.H.; et al. Human malaria diagnosis using a single-step direct-PCR based on the *Plasmodium* cytochrome oxidase III gene. *Malar. J.* **2016**, *15*, 128. [CrossRef] [PubMed]

111. Wichmann, D.; Poppert, S.; Von Thien, H.; Clerinx, J.; Dieckmann, S.; Jensenius, M.; Parola, P.; Richter, J.; Schunk, M.; Stich, A.; et al. Prospective European-wide multicentre study on a blood based real-time PCR for the diagnosis of acute schistosomiasis. *BMC Infect. Dis.* **2013**, *13*, 55. [CrossRef] [PubMed]

112. Wichmann, D.; Panning, M.; Quack, T.; Kramme, S.; Burchard, G.-D.; Grevelding, C.; Drosten, C. Diagnosing schistosomiasis by detection of cell-free parasite DNA in human plasma. *PLoS Negl. Trop. Dis.* **2009**, *3*, e422. [CrossRef] [PubMed]

113. Xu, J.; Liu, A.; Guo, J.; Wang, B.; Qiu, S.J.; Sun, H.; Guan, W.; Zhu, X.Q.; Xia, C.M.; Wu, Z.D. The sources and metabolic dynamics of *Schistosoma japonicum* DNA in serum of the host. *Parasitol. Res.* **2013**, *112*, 129–133. [CrossRef] [PubMed]

114. Weerakoon, K.G.; McManus, D.P. Cell-Free DNA as a diagnostic tool for human parasitic infections. *Trends Parasitol.* **2016**, *32*, 378–391. [CrossRef] [PubMed]

115. Suzuki, T.; Osada, Y.; Kumagai, T.; Hamada, A.; Okuzawa, E.; Kanazawa, T. Early detection of *Schistosoma mansoni* infection by touchdown PCR in a mouse model. *Parasitol. Int.* **2006**, *55*, 213–218. [CrossRef] [PubMed]

116. Xia, C.-M.; Rong, R.; Lu, Z.-X.; Shi, C.-J.; Xu, J.; Zhang, H.-Q.; Gong, W.; Luo, W. *Schistosoma japonicum*: A PCR assay for the early detection and evaluation of treatment in a rabbit model. *Exp. Parasitol.* **2009**, *121*, 175–179. [CrossRef] [PubMed]

117. Kato-Hayashi, N.; Kirinoki, M.; Iwamura, Y.; Kanazawa, T.; Kitikoon, V.; Matsuda, H.; Chigusa, Y. Identification and differentiation of human schistosomes by polymerase chain reaction. *Exp. Parasitol.* **2010**, *124*, 325–329. [CrossRef] [PubMed]

118. Kato-Hayashi, N.; Yasuda, M.; Yuasa, J.; Isaka, S.; Haruki, K.; Ohmae, H.; Osada, Y.; Kanazawa, T.; Chigusa, Y. Use of cell-free circulating schistosome DNA in serum, urine, semen, and saliva to monitor a case of refractory imported schistosomiasis hematobia. *J. Clin. Microbiol.* **2013**, *51*, 3435–3438. [CrossRef] [PubMed]

119. Kato-Hayashi, N.; Leonardo, L.R.; Arevalo, N.L.; Tagum, M.N.B.; Apin, J.; Agsolid, L.M.; Chua, J.C.; Villacorte, E.A.; Kirinoki, M.; Kikuchi, M.; et al. Detection of active schistosome infection by cell-free circulating DNA of *Schistosoma japonicum* in highly endemic areas in Sorsogon Province, the Philippines. *Acta Trop.* **2015**, *141*, 178–183. [CrossRef] [PubMed]

120. Härter, G.; Frickmann, H.; Zenk, S.; Wichmann, D.; Ammann, B.; Kern, P.; Fleischer, B.; Tannich, E.; Poppert, S. Diagnosis of neuroschistosomiasis by antibody specificity index and semi-quantitative real-time PCR from cerebrospinal fluid and serum. *J. Med. Microbiol.* **2014**, *63*, 309–312. [CrossRef] [PubMed]

121. Kincaid-Smith, J.; Rey, O.; Toulza, E.; Berry, A.; Boissier, J. Emerging schistosomiasis in Europe: A need to quantify the risks. *Trends Parasitol.* **2017**, *33*, 600–609. [CrossRef] [PubMed]

122. Leblanc, C.; Pham, L.L.; Mariani, P.; Titomanlio, L.; El Ghoneimi, A.; Paris, L.; Escoda, S.; Lottmann, H.; Toubiana, J.; Paugam, A.; et al. Imported schistosomiasis in children: Clinical, diagnostic aspects and outcome in 5 tertiary hospitals in France. *Pediatr. Infect. Dis. J.* **2017**, *36*, e349–e351. [CrossRef] [PubMed]

123. Olveda, D.U.; Li, Y.; Olveda, R.M.; Lam, A.K.; McManus, D.P.; Chau, T.N.P.; Harn, D.A.; Williams, G.M.; Gray, D.J.; Ross, A.G.P. Bilharzia in the Philippines: Past, present, and future. *Int. J. Infect. Dis.* **2014**, *18*, 52–56. [CrossRef] [PubMed]

124. Cao, Z.G.; Zhao, Y.E.; Lee Willingham, A.; Wang, T.P. Towards the elimination of schistosomiasis japonica through control of the disease in domestic animals in the People's Republic of China: A tale of over 60 years. *Adv. Parasitol.* **2016**, *92*, 269–306. [PubMed]

125. Wu, H.W.; Qin, Y.F.; Chu, K.; Meng, R.; Liu, Y.; McGarvey, S.T.; Olveda, R.; Acosta, L.; Ji, M.-J.; Fernandez, T.; et al. High prevalence of *Schistosoma japonicum* infection in water buffaloes in the Philippines assessed by real-time polymerase chain reaction. *Am. J. Trop. Med. Hyg.* **2010**, *82*, 646–652. [CrossRef] [PubMed]

126. Hamburger, J.; Hoffman, O.; Kariuki, H.C.; Muchiri, E.M.; Ouma, J.H.; Koech, D.K.; Sturrock, R.F.; King, C.H. Large-scale, polymerase chain reaction-based surveillance of *Schistosoma haematobium* DNA in snails from transmission sites in coastal Kenya: A new tool for studying the dynamics of snail infection. *Am. J. Trop. Med. Hyg.* **2004**, *71*, 765–773. [PubMed]

127. King, C.H.; Sturrock, R.F.; Kariuki, H.C.; Hamburger, J. Transmission control for schistosomiasis—Why it matters now. *Trends Parasitol.* **2006**, *22*, 575–582. [CrossRef] [PubMed]

128. Amarir, F.; Sebti, F.; Abbasi, I.; Sadak, A.; Fellah, H.; Nhammi, H.; Ameur, B.; El Idrissi, A.L.; Rhajaoui, M. *Schistosoma haematobium* detection in snails by *DraI* PCR and *Sh110/Sm-Sl* PCR: Further evidence of the interruption of schistosomiasis transmission in Morocco. *Parasit. Vectors* **2014**, *7*, 288. [CrossRef] [PubMed]

129. Tanaka, H.; Tsuji, M. From discovery to eradication of schistosomiasis in Japan: 1847–1996. *Int. J. Parasitol.* **1997**, *27*, 1465–1480. [CrossRef]

130. Abbasi, I.; King, C.H.; Muchiri, E.M.; Hamburger, J. Detection of *Schistosoma mansoni* and *Schistosoma haematobium* DNA by loop-mediated isothermal amplification: Identification of infected snails from early prepatency. *Am. J. Trop. Med. Hyg.* **2010**, *83*, 427–432. [CrossRef] [PubMed]

131. Abath, F.G.C.; Gomes, A.L.D.V.; Melo, F.L.; Barbosa, C.S.; Werkhauser, R.P. Molecular approaches for the detection of *Schistosoma mansoni*: Possible applications in the detection of snail infection, monitoring of transmission sites, and diagnosis of human infection. *Mem. Inst. Oswaldo Cruz* **2006**, *101* (Suppl. 1), 145–148. [CrossRef] [PubMed]

132. Melo, F.L.; Gomes, A.L.D.V.; Barbosa, C.S.; Werkhauser, R.P.; Abath, F.G.C. Development of molecular approaches for the identification of transmission sites of schistosomiasis. *Trans. R. Soc. Trop. Med. Hyg.* **2006**, *100*, 1049–1055. [CrossRef] [PubMed]

133. Caldeira, R.L.; Jannotti-Passos, L.K.; Dos Santos Carvalho, O. Use of molecular methods for the rapid mass detection of *Schistosoma mansoni* (Platyhelminthes: Trematoda) in *Biomphalaria* spp. (Gastropoda: Planorbidae). *J. Trop. Med.* **2017**, *2017*, 8628971. [CrossRef] [PubMed]

134. Gandasegui, J.; Fernández-Soto, P.; Hernández-Goenaga, J.; López-Abán, J.; Vicente, B.; Muro, A. Biompha-LAMP: A new rapid loop-mediated isothermal amplification assay for detecting *Schistosoma mansoni* in *Biomphalaria glabrata* snail host. *PLoS Negl. Trop. Dis.* **2016**, *10*, e0005225. [CrossRef] [PubMed]

135. Tong, Q.; Chen, R.; Zhang, Y.; Yang, G.-J.; Kumagai, T.; Furushima-Shimogawara, R.; Lou, D.; Yang, K.; Wen, L.; Lu, S.; et al. A new surveillance and response tool: Risk map of infected *Oncomelania hupensis* detected by loop-mediated isothermal amplification (LAMP) from pooled samples. *Acta Trop.* **2015**, *141*, 170–177. [CrossRef] [PubMed]

136. Jannotti-Passos, L.K.; Magalhães, K.G.; Carvalho, O.S.; Vidigal, T.H.D.A. Multiplex PCR for both identification of Brazilian *Biomphalaria* species (Gastropoda: Planorbidae) and diagnosis of infection by *Schistosoma mansoni* (Trematoda: Schistosomatidae). *J. Parasitol.* **2006**, *92*, 401–403. [CrossRef] [PubMed]

137. Muhoho, N.D.; Katsumata, T.; Kimura, E.; Migwi, D.K.; Mutua, W.R.; Kiliku, F.M.; Habe, S.; Aoki, Y. Cercarial density in the river of an endemic area of schistosomiasis haematobia in Kenya. *Am. J. Trop. Med. Hyg.* **1997**, *57*, 162–167. [CrossRef] [PubMed]

138. Aoki, Y.; Sato, K.; Muhoho, N.D.; Noda, S.; Kimura, E. Cercariometry for detection of transmission sites for schistosomiasis. *Parasitol. Int.* **2003**, *52*, 403–408. [CrossRef]

139. Hertel, J.; Kedves, K.; Hassan, A.H.M.; Haberl, B.; Haas, W. Detection of *Schistosoma mansoni* cercariae in plankton samples by PCR. *Acta Trop.* **2004**, *91*, 43–46. [CrossRef] [PubMed]

140. Worrell, C.; Xiao, N.; Vidal, J.E.; Chen, L.; Zhong, B.; Remais, J. Field detection of *Schistosoma japonicum* cercariae in environmental water samples by quantitative PCR. *Appl. Environ. Microbiol.* **2011**, *77*, 2192–2195. [CrossRef] [PubMed]

141. Hung, Y.W.; Remais, J. Quantitative detection of *Schistosoma japonicum* cercariae in water by real-time PCR. *PLoS Negl. Trop. Dis.* **2008**, *2*, e337. [CrossRef] [PubMed]

142. Utzinger, J.; Becker, S.L.; van Lieshout, L.; van Dam, G.J.; Knopp, S. New diagnostic tools in schistosomiasis. *Clin. Microbiol. Infect.* **2015**, *21*, 529–542. [CrossRef] [PubMed]

143. Hawkins, K.R.; Cantera, J.L.; Storey, H.L.; Leader, B.T.; de Los Santos, T. Diagnostic tests to support late-stage control programs for schistosomiasis and soil-transmitted helminthiases. *PLoS Negl. Trop. Dis.* **2016**, *10*, e0004985. [CrossRef] [PubMed]
144. Feldmeier, H.; Poggensee, G. Diagnostic techniques in schistosomiasis control. A review. *Acta Trop.* **1993**, *52*, 205–220. [CrossRef]
145. TchuemTchuenté, L.A. Control of soil-transmitted helminths in sub-Saharan Africa: Diagnosis, drug efficacy concerns and challenges. *Acta Trop.* **2011**, *120* (Suppl 1), S4–S11. [CrossRef] [PubMed]
146. Stothard, J.R.; Stanton, M.C.; Bustinduy, A.L.; Sousa-Figueiredo, J.C.; Van Dam, G.J.; Betson, M.; Waterhouse, D.; Ward, S.; Allan, F.; Hassan, A.A.; et al. Diagnostics for schistosomiasis in Africa and Arabia: A review of present options in control and future needs for elimination. *Parasitology* **2014**, *141*, 1947–1961. [CrossRef] [PubMed]

9

WIPO Re:Search—A Platform for Product-Centered Cross-Sector Partnerships for the Elimination of Schistosomiasis

Callie J. Weber, Joseph Hargan-Calvopiña, Katy M. Graef, Cathyryne K. Manner and Jennifer Dent *

BIO Ventures for Global Health, 2101 Fourth Avenue, Suite 1950, Seattle, WA 98121, USA; cweber@bvgh.org (C.J.W.); jhargan@bvgh.org (J.H.-C.); kgraef@bvgh.org (K.M.G.); cmanner@bvgh.org (C.K.M.)
* Correspondence: jdent@bvgh.org

Abstract: Schistosomiasis is an acute and chronic disease that affects over 200 million people worldwide, and with over 700 million people estimated to be at risk of contracting this disease, it is a pressing issue in global health. However, research and development (R&D) to develop new approaches to preventing, diagnosing, and treating schistosomiasis has been relatively limited. Praziquantel, a drug developed in the 1970s, is the only agent used in schistosomiasis mass drug administration (MDA) campaigns, indicating a critical need for a diversified therapeutic pipeline. Further, gaps in the vaccine and diagnostic pipelines demonstrate a need for early-stage innovation in all areas of schistosomiasis product R&D. As a platform for public-private partnerships (PPPs), the WIPO Re:Search consortium engages the private sector in early-stage R&D for neglected diseases by forging mutually beneficial collaborations and facilitating the sharing of intellectual property (IP) assets between the for-profit and academic/non-profit sectors. The Consortium connects people, resources, and ideas to fill gaps in neglected disease product development pipelines by leveraging the strengths of these two sectors. Using WIPO Re:Search as an example, this article highlights the opportunities for the PPP model to play a key role in the elimination of schistosomiasis.

Keywords: schistosomiasis; neglected tropical diseases; WIPO Re:Search; BIO Ventures for Global Health; cross-sector collaboration; capacity-building; drug discovery; public-private partnerships

1. The Multifaceted Impact of Schistosomiasis

Schistosomiasis is an acute and chronic disease that affects an estimated 219 million people worldwide [1] and results from infection by parasitic trematode worms of the genus *Schistosoma*. Initial infection occurs when humans come into contact with parasite-infested water sources, and the free-swimming larvae of the parasite, the cercariae, penetrate the skin and migrate into the blood in order to mature. Once inside the circulatory system, these juvenile worms mature into the adult stage [2]. In a study conducted by Warren K.S et al. on Yemeni agricultural workers, it was estimated that in the case of *S. mansoni*, adult worms can have a mean lifespan of five to ten years [3,4] and in some cases have been shown to live as long as 40 years [3,5]. While inside the host, the adult worms are capable of reproducing and laying eggs throughout their lifetimes, leading to a state of chronic infection for the host that, depending on the species, can result in symptoms such as abdominal pain, diarrhea, hepatosplenic inflammation, liver fibrosis, and rectal bleeding (*S. mansoni*, *S. japonicum*, and *S. mekongi*), or obstructive disease in the urinary system, haematuria, chronic fibrosis of the urinary tract, and potentially renal dysfunction (*S. haematobium*). In addition to these species-specific symptoms, all species of *Schistosoma* have been associated with co-morbidities such as anemia [4,6].

Schistosomiasis is endemic in 78 countries, 42 of which are in the World Health Organization (WHO) African Region [7]. It is estimated that over 700 million people are at risk of contracting schistosomiasis worldwide and over 200 million people are currently infected, making this a pressing issue in global health [8]. There are six species of *Schistosoma* that are largely responsible for human infection. *S. japonicum* occurs only in Asia and *S. mansoni* occurs in sub-Saharan Africa, the Middle East, South America, and the Caribbean; these two species are responsible for intestinal schistosomiasis. *S. mekongi* is primarily restricted to Laos and Cambodia [9], whereas *S. haematobium* occurs predominantly in Africa and the Middle East [4] and leads to various urogenital clinical presentations that include urinary tract fibrosis, obstructive renal failure, and squamous cell carcinoma (SCC) of the bladder [10,11]. The less common *S. intercalatum* [12] and *S. guineensis* live in the rectal veins and are also known to cause disease [13].

Due to the disabling systemic morbidities associated with schistosomiasis, such as anemia, malnutrition, and impaired childhood development [14], it is estimated that 18.3 age-standardized disability adjusted life years (DALYs) per 100,000 population were lost to schistosomiasis for both males and females in 2017 [15]. This not only places an enormous burden on healthcare systems in endemic countries, but also interferes with economic productivity due to the reduced ability of the affected population to perform physical activities and participate in the workforce [14,16,17]. In addition to the considerable impact schistosomiasis has on adult and working populations, it is also important to consider its long-term impacts on the next generation. Schistosomiasis has been associated with reduced functional scores and malnutrition [18]. This can severely affect a child's ability [19–21] to become educated [22], lead a productive life [21,22], and break out of the vicious cycle of disease-related poverty.

A growing threat to people living in *S. haematobium*-endemic countries is schistosomiasis-associated SCC of the bladder [23]. This disease is thought to be caused by the inflammatory reaction triggered by schistosomal eggs deposited in the bladder [24]. Eggs are typically excreted through urination but can remain lodged in the patient's bladder. The continued exposure to antigen-releasing eggs during the long lifespan of the adult schistosome [25], and the resulting chronic inflammation and augmented cellular proliferation [4,11,26], increase the likelihood of SCC of the urinary bladder [27], which is estimated to occur at a rate of three to four cases per 100,000 [28]. *S. haematobium* is classified as a carcinogenic agent to humans by the International Agency for Research on Cancer (IARC) [29], and thus it is of high priority to develop more efficacious drugs and better diagnostics to stop acute schistosomiasis from leading to other severe and non-reversible bladder pathologies such as cancer. When treated with praziquantel (PZQ), which is the only approved drug for schistosomiasis, pathological lesions present in the urinary tract are eliminated, indicating that the high cost of caring for patients with schistosomiasis-induced bladder cancer can be avoided by addressing schistosomiasis at an early stage [30]. For the purpose of their studies, Botelho et al. estimated that the current annual treatment cost of PZQ per schistosomiasis patient is $0.16 USD, or approximately $17.92 million USD globally [31]. By not addressing schistosomiasis infection at an early stage, it is estimated that *S. haematobium*-associated bladder cancer results in additional treatment costs of at least $20 million USD per year worldwide [31]. These numbers demonstrate the economic benefits that can result from the development of more efficacious drugs that target this disease.

S. haematobium infection has also been shown to be disproportionately detrimental to women's reproductive and sexual health [32]. Infection-associated genital tract damage can lead to infertility [33], stress incontinence, ectopic pregnancy, increased risk of abortion [4], adverse birth outcomes such as low birth weight, and increased infant and maternal mortality [34]. Further, in multiple population-based studies, *S. haematobium* infection has been linked to an increase in HIV infection in women [35,36], with evidence showing that CD4-positive cells in peripheral blood express increased concentrations of HIV co-receptors [37]. This data implies that cells from patients infected by schistosomiasis may be more susceptible to HIV-1 infection.

Although *S. haematobium* has been known to primarily affect the urinary tract, studies have also shown that in males, *S. haematobium* eggs are found in the seminal vesicles and prostate [38]. In a community-based study of genital schistosomiasis in men from Madagascar, *S. haematobium* eggs were detected in 43% of the semen samples, providing preliminary evidence that male genital organs can also be affected by schistosomiasis [39]. The authors of the study hypothesized that egg deposition in a male's genital organs could potentially lead to an increased accumulation of lymphocytes, eosinophils, and other white cells, which in turn could increase the viral load in semen from males infected with HIV. Along these lines, other population-based studies demonstrated that schistosomiasis has been linked to an increase in HIV infection due to increased concentrations of CD4-positive cells in semen of men with schistosomiasis compared to men who had been cleared of the infection [40]. By successfully detecting and treating schistosomiasis, the global health community is not only removing the burden of this debilitating disease from the population, but also reducing the chances of people suffering from other high-mortality co-morbidities such as HIV.

According to the 5th Progress Report on the London Declaration on Neglected Tropical Diseases (NTDs) [41], the WHO has set a goal of 75% of at-risk populations covered by schistosomiasis control efforts. Regrettably, there has been very little measurable progress made towards elimination [41]. Although strong evidence suggests that PZQ targets schistosome voltage-gated calcium channels, leading to calcium-dependent contraction and paralysis in treated worms [42,43], and the drug has proven to be very useful in controlling morbidity, it is not effective against immature schistosomes [44,45]. Further, it is currently the only drug that is being used in schistosomiasis mass drug administration (MDA) campaigns [46], thus increasing the risk that schistosomes will develop resistance. While it is imperative that new drugs be developed to continue treating infected and at-risk populations, there has not been significant progress in developing alternative treatments since the development of PZQ by Merck KGaA in the 1970s. In fact, due to limited commercial incentives, very little has been done by the for-profit sector in terms of developing new diagnostics, drugs, and vaccines and fueling the early-stage product development pipeline for schistosomiasis. Although these hurdles, among others, currently stand in the way of the elimination of schistosomiasis, the global community is determined to identify solutions through cross-sector partnerships that not only distribute the risk of product development over various stakeholders, but also engage worldwide expertise. While the barriers are high, and the challenge is significant, this article focuses on the incredible efforts being employed in product research and development (R&D) through cross-sector collaborations to make progress toward elimination of schistosomiasis, and the critical roles public-private partnerships (PPPs) play in making that a reality.

2. Limitations of Current Control Efforts and Product Gap Analysis

Current control efforts for schistosomiasis include education programs to promote preventive behavioral and lifestyle changes, such as limiting contact with infected waters, boiling fresh water prior to drinking or bathing, wearing DEET (diethyltoluamide) insect repellent, and implementing vigorous towel drying to prevent parasites from penetrating the skin [47]. However, such preventive strategies focus on decreasing the individual risk of infection, rather than prevention on a large scale. Another approach is to control the host snail population through the administration of effective molluscicides, habitat modification, and biologic control strategies such as introducing competing snail species or natural predators [48]. Despite resulting in high snail mortality, the administration of molluscicides must be replicated twice annually to be effective, and thus is both expensive and (along with habitat modification and biologic control strategies) potentially detrimental to the environment [48]. Concurrent with educational and host snail-targeted interventions, the expansion of the drug, diagnostic, and vaccine development pipelines are crucial to systematically prevent and combat schistosomiasis. These development efforts are the primary focus of this article.

Schistosomiasis is endemic in 78 countries, and mass-scale administration of PZQ is the primary method of both treatment and prevention in all of the affected nations. Since 2012, MDA, or preventive chemotherapy, has been mandated by the governments of 52 endemic countries, covering approximately 250 million people [47].

The MDA movement is rooted in the 2001 World Health Assembly (WHA) resolution calling for the global scale-up of preventive chemotherapy to at-risk population groups for the control of schistosomiasis morbidity [49]. At-risk population groups include school-aged children in endemic areas, adults with occupational risk due to contact with infested waters, and, in many instances, entire communities living in areas with high disease prevalence [47]. In the absence of a preventive vaccine, the annual administration of PZQ is recognized as an accepted schistosomiasis prevention strategy for both children and adults, even during pregnancy and lactation [50]. Further, Merck KGaA and others are reformulating PZQ to develop a pediatric PZQ to expand MDA coverage to include children as young as three to six months old [51]. Efforts to expand the reach of MDA programs to rural communities have received international support, with the objective of reducing schistosomiasis morbidity in school children and funding national control programs that have been widely adopted. For example, in 2012, a five-year grant from the END Fund and Children's Investment Fund Foundation (CIFF) supported the Kenyan government's implementation of a nationwide school-based deworming program that included annual administration of PZQ to all school children in schistosomiasis-endemic areas [52,53]. After just two years, the prevalence of *S. haematobium* fell from 18% to 7.6%, according to a 2014 survey that randomly tested students from 60 schools selected across 16 counties in the Nyanza, Rift Valley, Western, and Coast regions of Kenya [53]. All PZQ distributed through this program was donated by Merck KGaA, which recently committed to donate 250 million tablets of PZQ per year indefinitely to further support global MDA efforts [54,55].

Efforts put forth for MDA programs have not gone unrewarded. In combination with snail-population control efforts, MDA programs have resulted in the WHO declaring that schistosomiasis is no longer a significant public health issue in several countries including Iran, Japan, Jordan, Mauritius, Morocco, Puerto Rico, and Tunisia [47,48].

Despite such successes, MDA programs face significant challenges due to inadequate infrastructure and drug coverage in rural at-risk communities, poor drug compliance, and insufficient monitoring and evaluation [47,56]. A recent WHO publication capturing data from 38 endemic countries reported that 70.9 million school-age children and 18.3 million adults were treated with PZQ for schistosomiasis in 2016, although this only covers 53.7% and 14.3% of at-risk school-age children and adults respectively. The coverage was calculated by dividing the number of children requiring PZQ and treated, by the total number of children in need of PZQ ("WHO 2017 Report on 2016 Treatment of Schistosomiasis") [57].

Even with an unlimited supply, optimal distribution, and high patient compliance in MDA campaigns, PZQ itself has limitations. PZQ was selected as the best treatment option for MDA due to its mild side effects, affordability, single-dose administration, and proven efficacy against every human schistosome species [42,43,58,59]. However, it is important to note that to optimize efficacy, PZQ is recommended to be administered in three 20 mg/kg doses in a single day, but to promote single-dose administration, MDA campaigns supply a single 40 mg/kg daily dose, which contributes to lower treatment efficacy [58]. According to a meta-analysis of 55 published studies, the 40 mg/kg daily dose is justified as a reasonable compromise, although the cure rate varies significantly between species, ranging from 94.7% for *S. japonicum* and 63.5% for mixed *S. haematobium/S. mansoni* infections [60]. Multiple field studies over the last two decades have reported cure rates as low as 52% when administering the recommended 40 mg/kg single dose [56,61,62]. Mild side effects, which include dizziness, nausea, headaches, and diarrhea, further hinder patient compliance [47,56]. In a 2014 tolerability study involving 12,435 participants, incidence of adverse events ranged from 2.3% for urticaria to 31.1% for abdominal pain [60]. This is particularly important to note as children carry most of the schistosomiasis burden and PZQ MDA campaigns often target school-aged children [63]. Additionally, PZQ is not effective against juvenile schistosomes. To ensure parasite clearance and to combat reinfection, repeated treatments are common in endemic areas, although lower efficacy of PZQ is observed in subsequent treatments because surviving juvenile schistosomes experience reduced susceptibility to PZQ as adults [42,62].

Despite its drawbacks, PZQ remains the best available option for both prevention and treatment of schistosomiasis, and thus has global support to improve its access and distribution to all endemic populations. However, this complete reliance on a single drug has raised global concerns about the development of PZQ drug resistance [56,64]. The severity of this issue is compounded by the longevity of MDA programs, which may promote the persistence of drug resistance because reductions in PZQ susceptibility are heritable [43,65]. Adult worms with reduced PZQ susceptibility have been found to have higher basal levels of ABC multidrug transporters, suggesting that they remove PZQ along with metabolic toxins by translocating substrates across the cell membrane [43,62,65]. To combat this, studies suggest that co-administration of ABC multidrug transporter inhibitors with PZQ may restore the efficacy of PZQ against adult *S. mansoni* [43,62,65]. To continue to diversify treatment options beyond monotherapy PZQ, the co-administration of PZQ with artemisinin-based derivatives, such as artemether, artesunate, and dihydroartemisinin, are also being explored and have demonstrated higher efficacy than treatment with PZQ alone [66]. For example, a preclinical study in China found that the combined treatment of PZQ and artemether reduced total *S. japonicum* worm burdens by 79–92% compared to a total worm burden reduction of 28–66% when treated with PZQ alone. The study was conducted in rabbits infected with 7- to 12-day-old schistosomula and 42-day-old adult schistosomes [66]. Because PZQ and artemether target different developmental stages of the parasite (PZQ is only effective against adult-stage *Schistosoma* and artemether acts against juvenile worms), their combined administration targets both developmental stages and demonstrates higher efficacy than monotherapies with either drug [42,66]. However, the high inherent fail rate of PZQ (previously cited at 40%) makes it extremely difficult to accurately measure the efficacy of co-administered treatment regimens or the global prevalence of drug resistance.

Despite more than 30 years of scientific and technological advances, the management of schistosomiasis remains unchanged since the development of PZQ in the early 1970s [58]. There is a need to improve current approaches by developing an integrated and intersectional method to sustainably prevent, diagnose, and treat schistosomiasis [56,61]. An antischistosomal vaccine would halt the overuse of PZQ as both a method of prevention and treatment, limit the geographic spread of schistosomiasis, and reduce the high rates of reinfection. Concurrently, the drug development pipeline must be expanded to include a diversified set of compounds that perturb novel molecular targets of PZQ-resistant parasites and that are active against both adult and immature schistosomes. To permit detection of lower-level infections as disease burden and intensity decrease due to successful interventions, highly sensitive, point-of-care (POC) diagnostics are needed. Accurate diagnostics are required for on-site detection of infection before administering treatment, as well as for certification of parasite clearance to avoid unnecessary and prolonged treatment regimens. This two-pronged diagnostic approach will maximize the efficiency of drug administration and distribution.

3. Product Development Pipelines

3.1. Vaccine Development

Despite increased education and MDA efforts, parasite transmission models predict that, based on the current levels of disease prevalence, the WHO's goal to control schistosomiasis morbidity by 2020 will not be attainable through MDA efforts alone [67]. Incidence rates could be significantly reduced by implementing strategies to prevent initial infection and reinfection. Thus, there is a need for a more permanent method of prevention than mass administration of PZQ. In recognition of this high-need, high-impact development gap, there have been increased efforts toward the development of an antischistosomal vaccine over the past two decades. In a 2013 meeting to develop Preferred Product Characteristics (PPC) for a schistosomiasis vaccine held by the National Institute of Allergy and Infectious Diseases (NIAID), it was agreed that a vaccine should reduce the overall worm burden by at least 75% and reduce egg excretion by close to 75% in order to be considered effective [68].

Currently, there are 10 vaccines in the development pipeline: Five in preclinical; three in Phase I; one in Phase II; and one in Phase III (Table 1) [69–71].

Table 1. Vaccines in development (Phase I-III clinical trials).

Product	Antigen	Phase of Clinical Development [1]	Targeted Species
Bilhvax®	Sh-GST28	Phase III	S. haematobium
Sm-14	Sm-14	Phase II	S. haematobium S. mansoni
Alhydrogel®	Sm-TSP-2	Phase Ib	S. mansoni
Sm-97 paramyosin	Sm-97	Phase I	S. mansoni
Calpain®	Sm-p80	Phase I	S. mansoni

[1] Vaccines in preclinical stages of development are not included.

The French National Institute of Health and Medical Research (INSERM) and Institut Pasteur took Bilhvax® (Sh-GST28; Phase III), a recombinant *S. haematobium* vaccine, through Phase I clinical testing at Lille University Hospital in France and Phase II in Saint-Louis, Senegal [72,73]. Following positive results, Bilhvax® has progressed into Phase III clinical studies, sponsored by INSERM, in the Saint-Louis Region of Senegal as a potential pediatric vaccine candidate against urinary schistosomiasis, with publication of the trial results pending [74].

Sm-14 (Phase II) is being developed in partnership between the Oswaldo Cruz Foundation (FIOCRUZ), the Brazilian governmental financial agency (FINEP), and Alvos Biotecnologia as a vaccine candidate against both *S. mansoni* and *S. haematobium* [72,75]. The Phase I clinical trial was completed in 2014 in Rio de Janeiro, Brazil, and the candidate advanced into Phase II clinical trials in the Saint-Louis Region of Senegal in collaboration with the Infectious Disease Research Institute (IDRI). The Phase II study was completed in June 2017, with publication pending [75,76].

Alhydrogel® (Sm-TSP-2; Phase I), and Sm-97 paramyosin (Phase I), are both recombinant *S. mansoni* vaccines. Alhydrogel® was developed in partnership between the Sabin Vaccine Institute and Texas Children's Hospital Center for Vaccine Development to target intestinal schistosomiasis caused by *S. mansoni* [77,78]. After 18 years of combined efforts, the vaccine is now entering Phase Ib development with continued efforts to be led by the Baylor College of Medicine and Texas Children's Hospital Center for Vaccine Development [77,78]. The ongoing Phase Ib dose-escalating clinical trial, sponsored by the NIAID, is currently in recruitment phase and will be conducted in the *S. mansoni*-endemic area of Americaninhas, Brazil [79].

Calpain® (Sm-p80; Phase I) has been rapidly progressing through the development pipeline due to the targeted efforts of a team of researchers at Texas Tech University, and is poised to enter Phase I clinical trials in 2019 [80]. Sm-p80 is a highly immunodominant antigen in the surface membranes of the worms, and the vaccine works by disrupting the schistosome's mechanisms to evade the host's natural immune response [81]. A recent study demonstrated that Calpain® significantly reduced both the quantity and size of the *S. mansoni* hepatic egg load in vaccinated baboons, and investigators are moving forward to conduct a large-scale double-blinded experiment to validate the vaccine's transmission-blocking potential in baboons [80,81].

Although the vaccine development pipeline is expanding, the established pathway to market is both expensive and time-consuming. At the moment, the majority of pipeline vaccines only target a single species of schistosome (primarily *S. mansoni*). Ideally, the development pipeline would feature a vaccine effective against the infective form of the parasite for all schistosome species found in humans. However, until such a product has been discovered, there is a continued need to expand and diversify the vaccine pipeline to include products targeting immunogenic antigens that are conserved across all species.

3.2. Diagnostic Development

Innovative, effective, and precise diagnostics are particularly important during schistosomiasis elimination, when it is necessary to identify geographic areas where transmission has been interrupted and ensure that the disease is no longer present in the population. Paralleling the vaccine development pipeline, efforts have also been made to improve the accurate diagnosis of schistosomiasis at low levels of infection to best direct and inform key decisions throughout elimination programs: (1) Mapping prevalence—establish a baseline disease prevalence to inform MDA strategy; (2) monitoring the impact of MDA—track disease prevalence; (3) inform reduction/stopping of MDA—determine when morbidity reduction targets have been achieved; (4) post-elimination surveillance—detect the re-emergence of the disease (PATH, Diagnostics for Neglected Tropical Diseases). A single universal diagnostic is unable to inform the entire elimination process, thus there is a need to develop diagnostic tools of varying levels of field implementation and sensitivity to be effectively partnered and applied with each step of schistosome elimination programs (Table 2) [82] (PATH, Diagnostics for Neglected Tropical Diseases).

Table 2. Applications of diagnostic platforms.

Diagnostic Platform	Qualities	Mechanism of Detection	Stage of Elimination Program for Application
Microscopic Detection	Recommended by WHO Low sensitivity: egg shedding is often not observed upon infection or in instances of low infection	Microscopic egg counting from fecal or urine sample	Mapping prevalence
Lateral flow test	Field deployable Minimal training requirements Relatively low cost Incorporating a reader may improve test performance metrics	Antigen detection: indication of active infection	Mapping prevalence Monitoring the impact of MDA Informing reduction/stopping of MDA
		Antibody detection: indication of past or present exposure to disease	Post-elimination surveillance [1]
Molecular Diagnostic Testing	Implementation is limited to a laboratory setting Requires sample preparation Highly sensitive and specific Too expensive for mass distribution Ability for multiplex pathogen detection Rapid turnaround time	Nucleic acid detection: indication of active infection	Informing reduction/stopping of MDA

[1] Antibody-based technology is limited due to its inability to differentiate between ongoing and previous infections, as the detected antibodies remain present even after clearance of parasites. Antibody-based diagnostics have application for post-elimination surveillance by monitoring antibody prevalence in age cohorts that were born after elimination was certified; if antibodies are detected in this youth population, then there has been a re-emergence of the disease [70] (PATH, Diagnostics for Neglected Tropical Diseases).

The below analysis focuses on clinically available diagnostic tests. Currently, the most commonly practiced method of diagnosis for all schistosome species is microscopic evaluation and detection of parasite eggs in human urine or stool, for which WHO recommends a polycarbonate filtration technique or the Kato-Katz (KK) fecal smear, respectively [83–85]. However, the KK technique is not sufficiently sensitive for low-grade infections and has been repeatedly shown to underestimate disease burden in areas where transmission has declined, and egg burdens are low [85]. Further, egg shedding is often not observed during an initial infection or in cases of low-level infection, due to the PZQ-induced sterilization of worm pairs or the survival of single-sex worm populations following PZQ treatment [83]. Following multiple rounds of PZQ MDA, low levels of infection will become more common, and thus new diagnostic tools with higher specificity and sensitivity are needed to ensure the accurate detection of schistosomiasis. For instance, following a very successful MDA program in Morocco, there have been zero reported cases of urogenital schistosomiasis from *S. haematobium* since 2004. However, when testing the efficacy of three newly developed diagnostic methods—two commercially available antibody tests (haemagglutination and enzyme-linked immunosorbent assay [ELISA] formats) and a lateral flow antigen strip—it was found that some citizens remained infected with *S. haematobium* worms that were simply not producing eggs [83]. There is a need to develop and validate monitoring diagnostics to accurately detect the re-emergence of schistosomiasis in areas where previous MDA campaigns have been successful. Moreover, there remains a need for the development of highly sensitive diagnostics to complement MDA programs that often result in lower levels of eggs in order to inform the decisions to stop MDA.

To identify the best technology to fill the need for accurate disease monitoring, recent studies have conducted comparative analyses of available molecular and immunological diagnostic methods that do not rely on egg counting [83,85,86]. ELISAs are able to accurately monitor low-grade infection through the detection of antibodies or antigens and can be adapted for large-scale implementation. Antibody-based technology is limited due to its inability to differentiate between ongoing and previous infections, as the detected antibodies remain present even after the clearance of parasites [86]. However, this may be useful for post-elimination surveillance by monitoring antibody prevalence in age cohorts that were born after elimination was certified; if antibodies are detected in this youth population, then there has been a re-emergence of the disease [82]. An alternative approach is the development of molecular diagnostics to detect *Schistosoma* DNA. Although PCR-based diagnostics have been developed with the ability to detect the four main human *Schistosoma* species with high sensitivity and specificity, PCR technology remains too expensive for mass distribution, and implementation is limited to laboratory settings [86,87]. Although ELISA and PCR technologies have promising features, POC immunodiagnostics have been adopted as the most common alternatives to the KK fecal smear. One of the most promising diagnostics is the POC-CCA developed by Rapid Medical Diagnostics [84]. POC-CCA is a commercially available serological assay that is able to detect *Schistosoma* circulating cathodic antigen (CCA), which is produced by adult schistosomes, in either human blood or urine samples [86]. As CCA is a genus-specific glycan, this method is able to detect active infections caused by the four main species of schistosome that infect humans—excluding urogenital schistosomiasis—and has consistently been identified as a more sensitive substitute for KK when estimating a region's schistosomiasis prevalence [83–86,88]. However, the POC-CCA diagnostic has high rates of false negatives due to frequent trace CCA results on the test strip. In a 2017 comparative study in Brazil, 461 participants donated feces, blood, and urine samples to comparatively map schistosomiasis prevalence using three diagnostic mechanisms, including the KK fecal smear and POC-CCA diagnostic [83]. The POC-CCA method produced the highest proportion of false-negative results and the lowest proportion of true-positive results, thus demonstrating the need for expanding the product development pipeline and continuing sensitivity testing and validation of available immunodiagnostics [83–85].

Through improved access to sequencing technology, the *S. mansoni* genome has been successfully assembled and new secretion proteins from both adult worms and eggs have been identified as new potential diagnostic targets [86]. This presents opportunities for continued development and improvement of multiplex serological assays to simultaneously detect *S. haematobium*, *S. mansoni*, and *S. japonicum*. Continued development of accurate diagnostics will also improve the detection of reduced drug efficacy and the subsequent monitoring of the development of PZQ resistance. To date, the development of new diagnostics for schistosomiasis has been primarily driven by the academic sector, and there is a need to also engage and incentivize the private sector to drive pipeline expansion and product development.

3.3. Drug Development

Due to the widespread dependence on PZQ to combat schistosomiasis, the therapeutic development pipeline is critically limited (Table 3). The only candidate in clinical trials is Co-Arinate FDC®, an artemisinin-based combination therapy (ACT) consisting of artesunate and sulfamethoxypyrazine/pyrimethamin that was developed by Dafra Pharmaceuticals as an antimalarial drug [89]. Due to the high rates of co-infection of malaria and *S. haematobium*, artemisinins have been observed to have unexpected antischistosomal effects, particularly against juvenile parasites [89]. Thus, Co-Arinate FDC® was tested in a Phase III clinical trial to compare its efficacy to that of PZQ against *S. haematobium* in children [90]. Although it has a strong safety profile, Co-Arinate FDC® has only partial efficacy against *S. haematobium*, with a 43.9% cure rate, which was lower than the 53% cure rate observed in patients receiving PZQ [89]. These findings indicate the need for the further exploration of the efficacy of various ACT formulations against *Schistosoma* species. Alternative preclinical and discovery stage therapeutic programs include the repurposing of miltefosine (MFS), which is currently a widely adopted treatment for leishmaniasis, and evaluating the efficacy of thioredoxin glutathione reductase (TGR) inhibitors through high-throughput screening [91,92]. MFS was reported to have significant activity against various stages of *S. mansoni* in in vitro studies, thus spurring further exploration of repurposing that drug for the treatment of schistosomiasis [91]. A 2015 preclinical study reported that delivering MFS in lipid nanocapsules allowed for single-dose oral delivery in mice [91].

Table 3. Therapeutics in development.

Product	Phase of Development	Targeted Species
Co-Arinate FDC®	Phase III	*S. haematobium*
Pediatric PZQ	Preclinical	*S. haematobium* *S. mansoni* *S. japonicum*
Miltefosine (MFS)	Preclinical	*S. mansoni*

To date, the majority of drug development efforts have focused on developing derivatives of PZQ, including the development of a PZQ pediatric formulation and deuterated PZQ analogs [93]. However, to prepare for the risk of widespread drug resistance, there is a critical need for a diversified therapeutic pipeline with novel drug targets.

3.4. Call to Action: Expanding Product Development Pipelines

To effectively combat schistosomiasis on a population-wide basis, intersectional technological innovations—new drugs with novel molecular targets and activity against immature schistosomes; POC diagnostics to detect low-level infections, assess treatment efficacy, and inform treatment decisions; and effective vaccines to prevent initial infection and reinfection—must be developed and made broadly accessible.

With over 700 million people at risk for infection, there is a clear and pressing need to develop new tools that make schistosomiasis elimination a reality. However, since schistosomiasis largely affects the world's poorest populations, consumers are unable to pay high prices for new products. This has resulted in limited commercial incentives to develop innovative vaccines, diagnostics, and drugs for schistosomiasis and other diseases of poverty. To develop new products, companies must make substantial monetary investments during the discovery, preclinical, and clinical stages of development [94], and must bear the risk that the resulting product may not receive U.S. Food and Drug Administration (FDA) approval and may fail to make it to market. In order for a company to remain profitable, its products must generate a margin of profit that returns the initial investments made during R&D. In comparison to "high-incentive" diseases with profitable markets such as cancer, hypercholesterolemia, and other cardiovascular diseases, the profitability of the schistosomiasis market and the socioeconomic status of its customers do not align particularly well with the business models of most pharmaceutical and biotechnology companies, particularly if the companies are expected to shoulder the financial risk and resource-heavy investment associated with de novo product development. Although schistosomiasis is a high-priority disease to the WHO due to the number of people who are currently infected and are at risk for infection, the commercial incentives to invest resources into product development for this disease are low and not compatible with many business models.

Along these lines, a study that profiled the drug and vaccine landscape for neglected diseases between 2000 and 2011 found that out of 850 new registered products, only 4% were indicated for neglected diseases [95], illustrating the massive gaps in product development for neglected diseases. In order to incentivize the private sector and distribute the financial risk associated with bringing a healthcare product to the market for high-priority, low-incentive indications, new product development models have emerged. One such model is the PPP, in which the strengths of the public and private sectors are combined and leveraged to develop breakthrough products while simultaneously redistributing the financial risk involved with product development [96]. An example of a PPP focused on schistosomiasis is the Pediatric Praziquantel Consortium, which is working to develop a pediatric formulation of PZQ for preschool-aged children. The Pediatric Praziquantel Consortium was launched in 2012 by Astellas Pharma, Merck KGaA, the Swiss Tropical and Public Health Institute (TPH), and Lygature. Armed with funding from the Bill & Melinda Gates Foundation and the Global Health Innovative Technology Fund (GHIT), the Consortium identified promising candidates and is currently optimizing its formulation before moving into clinical trials [97]. Having the capabilities for a Phase I-III clinical development program that includes FDA recommendations for pediatric development, the Consortium aims to have its pediatric-specific product available by 2020 [97]. With approximately 25 million preschool-aged children requiring treatment for schistosomiasis [97], the need for a pediatric formulation of PZQ is pressing, but not highly profitable. Through the Pediatric Praziquantel Consortium, the private and public sectors are working together to fill this high-priority product development gap by contributing specific know-how. Merck KGaA is the sponsor of the clinical trials and will be providing support and resources in the areas of preclinical, clinical, manufacturing, regulatory, and access, while Astellas provides advice on clinical development and pharmacokinetic modeling. Scientists from Swiss TPH, as well as other academic institutions, will contribute extensive experience in helminth biological and pharmacological research; epidemiology; and clinical research in endemic regions. Further, by pivoting from the current donation-based PZQ-MDA model towards a more sustainable pricing model, the Pediatric Praziquantel Consortium plans to make the product available on a not-for-profit basis. The Pediatric Praziquantel Consortium is exploring alternative business models and will work with relevant stakeholders to examine ways of providing access to its novel formulation in an affordable manner. This type of partnership demonstrates that, through the sharing of resources and expertise between the private and public sectors, it is possible to develop products for a market that historically has not been highly profitable.

Another type of collaborative model that fits under the umbrella of a PPP is the not-for-profit product development partnership (PDP). PDPs focus on product development and uncoupling the cost of R&D from the price of medicines, thereby resulting in a more affordable product [98]. Many PDPs are also PPPs, as they work with the pharmaceutical industry, academic research institutions, and other not-for-profit organizations. PDPs such as the Drugs for Neglected Diseases *initiative* (DNDi), PATH, Medicines for Malaria Venture (MMV), Global Alliance for Tuberculosis Drug Development (TB Alliance), and the Foundation for Innovative New Diagnostics (FIND) tackle the traditionally high cost of R&D and work to bring new NTD, malaria, and tuberculosis products to the market at affordable prices. In contrast to private industry, which funds its R&D through revenues from marketed products as well as investors, PDPs are supported through various mechanisms that include public funding and philanthropy. This funding mechanism allows PDPs to decouple the price of medicines developed from the cost of R&D. Pharmaceutical companies generally employ cost-based pricing to cover the costs of R&D and to generate a profit. Not only do PDPs keep their costs low through efficient collaborations, and smaller clinical trials [98], but once a product is developed, PDPs are not under pressure to generate high-margin profits to cover development costs. Consequently, PDPs can price products in a manner that can be afforded by those in need. In addition to this, by establishing strong partnerships with private industry, PDPs benefit from access to resources such as compound libraries and the pharmaceutical industry's expertise in getting a product to market. Through this collaborative model, it has been possible to reduce development costs and set prices that can be afforded by low- and middle- income countries (LMICs), thus demonstrating that alternative models for neglected disease R&D are possible [98].

By leveraging world-class infectious disease and biological expertise as well as innovative thinking from various research institutions, and by maximizing the use of the material assets and product development know-how of global pharmaceutical and biotechnology companies, PDPs have made it possible to streamline drug discovery to target diseases of poverty in a coordinated and efficient manner. Not only does this incentivize the sharing of ideas and resources across various sectors as outlined in United Nations Sustainable Development Goal (SDG) 3, but it also successfully addresses SDG 17 by directly engaging the private and public sectors in global partnerships and cooperation. However, due to the limited resources available to support product development for neglected diseases, additional collaborative efforts are needed to fill R&D gaps. Although the Pediatric Praziquantel Consortium is working towards a new pediatric formulation of PZQ, there are currently no PDPs focused on novel schistosomiasis drug discovery, thus necessitating other collaborative models. It is such collaborative agreements and cross-sector-inspired business models that will create a sustainable framework for product development in schistosomiasis and other diseases of poverty.

4. WIPO Re:Search as a Platform for Cross-Sector Collaborations That Accelerate Drug Discovery

New and creative collaborative approaches involving both the for-profit and academic/non-profit sectors are required to catalyze product development for schistosomiasis and other high-priority, low-incentive medical needs. Although many pharmaceutical companies have demonstrated commitment to corporate social responsibility (CSR) through drug donation programs for schistosomiasis and other diseases of poverty, as well as through participation in PDPs and PPPs, additional models that complement those efforts and have a longer-term and more sustainable impact on affected populations are needed. Such models need to not only put in place access plans, so that the resulting products are available to the world's poorest populations (as is done with PDPs), but also continue to drive innovation and product development through alternative frameworks that build the capacity for researchers in endemic countries to jumpstart their own R&D efforts.

One such collaborative model, WIPO Re:Search, was established in 2011 by the World Intellectual Property Organization (WIPO) and BIO Ventures for Global Health (BVGH), and is supported by eight pharmaceutical companies (Eisai Co., Ltd., GlaxoSmithKline, Johnson & Johnson, Merck KGaA, Merck Sharp & Dohme [MSD; known as Merck & Co., Inc. in the U.S. and Canada], Novartis, Pfizer, and Takeda Pharmaceutical Company, Ltd.). WIPO Re:Search is a global initiative that connects people, resources, and ideas across biotechnology and pharmaceutical companies, governments, and non-profits to accelerate drug, diagnostic, and vaccine development for schistosomiasis, other NTDs, malaria, and tuberculosis [99]. WIPO Re:Search operations are supported by the financial contributions of the eight participating companies. While the companies may have internal R&D programs focused on neglected diseases, they have also made commitments to sharing their intellectual property (IP) assets with WIPO Re:Search investigators all over the world, to accelerate the development of novel products that can one day play a critical role in eliminating diseases of poverty. To date, WIPO Re:Search has 140 members in 40 countries across six continents, and has established 140 collaborations, with 14 of them focused on schistosomiasis.

The WIPO Re:Search consortium is a global PPP platform, which, through BVGH's targeted partnering approach, catalyzes product development for neglected diseases. BVGH recruits targeted member organizations based on strategic considerations, which may include the need for additional corporate engagement, specialized subject matter expertise, or other resources such as specific screening assays or animal models. Once an academic/non-profit institution joins the Consortium, BVGH reviews its assets, and identifies and connects with researchers who work on neglected diseases.

The researchers share their partnering interests with BVGH during introductory calls, enabling the identification of potential collaborators with aligned interests. Once mutual interest in collaborating is established, BVGH introduces the parties to each other and coordinates communications between partners to solidify collaboration details, roles, and responsibilities. Once milestones, timelines, deliverables, and action items are developed and agreed upon, the participating organizations execute material transfer agreements (MTAs) or other legal agreements to begin the collaboration. Once an agreement is in place, BVGH provides partnership support and alliance management to help ensure project success.

WIPO Re:Search uses IP sharing to incentivize and promote innovative product development and access in areas that have traditionally yielded low profitability, such as neglected diseases. It is through the sharing of IP assets for neglected disease R&D at no cost to the user organization, and by having members agree to the WIPO Re:Search Guiding Principles (detailed below) [100], that the Consortium promotes the accessibility of the resulting products to populations that are disproportionately affected by those diseases. Each legal agreement is executed in accordance with the Guiding Principles, which state that IP is to be shared on a royalty-free basis for R&D of products, technologies, and services to address public health needs for neglected diseases in least developed countries (LDCs), which are low-income countries currently confronting severe structural impediments to sustainable development that are also highly vulnerable to economic and environmental shocks [101]. Further, the Guiding Principles state that, for any products resulting from WIPO Re:Search collaborations, IP owners agree to provide royalty-free licenses for their use and sale in LDCs. IP owners also agree to consider in good faith the issue of product access for all developing countries. Finally, the institution that is using the shared IP is allowed to retain ownership of any new IP that results from WIPO Re:Search collaborations and is encouraged to share those assets with other members of the Consortium.

Through WIPO Re:Search, the most commonly shared IP assets are pharmaceutical company compounds (both targeted libraries and diversity sets) that have the potential to be repurposed as new drugs for schistosomiasis and other neglected diseases. Compounds provided by pharmaceutical companies may have already undergone preclinical or early-stage clinical testing, thereby reducing the number of experiments that need to be conducted to validate the compounds' safety or metabolic properties. This adds value, as it allows scientists to prioritize compounds with good metabolic and safety data that are more likely to move forward through the drug development pipeline. Alternatively, if a compound has a poor toxicity/safety profile, investigators can save valuable time and resources by focusing their efforts on compounds with better profiles. Further, during the drug development process, pharmaceutical companies synthesize large sets of compounds and structurally similar analogs as inhibitors of human target proteins. Like humans, *Schistosoma* are eukaryotes and thus have similar, yet distinct, cellular targets. Thus, compounds targeting human molecules with weak affinity/activity may have the potential to bind to and inhibit homologous proteins found in parasites such as *Schistosoma*. Such large target-specific compound libraries can be repurposed for schistosomiasis as well as many other diseases. Given that the average time required for a drug to reach the market is 12 years [102], it is important to not only identify ways to reduce the time it takes for that drug to get to market (and potentially the cost of the final product), but also reposition important resources such as compounds, technology platforms, and funding in a way that maximizes the strengths of industry and academic/non-profit scientists.

Since companies are likely to have invested significant time and money in developing compounds that target proteins that are dysregulated in non-communicable diseases such as cancer and hypercholesterolemia, targeting the parasitic homologs of those human proteins can be especially promising for neglected disease drug discovery. The key is to identify homologous target proteins that are essential to the survival of the parasite, and pharmaceutical compounds with biological activity against those homologous targets. One of the earliest schistosomiasis-related collaborations established through WIPO Re:Search began in 2013. Through phenotypic whole-organism screens of various compounds, Dr. Conor Caffrey, then at the University of California, San Francisco (UCSF), found that commercial anti-hypercholesterolemia statin drugs were potent schistosomicidal compounds [103]. The statins had been initially developed to treat patients who suffered from elevated cholesterol levels, but as inhibitors of HMG-CoA reductase (3-hydroxy-3-methyl-glutaryl-CoA reductase or HMGR), they also had the potential to be repurposed to inhibit HMG-CoA reductase activity in other organisms. In particular, S. mansoni's survival and egg-producing abilities had been shown to be dependent on schistosomal HMG-CoA reductase (SmHMGR) activity both in vivo and in vitro [104], and Dr. Caffrey was looking to exploit that vulnerability with inhibitors that specifically targeted this protein.

In order to screen chemical analogs that could prove to be even more potent against SmHMGR and develop a drug discovery program around this promising validated target, BVGH connected Dr. Caffrey with MSD. As a successful manufacturer of statin drugs, MSD was able to provide a select set of statin analogs to support Dr. Caffrey's efforts. BVGH also connected Dr. Caffrey with investigators from the Center for Infectious Disease Research (CIDR), and the NIAID-funded Seattle Structural Genomics Center for Infectious Disease (SSGCID) to solve the crystal structure for SmHMGR. In addition, MSD scientists provided scientific input on optimized SmHMGR gene expression methodologies that are being used to express the SmHMGR protein so that the crystal structure can be elucidated. With the crystal structure, Dr. Caffrey, now at the Center for Discovery and Innovation in Parasitic Diseases (CDIPD) at the University of California, San Diego (UCSD), and his collaborators will have the option to optimize the hit compounds utilizing a structure-guided medicinal chemistry approach.

Based on the model of directing drug discovery efforts by using validated targets essential to parasite survival, BVGH has continued to establish fruitful collaborations that involve the sharing of targeted compounds from WIPO Re:Search company members. Eisai Co., Ltd. has also become involved in schistosomiasis R&D by agreeing to provide an investigator with a calcium channel antagonist, as it has been shown that this type of inhibitor has activity against schistosomula and is capable of significantly reducing the viability of adult worms, alone or in combination with PZQ [105]. Further, in line with the hypothesis that polo-like kinases play an important role in S. mansoni gametogenesis [106], Takeda Pharmaceutical Company, Ltd., agreed to support efforts surrounding this target by providing a selective polo-like kinase inhibitor that was originally developed to treat solid tumors. By sharing compounds that have selective activity against a verified target, companies are not only providing chemical analogs that researchers would typically have difficulty accessing, they are also directly accelerating the drug discovery process by avoiding the use of compounds with unknown activities, properties, and targets. The use of natural products is also an area that is quite active for drug discovery. Due to the need for novel drugs against schistosomiasis, screening natural products for schistosomicidal activity could potentially lead to the identification of interesting starting points for further drug development, such as novel chemistry or mechanisms of action. For this reason, BVGH connected a researcher at Swiss TPH with the Griffith Institute for Drug Discovery (GRIDD) to gain access to GRIDD's Nature Bank [107] and screen natural product extracts for activity against S. mansoni.

Although repurposing pharmaceutical compounds is an important strategy for developing novel therapeutics in a cost-effective way, the value of the WIPO Re:Search IP-sharing model in advancing R&D for schistosomiasis and other diseases of poverty goes beyond compounds. The model also involves the sharing of knowledge and expertise. Such sharing is especially impactful when it involves scientists from LMICs, as it not only incentivizes innovation in neglected disease-endemic countries, but it also promotes R&D capacity building. This type of capacity building plays an essential role in changing the global development landscape from donation-based programs to long-term sustainable R&D models in countries that currently lack the necessary resources to successfully jumpstart their own product development efforts. Many LMIC researchers focus their efforts on diseases that affect their countries, but they may not have the product development know-how or infrastructure to advance those efforts to the clinic. WIPO Re:Search provides LMIC scientists with a platform that reduces the access barrier to industry and academic/non-profit IP assets and facilitates the necessary knowledge transfer that will eventually empower and strengthen the scientists' ability to contribute to product development for diseases that challenge their populations.

WIPO Re:Search collaborations are enabling knowledge and technology transfer between high-income country organizations and LMIC institutions to bolster schistosomiasis R&D capacity in the latter. In one instance, an investigator from Ghana's Kwame Nkrumah University of Science and Technology (KNUST) was interested in receiving training in *S. mansoni* cultivation and maintenance and screening of Ghanaian medicinal plants for antiparasitic activity, to enhance KNUST's research and education programs. BVGH connected the researcher with a faculty member who was at UCSF at the time, and the visiting scientist was able to receive the desired training from a world-renowned schistosomiasis researcher. The collaborative work between these two investigators resulted in a *Journal of Parasitology Research* publication [108]. Other WIPO Re:Search collaborations involve the sharing of reagents critical to LMIC investigators' work plans. For example, Dr. Floriano Paes Silva Junior, an investigator at FIOCRUZ (Brazil), was interested in validating a group of genes as essential to *S. mansoni* through RNA interference (RNAi) and determining whether those proteins could be potential drug discovery targets. BVGH connected the researcher to Alnylam, a pharmaceutical company focused on RNAi therapeutics. Alnylam agreed to design and synthesize optimized siRNAs that would enable the FIOCRUZ team to knock down the genes and determine whether their loss affects parasite viability. An additional example involved the sharing of a recombinant schistosome protein that Dr. Moustapha Mbow at Cheikh Anta Diop University (Senegal) was interested in using to assess in vitro immune responses to the protein. BVGH connected Dr. Mbow to Dr. Michael Hsieh at the Biomedical Research Institute (BRI), who expressed, purified, and shared the protein. This collaboration has led to a joint grant submission.

5. Conclusions

To boost the number of quality novel candidates that enter clinical-stage development, the schistosomiasis product development pipeline needs to be continuously fueled by early-stage research. It is during this stage of the product development process that WIPO Re:Search can have the greatest impact by establishing collaborations between for-profit and academic/non-profit institutions. The pharmaceutical industry not only engages in global health initiatives through its drug donation programs, but it also plays an important role in driving R&D for diseases of poverty. However, many academic/non-profit researchers remain unaware of the partnership opportunities that are available to them to drive their own research forward. The WIPO Re:Search consortium can bridge the gap between academic/non-profit and industry scientists to reduce duplicative efforts and encourage synergy to develop vaccines, diagnostics, and drugs for schistosomiasis and other neglected diseases. Furthermore, through the capacity building activities of WIPO Re:Search, LMIC scientists are not only able to gain valuable expertise, but also to use that expertise to develop new skills, accelerate their research, and advance their careers. The expertise gained through such collaborations provides scientists with a distinct advantage that can result in additional funding to reach important milestones. It is through the mutually beneficial model of WIPO Re:Search, where product development risk and cost are distributed among various key stakeholders, that a tangible and significant impact can be made to eliminate schistosomiasis and other diseases of poverty.

As the fight against schistosomiasis continues, the involvement of private industry and their critical contributions of assets and expertise should be causes for optimism. While promising industry collaborations continue to advance towards novel products and tools that will play a key role in the elimination of schistosomiasis, it is important to remember that this task is too great to be overcome by a single sector. As pharmaceutical companies continue to invest resources and funding to combat schistosomiasis, it is important for these efforts to receive the support of various stakeholders such as governments and international funding agencies. Through a concerted effort that distributes risk, and leverages the strengths and resources of the private and public sectors, every day brings us closer to winning the fight against schistosomiasis.

Author Contributions: C.J.W. and J.H.-C. wrote the manuscript. K.M.G. and C.K.M. reviewed the manuscript and provided valuable feedback. J.D. oversaw operations.

Acknowledgments: The authors thank Alnylam, Biomedical Research Institute, Center for Infectious Disease Research, Cheikh Anta Diop University, Eisai Co., Ltd., Griffith Institute for Drug Discovery, Oswaldo Cruz Foundation, Kwame Nkrumah University of Science and Technology, MSD, Swiss TPH, Takeda Pharmaceutical Company, Ltd., and University of California, San Diego for their review and helpful suggestions.

References

1. World Health Organization. Schistosomiasis and soil-transmitted helminthiases: Number of people treated in 2017. *WHO Wkly. Epidemiological Rec.* **2018**, *93*, 681–692.

2. Nour, N.M. Schistosomiasis: Health Effects on Women. *Rev. Obsterics Gynecol.* **2010**, *3*, 28–32.

3. Warren, K.S.; Mahmoud, A.A.; Cummings, P.; Murphy, D.J.; Houser, H.B. Schistosomiasis mansoni in Yemeni in California: Duration of infection, presence of disease, therapeutic management. *Am. J. Trop. Med. Hyg.* **1974**, *23*, 902–909. [CrossRef] [PubMed]

4. Colley, D.G.; Bustinduy, A.L.; Secor, W.E.; King, C.H. Human schistosomiasis. *Lancet* **2014**, *383*, 2253–2264. [CrossRef]

5. Chabasse, D.; Bertrand, G.; Leroux, J.P.; Gauthey, N.; Hocquet, P. Developmental bilharziasis caused by Schistosoma mansoni discovered 37 years after infestation. *Bull. Soc. Pathol. Exot.* **1985**, *78*, 643–647.

6. Gryseels, B.; Polman, K.; Clerinx, J.; Kestens, L. Human Schistosomiasis. *Lancet* **2006**, *368*, 23–29. [CrossRef]

7. World Health Organization. *Schistosomiasis: Progress Report 2001–2011, Strategic Plan 2012–2020*; World Health Organization: Geneva, Switzerland, 2013.

8. Steinmann, P.; Keiser, J.; Bos, R.; Tanner, M.; Utzinger, J. Schistosomiasis and water resources development: Systematic review, meta-analysis, and estimates of people at risk. *Lancet Infect. Dis.* **2006**, *6*, 411–425. [CrossRef]

9. Elbaz, T.; Esmat, G. Hepatic and intestinal schistosomiasis: Review. *J. Adv. Res.* **2013**, *4*, 445–452. [CrossRef]

10. Rambau, P.F.; Chalya, P.L.; Jackson, K. Schistosomiasis and urinary bladder cancer in North Western Tanzania: A retrospective review of 185 patients. *Infect. Agents Cancer* **2013**, *8*, 1–6. [CrossRef]

11. Ray, D.; Nelson, T.A.; Fu, C.L.; Patel, S.; Gong, D.N.; Odegaard, J.I.; Hsieh, M.H. Transcriptional profiling of the bladder in urogenital schistosomiasis reveals pathways of inflammatory fibrosis and urothelial compromise. *PLoS Negl. Trop. Dis.* **2012**, *6*, e1912. [CrossRef] [PubMed]

12. Center For Disease Control and Prevention/Schistosomiasis FAQ. Available online: https://www.cdc.gov/parasites/schistosomiasis/gen_info/faqs.html (accessed on 17 September 2018).

13. Moné, H.; Minguez, S.; Ibikounlé, M.; Allienne, J.F.; Massougbodji, A.; Mouahid, G. Natural Interactions between *S. haematobium* and *S. guineensis* in the Republic of Benin. *Sci. World J.* **2012**, *2012*. [CrossRef] [PubMed]

14. King, C.H.; Dangerfield-Cha, M. The unacknowledged impact of chronic schistosomiasis. *Chronic Illn* **2008**, *4*, 65–79. [CrossRef] [PubMed]

15. GBD 2017 DALYs and HALE Collaborators. Global, regional, and national disability-adjusted life-years (DALYs) for 359 diseases and injuries and healthy life expectancy (HALE) for 195 countries and territories, 1990–2017: A systematic analysis for the Global Burden of Disease Study 2017. *Lancelet* **2018**, *392*, 859–922.

16. King, C.H. Parasites and poverty: The case of schistosomiasis. *Acta Trop.* **2010**, *113*, 95–104. [CrossRef] [PubMed]

17. Ndamba, J.; Makaza, N.; Munjoma, M.; Gomo, E.; Kaondera, K.C. The physical fitness and work performance of agricultural workers infected with Schistosoma mansoni in Zimbabwe. *Anal. Trop. Med. Parasitol.* **1993**, *87*, 553–561. [CrossRef]

18. Friedman, J.F.; Kanzaria, H.K.; Acosta, L.P.; Langdon, G.C.; Manalo, D.L.; Wu, H.; Olveda, R.M.; McGarvey, S.T.; Kurtis, J.D. Relationship between Schistosoma japonicum and nutritional status among children and young adults in Leyte, the Philippines. *Am. J. Trop. Med. Hyg.* **2005**, *72*, 527–533. [CrossRef] [PubMed]

19. McDonald, E.A.; Cheng, L.; Jarilla, B.; Sagliba, M.J.; Gonzal, A.; Amoylen, A.J.; Olveda, R.; Acosta, L.; Baylink, D.; White, E.S.; et al. Maternal infection with Schistosoma japonicum induces a profibrotic response in neonates. *Infect. Immun.* **2014**, *82*, 350–355. [CrossRef]

20. Kurtis, J.D.; Higashi, A.; Wu, H.W.; Gundogan, F.; McDonald, E.A.; Sharma, S.; PondTor, S.; Jarilla, B.; Sagliba, M.J.; Gonzal, A.; et al. Maternal Schistosomiasis japonica is associated with maternal, placental, and fetal inflammation. *Infect. Immun.* **2011**, *79*, 1254–1261. [CrossRef]

21. Sacko, M.; Magnussen, P.; Keita, A.D.; Traore, M.S.; Landoure, A.; Doucoure, A.; Madsen, H.; Vennervald, B.J. Impact of Schistosoma haematobium infection on urinary tract pathology, nutritional status and anaemia in school-aged children in two different endemic areas of the Niger River Basin, Mali. *Acta Trop.* **2011**, *120* (Suppl. 1), S142–S150. [CrossRef]

22. Stothard, J.R.; Sousa-Figueiredo, J.C.; Betson, M.; Bustinduy, A.; Reinhard-Rupp, J. Schistosomiasis in African infants and preschool children: Let them now be treated! *Trends Parasitol.* **2013**, *29*, 197–205. [CrossRef]

23. Mostafa, M.H.; Sheweita, S.A.; O'Connor, P.J. Relationship between Schistosomiasis and Bladder Cancer. *Clin. Microbiol. Rev.* **1999**, *12*, 97–111. [CrossRef] [PubMed]

24. Parkin, D.M. The global health burden of infection-associated cancers in the year 2002. *Int. J. Cancer* **2006**, *118*, 3030–3044. [CrossRef] [PubMed]

25. Adenowo, A.F.; Oyinloye, B.E.; Ogunyinka, B.I.; Kappo, A.P. Impact of human schistosomiasis in sub-Saharan Africa. *Braz. J. Infect. Dis.* **2015**, *19*, 196–205. [CrossRef] [PubMed]

26. Dematei, A.; Fernandes, R.; Soares, R.; Alves, H.; Richter, J.; Botelho, M.C. Angiogenesis in Schistosoma haematobium-associated urinary bladder cancer. *APMIS* **2017**, *125*, 1056–1062. [CrossRef]

27. Rosin, M.P.; Zaki, S.S.E.D.; Ward, A.J.; Anwar, W.A. Involvement of inflammatory reactions and elevated cell proliferation in the development of bladder cancer in schistosomiasis patients. *Mut. Res.* **1994**, *305*, 283–292. [CrossRef]

28. Shiff, C.; Veltri, R.; Naples, J.; Quartey, J.; Otchere, J.; Anyan, W.; Marlow, C.; Wiredu, E.; Adjei, A.; Brakohiapa, E.; et al. Ultrasound verification of bladder damage is associated with known biomarkers of bladder cancer in adults chronically infected with Schistosoma haematobium in Ghana. *Trans. R. Soc. Trop. Med. Hyg.* **2006**, *100*, 847–854. [CrossRef]

29. International Agency for Research on Cancer. Biological Agents. Volume 100B. A Review of Human Carcinogenesis. *IARC Monogr. Evalutation Carcinogenic Risks Hum.* **2012**, *100*, 1–441.

30. Doehring, E.; Ehrich, J.H.; Bremer, H.J. Reversibility of urinary tract abnormalities due to Schistosoma haematobium infection. *Kidney Int.* **1986**, *30*, 582–585. [CrossRef]

31. Botelho, M.C.; Alves, H.; Richter, J. Halting Schistosoma haematobium—Associated bladder cancer. *Int. J. Cancer Manag.* **2017**, *10*, e9430. [CrossRef]

32. Kjetland, E.F.; Leutscher, P.D.; Ndhlovu, P.D. A Review of Female Genital Schistosomiasis. *Trends Parasitol.* **2012**, *28*, 58–65. [CrossRef]

33. Santos, J.; Gouveia, M.J.; Vale, N.; Delgado Mde, L.; Goncalves, A.; da Silva, J.M.; Oliveira, C.; Xavier, P.; Gomes, P.; Santos, L.L.; et al. Urinary Estrogen Metabolites and Self-Reported Infertility in Women Infected With Schistosoma Haematobium. *PLoS ONE* **2014**, *9*, e96774. [CrossRef] [PubMed]

34. Friedman, J.; Mital, P.; Kanzaria, H.K.; Olds, G.R.; Kurtis, J.D. Schistosomiasis and pregnancy. *Trends Parasitol.* **2007**, *23*, 159–164. [CrossRef] [PubMed]

35. Kjetland, E.F.; Ndhlovu, P.D.; Gomo, E.; Mduluza, T.; Midzi, N.; Gwanzura, L.; Mason, P.R.; Sandvik, L.; Friis, H.; Gundersen, S.G. Association between genital schistosomiasis and HIV in rural Zimbabwean women. *AIDS* **2006**, *20*, 593–600. [CrossRef] [PubMed]

36. Brodish, P.H.; Singh, K. Association Between Schistosoma haematobium Exposure and Human Immunodeficiency Virus Infection Among Females in Mozambique. *Am. J. Trop. Med. Hyg.* **2016**, *94*, 1040–1044. [CrossRef] [PubMed]

37.   Secor, W.E.; Shah, A.; Mwinzi, P.M.N.; Ndenga, B.A.; Watta, C.O.; Karanja, D.M.S. Increased Density of Human Immunodeficiency Virus Type 1 Coreceptors CCR5 and CXCR4 on the Surfaces of CD4+ T Cells and Monocytes of Patients with Schistosoma mansoni Infection. *Infect. Immun.* **2003**, *71*, 6668–6671. [CrossRef] [PubMed]

38.   Gelfand, M.; Ross, C.M.; Blair, D.M.; Castle, W.M.; Weber, M.C. Schistosomiasis of the male pelvic organs. Severity of infection determined by digestion of tissue and histologic methods in 300 cadavers. *Am. J. Trop. Med. Hyg.* **1970**, *19*, 779–784. [CrossRef] [PubMed]

39.   Leutscher, P.; Ramarokoto, C.E.; Reimert, C.; Feldmeier, H.; Esterre, P.; Vennervald, B.J. Community-based study of genital schistosomiasis in men from Madagascar. *Lancet* **2000**, *355*, 117–118. [CrossRef]

40.   Leutscher, P.D.; Pedersen, M.; Raharisolo, C.; Jensen, J.S.; Hoffmann, S.; Lisse, I.; Ostrowski, S.R.; Reimert, C.M.; Mauclere, P.; Ullum, H. Increased prevalence of leukocytes and elevated cytokine levels in semen from Schistosoma haematobium-infected individuals. *J. Infect. Dis.* **2005**, *191*, 1639–1647. [CrossRef]

41.   Reaching a Billion. Fifth Progress Report on the London Declaration on NTDs. 2017. Available online: https://unitingtocombatntds.org/reports/5th-report/ (accessed on 7 January 2019).

42.   Greenberg, R.M. New approaches for understanding mechanisms of drug resistance in schistosomes. *Parasitology* **2013**, *140*, 1534–1546. [CrossRef]

43.   Greenberg, R.M. ABC multidrug transporters in schistosomes and other parasitic flatworms. *Parasitol. Int.* **2013**, *62*, 647–653. [CrossRef]

44.   Cioli, D.; Pica-Mattoccia, L.; Basso, A.; Guidi, A. Schistosomiasis control: Praziquantel forever? *Mol. Biochem. Parasitol.* **2014**, *195*, 23–29. [CrossRef] [PubMed]

45.   Caffrey, C.R. Chemotherapy of schistosomiasis: Present and future. *Curr. Opin. Chem. Biol.* **2007**, *11*, 433–439. [CrossRef] [PubMed]

46.   World Health Organization: Schistosomiasis Strategy. Available online: http://www.who.int/schistosomiasis/strategy/en/ (accessed on 14 September 2018).

47.   Inobaya, M.T.; Olveda, R.M.; Chau, T.N.; Olveda, D.U.; Ross, A.G. Prevention and control of schistosomiasis: A current perspective. *Res. Rep. Trop. Med.* **2014**, *2014*, 65–75.

48.   Sokolow, S.H.; Wood, C.L.; Jones, I.J.; Lafferty, K.D.; Kuris, A.M.; Hsieh, M.H.; De Leo, G.A. To Reduce the Global Burden of Human Schistosomiasis, Use 'Old Fashioned' Snail Control. *Trends Parasitol.* **2018**, *34*, 23–40. [CrossRef] [PubMed]

49.   Lo, N.C.; Addiss, D.G.; Hotez, P.J.; King, C.H.; Stothard, J.R.; Evans, D.S.; Colley, D.G.; Lin, W.; Coulibaly, J.T.; Bustinduy, A.L.; et al. A call to strengthen the global strategy against schistosomiasis and soil-transmitted helminthiasis: The time is now. *Lancet Infect. Dis.* **2017**, *17*, e64–e69. [CrossRef]

50.   Olds, G.R. Administration of Praziquantel to pregnant and lactating women. *Acta Trop.* **2003**, *86*, 185–195. [CrossRef]

51.   Reinhard-Rupp, J.; Klohe, K. Developing a comprehensive response for treatment of children under 6 years of age with schistosomiasis: Research and development of a pediatric formulation of praziquantel. *Infect. Dis. Poverty* **2017**, *6*, 122. [CrossRef] [PubMed]

52.   Abudho, B.O.; Ndombi, E.M.; Guya, B.; Carter, J.M.; Riner, D.K.; Kittur, N.; Karanja, D.M.S.; Secor, W.E.; Colley, D.G. Impact of Four Years of Annual Mass Drug Administration on Prevalence and Intensity of Schistosomiasis among Primary and High School Children in Western Kenya: A Repeated Cross-Sectional Study. *Am. J. Trop. Med. Hyg.* **2018**, *98*, 1397–1402. [CrossRef]

53.   Kenya National School-Based Deworming Programme: Year 2 Report (April 2013–March 2014). Available online: https://ciff.org/documents/16/Kenya_National_SchoolBased_Deworming_Programme_Year2_evaluation.pdf (accessed on 6 January 2019).

54.   Savioli, L.; Albonico, M.; Colley, D.G.; Correa-Oliveira, R.; Fenwick, A.; Green, W.; Kabatereine, N.; Kabore, A.; Katz, N.; Klohe, K.; et al. Building a global schistosomiasis alliance: An opportunity to join forces to fight inequality and rural poverty. *Infect. Dis. Poverty* **2017**, *6*, 65. [CrossRef]

55.   World Health Organization. *Crossing the Billion. Lymphatic Filariasis, Onchocerciasis, Schistosomiasis, Soil-Transmitted Helminthiases and Trachoma: Preventive Chemotherapy for Neglected Tropical Diseases*; World Health Organization: Geneva, Switzerland, 2017.

56.   Ross, A.G.; Chau, T.N.; Inobaya, M.T.; Olveda, R.M.; Li, Y.; Harn, D.A. A new global strategy for the elimination of schistosomiasis. *Int. J. Infect. Dis.* **2017**, *54*, 130–137. [CrossRef]

57. World Health Organization. Schistosomiasis and soil-transmitted helminthiases: Number of people treated in 2016. *WHO Wkly. Epidemiological Rec.* **2017**, *92*, 749–760.

58. Caffrey, C.R. Schistosomiasis and its treatment. *Future Med. Chem.* **2015**, *7*, 675–676. [CrossRef] [PubMed]

59. Doenhoff, M.J.; Hagan, P.; Cioli, D.; Southgate, V.; Pica-Mattoccia, L.; Botros, S.; Coles, G.; Tchuem Tchuente, L.A.; Mbaye, A.; Engels, D. Praziquantel: Its use in control of schistosomiasis in sub-Saharan Africa and current research needs. *Parasitology* **2009**, *136*, 1825–1835. [CrossRef] [PubMed]

60. Zwang, J.; Olliaro, P.L. Clinical efficacy and tolerability of praziquantel for intestinal and urinary schistosomiasis-a meta-analysis of comparative and non-comparative clinical trials. *PLoS Negl. Trop. Dis.* **2014**, *8*, e3286. [CrossRef] [PubMed]

61. Liu, R.; Dong, H.F.; Guo, Y.; Zhao, Q.P.; Jiang, M.S. Efficacy of praziquantel and artemisinin derivatives for the treatment and prevention of human schistosomiasis: A systematic review and meta-analysis. *Parasit Vectors* **2011**, *4*, 201. [CrossRef] [PubMed]

62. Kasinathan, R.S.; Sharma, L.K.; Cunningham, C.; Webb, T.R.; Greenberg, R.M. Inhibition or knockdown of ABC transporters enhances susceptibility of adult and juvenile schistosomes to Praziquantel. *PLoS Negl. Trop. Dis.* **2014**, *8*, e3265. [CrossRef] [PubMed]

63. Zwang, J.; Olliaro, P. Efficacy and safety of praziquantel 40 mg/kg in preschool-aged and school-aged children: A meta-analysis. *Parasit Vectors* **2017**, *10*, 47. [CrossRef]

64. Doenhoff, M.J.; Cioli, D.; Utzinger, J. Praziquantel: Mechanisms of action, resistance and new derivatives for schistosomiasis. *Curr. Opin. Infect. Dis.* **2008**, *21*, 659–667. [CrossRef]

65. Pinto-Almeida, A.; Mendes, T.; Armada, A.; Belo, S.; Carrilho, E.; Viveiros, M.; Afonso, A. The Role of Efflux Pumps in Schistosoma mansoni Praziquantel Resistant Phenotype. *PLoS ONE* **2015**, *10*, e0140147. [CrossRef]

66. Liu, Y.X.; Wu, W.; Liang, Y.J.; Jie, Z.L.; Wang, H.; Wang, W.; Huang, Y.X. New uses for old drugs: The tale of artemisinin derivatives in the elimination of schistosomiasis japonica in China. *Molecules* **2014**, *19*, 15058–15074. [CrossRef]

67. Toor, J.; Alsallaq, R.; Truscott, J.E.; Turner, H.C.; Werkman, M.; Gurarie, D.; King, C.H.; Anderson, R.M. Are We on Our Way to Achieving the 2020 Goals for Schistosomiasis Morbidity Control Using Current World Health Organization Guidelines? *Clin. Infect. Dis.* **2018**, *66*, S245–S252. [PubMed]

68. Mo, A.X.; Colley, D.G. Workshop report: Schistosomiasis vaccine clinical development and product characteristics. *Vaccine* **2016**, *34*, 995–1001. [CrossRef] [PubMed]

69. Policy Cures Research. Neglected Disease R&D Product Pipeline. Available online: https://www.pipeline.policycuresresearch.org/august2017 (accessed on 14 September 2018).

70. Hotez, P.J. The global fight to develop antipoverty vaccines in the anti-vaccine era. *Hum. Vaccin. Immunother.* **2018**, 1–4. [CrossRef] [PubMed]

71. Tendler, M.; Almeida, M.; Simpson, A. Development of the Brazilian Anti Schistosomiasis Vaccine Based on the Recombinant Fatty Acid Binding Protein Sm14 Plus GLA-SE Adjuvant. *Front. Immunol.* **2015**, *6*, 218. [CrossRef] [PubMed]

72. Ricciardi, A.; Ndao, M. Still hope for schistosomiasis vaccine. *Hum. Vaccin. Immunother.* **2015**, *11*, 2504–2508. [CrossRef] [PubMed]

73. Riveau, G.; Deplanque, D.; Remoue, F.; Schacht, A.M.; Vodougnon, H.; Capron, M.; Thiry, M.; Martial, J.; Libersa, C.; Capron, A. Safety and immunogenicity of rSh28GST antigen in humans: Phase 1 randomized clinical study of a vaccine candidate against urinary schistosomiasis. *PLoS Negl. Trop. Dis.* **2012**, *6*, e1704. [CrossRef]

74. Efficacy of Bilhvax in Association With Praziquantel for Prevention of Clinical Recurrences of Schistosoma Haematobium (Bilhvax3). Available online: https://clinicaltrials.gov/ct2/show/NCT00870649?term=Bilhvax&rank=2 (accessed on 14 September 2018).

75. Study of Safety and Immune Response of the Sm14 Vaccine in Adults of Endemic Regions. Available online: https://clinicaltrials.gov/ct2/show/NCT03041766?term=sm-14&cond=Schistosomiasis&rank=2 (accessed on 14 September 2018).

76. Santini-Oliveira, M.; Coler, R.N.; Parra, J.; Veloso, V.; Jayashankar, L.; Pinto, P.M.; Ciol, M.A.; Bergquist, R.; Reed, S.G.; Tendler, M. Schistosomiasis vaccine candidate Sm14/GLA-SE: Phase 1 safety and immunogenicity clinical trial in healthy, male adults. *Vaccine* **2016**, *34*, 586–594. [CrossRef]

77. Merrifield, M.; Hotez, P.J.; Beaumier, C.M.; Gillespie, P.; Strych, U.; Hayward, T.; Bottazzi, M.E. Advancing a vaccine to prevent human schistosomiasis. *Vaccine* **2016**, *34*, 2988–2991. [CrossRef]

78. Sabin Vaccine Institute. Available online: https://www.sabin.org/programs/schistosomiasis (accessed on 14 September 2018).

79. A Phase Ib Study of the Safety, Reactogenicity, and Immunogenicity of Sm-TSP-2/Alhydrogel)(R) with or without AP 10-701 for Intestinal Schistosomiasis in Healthy Exposed Adults. Available online: https://clinicaltrials.gov/ct2/show/NCT03110757?term=Alhydrogel&rank=8 (accessed on 14 September 2018).

80. Le, L.; Molehin, A.J.; Nash, S.; Sennoune, S.R.; Ahmad, G.; Torben, W.; Zhang, W.; Siddiqui, A.A. Schistosoma egg-induced liver pathology resolution by Sm-p80-based schistosomiasis vaccine in baboons. *Pathology* **2018**, *50*, 442–449. [CrossRef]

81. Siddiqui, A.A.; Siddiqui, S.Z. Sm-p80-Based Schistosomiasis Vaccine: Preparation for Human Clinical Trials. *Trends Parasitol.* **2017**, *33*, 194–201. [CrossRef]

82. Faulx, D.; Storey, H.L.; Murray, M.A.; Cantera, J.L.; Hawkins, K.R.; Leader, B.T.; Gallo, K.L.; de los Santntos, T. PATH. Diagnostics for Neglected Tropical Diseases: Defining the Best Tools through Target Product Profiles. 2015. Available online: https://www.finddx.org/wp-content/uploads/2016/03/PATH-2015_Dx-for-NTDs-Target-Products-Profile-report.pdf (accessed on 8 January 2019).

83. Balahbib, A.; Amarir, F.; Corstjens, P.L.; de Dood, C.J.; van Dam, G.J.; Hajli, A.; Belhaddad, M.; El Mansouri, B.; Sadak, A.; Rhajaoui, M.; et al. Selecting accurate post-elimination monitoring tools to prevent reemergence of urogenital schistosomiasis in Morocco: A pilot study. *Infect. Dis. Poverty* **2017**, *6*, 75. [CrossRef] [PubMed]

84. Foo, K.T.; Blackstock, A.J.; Ochola, E.A.; Matete, D.O.; Mwinzi, P.N.; Montgomery, S.P.; Karanja, D.M.; Secor, W.E. Evaluation of point-of-contact circulating cathodic antigen assays for the detection of Schistosoma mansoni infection in low-, moderate-, and high-prevalence schools in western Kenya. *Am. J. Trop. Med. Hyg.* **2015**, *92*, 1227–1232. [CrossRef] [PubMed]

85. Lindholz, C.G.; Favero, V.; Verissimo, C.M.; Candido, R.R.F.; de Souza, R.P.; Dos Santos, R.R.; Morassutti, A.L.; Bittencourt, H.R.; Jones, M.K.; St Pierre, T.G.; et al. Study of diagnostic accuracy of Helmintex, Kato-Katz, and POC-CCA methods for diagnosing intestinal schistosomiasis in Candeal, a low intensity transmission area in northeastern Brazil. *PLoS Negl. Trop. Dis.* **2018**, *12*, e0006274. [CrossRef] [PubMed]

86. Ogongo, P.; Kariuki, T.M.; Wilson, R.A. Diagnosis of schistosomiasis mansoni: An evaluation of existing methods and research towards single worm pair detection. *Parasitology* **2018**, *145*, 1355–1366. [CrossRef] [PubMed]

87. Sandoval, N.; Siles-Lucas, M.; Perez-Arellano, J.L.; Carranza, C.; Puente, S.; Lopez-Aban, J.; Muro, A. A new PCR-based approach for the specific amplification of DNA from different Schistosoma species applicable to human urine samples. *Parasitology* **2006**, *133*, 581–587. [CrossRef] [PubMed]

88. Field Evaluations of the Point-of-Care (POC) Circulating Cathodic Antigen (CCA) Urine Assay for Detection of *S. mansoni* infection. Available online: https://score.uga.edu/projects/poc-cca/ (accessed on 14 September 2018).

89. Sissoko, M.S.; Dabo, A.; Traore, H.; Diallo, M.; Traore, B.; Konate, D.; Niare, B.; Diakite, M.; Kamate, B.; Traore, A.; et al. Efficacy of artesunate + sulfamethoxypyrazine/pyrimethamine versus praziquantel in the treatment of Schistosoma haematobium in children. *PLoS ONE* **2009**, *4*, e6732. [CrossRef]

90. Comparing Praziquantel Versus Artesunate + Sulfamethoxypyrazine/Pyrimethamine for Treating Schistosomiasis. Available online: https://clinicaltrials.gov/ct2/show/NCT00510159?term=Co-Arinate&cond=schistosomiasis&rank=1 (accessed on 14 September 2018).

91. Eissa, M.M.; El-Moslemany, R.M.; Ramadan, A.A.; Amer, E.I.; El-Azzouni, M.Z.; El-Khordagui, L.K. Miltefosine Lipid Nanocapsules for Single Dose Oral Treatment of Schistosomiasis Mansoni: A Preclinical Study. *PLoS ONE* **2015**, *10*, e0141788. [CrossRef] [PubMed]

92. Simeonov, A.; Jadhav, A.; Sayed, A.A.; Wang, Y.; Nelson, M.E.; Thomas, C.J.; Inglese, J.; Williams, D.L.; Austin, C.P. Quantitative high-throughput screen identifies inhibitors of the Schistosoma mansoni redox cascade. *PLoS Negl. Trop. Dis.* **2008**, *2*, e127. [CrossRef]

93. TI Pharma Pediatric Praziquantel Consortium. Available online: https://www.tipharma.com/pharmaceutical-research-projects/neglected-diseases/pediatric-praziquantel-consortium/ (accessed on 14 September 2018).

94. The Truly Staggering Cost of Inventing New Drugs. Available online: https://www.forbes.com/sites/matthewherper/2012/02/22/the-truly-staggering-cost-of-inventing-new-drugs-the-print-version/#6a1435725f81 (accessed on 19 September 2018).

95. Pedrique, B.; Strub-Wourgaft, N.; Some, C.; Olliaro, P.; Trouiller, P.; Ford, N.; Pécoul, B.; Bradol, J.-H. The drug and vaccine landscape for neglected diseases (2000–2011): A systematic assessment. *Lancet Glob. Health* **2013**, *1*, e371–e379. [CrossRef]

96. Goldman, M.; Compton, C.; Mittleman, B.B. Public-private partnerships as driving forces in the quest for innovative medicines. *Clin. Transl. Med.* **2013**, *2*, 2. [CrossRef]

97. Pediatric Praziquantel Consortium. Available online: https://www.pediatricpraziquantelconsortium.org/ (accessed on 14 September 2018).

98. Maxmen, A. Big Pharma's Cost Cutting Challenger. *Nature* **2016**, *536*, 388–390. [CrossRef] [PubMed]

99. Dent, J.; Ramamoorthi, R.; Graef, K.; Nelson, L.M.; Wichard, J.C. WIPO Re:Search: A consortium catalyzing research and product development for neglected tropical diseases. *Pharm. Patent Anal.* **2013**, *2*, 591–596. [CrossRef] [PubMed]

100. WIPO Re:Search Guiding Principles. Available online: http://www.wipo.int/export/sites/www/research/docs/guiding_principles.pdf (accessed on 18 September 2018).

101. Economic Analysis and Policy Division, United Nations. Available online: https://www.un.org/development/desa/dpad/least-developed-country-category.html (accessed on 18 September 2018).

102. Van Norman, G.A. Drugs, Devices, and the FDA: Part 1: An Overview of Approval Processes for Drugs. *JACC Basic Transl. Sci.* **2016**, *1*, 170–179. [CrossRef] [PubMed]

103. Rojo-Arreola, L.; Long, T.; Asarnow, D.; Suzuki, B.M.; Singh, R.; Caffrey, C.R. Chemical and genetic validation of the statin drug target to treat the helminth disease, schistosomiasis. *PLoS ONE* **2014**, *9*, e87594. [CrossRef] [PubMed]

104. Chen, G.Z.; Foster, L.; Bennett, J.L. Antischistosomal action of mevinolin: Evidence that 3-hydroxy-methylglutaryl-coenzyme a reductase activity in Schistosoma mansoni is vital for parasite survival. *N-S Arch. Pharmacol.* **1990**, *324*, 477–482. [CrossRef]

105. Silva-Moraes, V.; Couto, F.F.B.; Vasconcelos, M.M.; Araújo, N.; Coelho, P.M.Z.; Katz, N.; Grenfell, R.F.Q. Antischistosomal activity of a calcium channel antagonist on schistosomula and adult Schistosoma mansoni worms. *Mem. Inst. Oswaldo Cruz* **2013**, *108*, 600–604. [CrossRef] [PubMed]

106. Dissous, C.; Grevelding, C.; Long, T. Schistosoma mansoni Polo-like kinases and their function in control of mitosis and parasite reproduction. *An. Acad. Brasil. Cienc.* **2011**, *83*, 627–635. [CrossRef]

107. Camp, D.; Newman, S.; B Pham, N.; J Quinn, R. Nature Bank and the Queensland Compound Library: Unique international resources at the Eskitis Institute for Drug Discovery. *Comb. Chem. High Throughput Screen.* **2014**, *17*, 201–209. [CrossRef]

108. Kyere-Davies, G.; Agyare, C.; Boakye, Y.D.; Suzuki, B.M.; Caffrey, C.R. Effect of Phenotypic Screening of Extracts and Fractions of Erythrophleum ivorense Leaf and Stem Bark on Immature and Adult Stages of Schistosoma mansoni. *J. Parasitol. Res.* **2018**, *2018*, 1–7. [CrossRef]

10

Schistosome Vaccines for Domestic Animals

Hong You, Pengfei Cai, Biniam Mathewos Tebeje, Yuesheng Li and Donald P. McManus *

Molecular Parasitology Laboratory, QIMR Berghofer Medical Research Institute, Brisbane, QLD 4006, Australia;
Hong.You@qimrberghofer.edu.au (H.Y.); Pengfei.Cai@qimrberghofer.edu.au (P.C.);
Biniam.Tebeje@qimrberghofer.edu.au (B.M.T.); Yuesheng.Li@qimrberghofer.edu.au (Y.L.)
* Correspondence: Don.McManus@qimrberghofer.edu.au

Abstract: Schistosomiasis is recognized as a tropical disease of considerable public health importance, but domestic livestock infections due to *Schistosoma japonicum, S. bovis, S. mattheei* and *S. curassoni* are often overlooked causes of significant animal morbidity and mortality in Asia and Africa. In addition, whereas schistosomiasis japonica is recognized as an important zoonosis in China and the Philippines, reports of viable schistosome hybrids between animal livestock species and *S. haematobium* point to an underappreciated zoonotic component of transmission in Africa as well. Anti-schistosome vaccines for animal use have long been advocated as part of the solution to schistosomiasis control, benefitting humans and animals and improving the local economy, features aligning with the One Health concept synergizing human and animal health. We review the history of animal vaccines for schistosomiasis from the early days of irradiated larvae and then consider the recombinant DNA technology revolution and its impact in developing schistosome vaccines that followed. We evaluate the major candidates tested in livestock, including the glutathione S-transferases, paramyosin and triose-phosphate isomerase, and summarize some of the future challenges that need to be overcome to design and deliver effective anti-schistosome vaccines that will complement current control options to achieve and sustain future elimination goals.

Keywords: schistosomiasis; *Schistosoma*; vaccine; zoonosis; Asia; Africa; domestic animals; buffalo; cattle; sheep; goats

1. Introduction

As well as being a disease of great public health importance, schistosomiasis can also be a chronic debilitating infection of animals and a problem of considerable economic significance in Asia and many parts of Africa. It has been estimated, for example, that 165 million cattle are infected with schistosomiasis worldwide [1]. Schistosome infections of livestock are very important, if often underappreciated, and they are often causes of serious animal mortality and morbidity with several species incriminated. In South and South-East Asia, schistosomiasis is caused by the highly zoonotic *Schistosoma japonicum* and/or *S. mekongi. S. mattheei* and/or *S. curassoni* infect cattle, sheep and goats in southern and Central Africa, whereas *S. bovis* is a major veterinary problem in many Mediterranean and African countries, causing high levels of morbidity among susceptible ruminants (cattle, goats, sheep, horses, camels and pigs), resulting in considerably reduced economic output due to liver condemnation, reduced productivity, poor subsequent reproductive performance, increased susceptibility to other infectious agents, and death [1,2].

It has been shown also that uninfected animals grow and gain weight faster and are overall healthier than schistosome-infected animals. *S. bovis* has recently come into the spotlight as an emerging clinical health threat as well following the isolation of *S. haematobium-S. bovis* hybrids from children in Senegal [3] and after a recent schistosomiasis outbreak in France [4]. There are also reports of eggs indicative of potential *S. haematobium-S. mattheei* hybrids in Zimbabwe and in southern

African ruminants [5]. The hybridization between human and ruminant schistosomes is of particular importance as inter-species hybridization may have a considerable impact on parasite evolution, disease dynamics, transmission rates and control interventions. Laboratory hybrids acquire enhanced characteristics, including infectivity, growth rates, maturation and egg production and, in cattle, it has been reported that introgressive *Schistosoma* hybrids may affect the success of drug treatment and can cause severe disease outbreaks [6]. The zoonotic component of transmission in sub-Saharan Africa does appear to be more significant than previously assumed, and may thereby affect the recently revised WHO vision to eliminate schistosomiasis as a public health problem by 2025. Moreover, animal schistosomiasis is likely to be a significant cost to affected communities due to its direct and indirect impacts on livelihoods. These findings underscore the need for improved disease control in animals, to reduce the zoonotic transmission of *S. japonicum* and *S. mekongi*, and to prevent the spread of hybrid schistosomes to humans from animal reservoirs.

The deployment of suitable anti-schistosome vaccines for use in animals has long been advocated as part of the solution to control and eliminate schistosomiasis. Indeed, a vaccine-directed control program that reduces prevalence, intensity and transmission of the disease in animals can directly benefit both humans and animals in endemic sites and improve the local economy, features that are in clear alignment with the One Health concept synergizing human and animal health. Furthermore, genuine change of the disease spectrum in endemic areas demands lasting results and the development and positioning of an effective vaccine represents an option for long-term protection. An entirely vaccine-based approach targeting humans and animals for schistosomiasis control is unrealistic, but acceptable protection could be achieved by chemotherapy treatment followed by vaccination aimed at reducing, or markedly delaying, the development of pathology and morbidity and limiting the impact of re-infection [7,8]. Thus, the issue is not drugs competing with vaccines, but how to graft a vaccine approach onto current schistosomiasis control programs [7,8]. Mathematical modelling of schistosome transmission supports this concept, predicting that a schistosome vaccine capable of reducing the faecal egg output in bovines by 45% in conjunction with praziquantel treatment would lead to a significant reduction in the transmission of schistosomiasis japonica almost to the point of elimination [9,10]. Domesticated animals represent significant reservoirs of *S. japonicum*, and their vaccination offers an approach to control schistosomiasis by interrupting its zoonotic transmission. Pertinent to this are studies undertaken in China [11] and the Philippines [12], which showed that bovines, in particular, are major animal reservoir hosts for *S. japonicum*, responsible for up to 90% of environmental egg contamination.

2. The Early Days—Irradiated Larval Vaccines

The immunological control of animal schistosomiasis was first advanced as an option in the 1970s as in many endemic areas, particularly in Africa, the use of molluscicides or chemotherapy as interventions was either too expensive or impractical [13]. Further, cattle had been shown to develop partial immunity to reinfection with *S. bovis* and *S. mattheei*, and sheep had been shown to develop some resistance to reinfection with *S. mattheei* [13]. As well, results of experiments in calves, cattle and sheep with harmless heterologous schistosome species suggested that the presence of adult egg-producing worms was not necessary for the development of acquired immunity to reinfection; these observations suggested the possibility of developing a vaccine incorporating either non-pathogenic heterologous larvae or, alternatively, larvae of the homologous species attenuated by irradiation to prevent them reaching full maturity [13]. Cercariae and schistosomula, attenuated with gamma rays, X-rays, or ultraviolet (UV) irradiation, were subsequently reported to elicit protective immunity against schistosomiasis. Indeed, the radiation attenuated vaccine approach provided protective efficacy against *Schistosoma* species in many different host species, including mice, rats, chimpanzees and baboons. The radiation attenuated vaccine also proved to be highly effective in livestock (cattle, buffaloes, sheep and pigs), thereby establishing the potential of developing irradiated live schistosome veterinary vaccines in the laboratory and their extended application to the field.

In a pioneering study in 1976, Taylor et al. [13] demonstrated that sheep could be partially protected against *S. mattheei* by prior immunisation with live cercariae or schistosomula of *S. mattheei* irradiated at 6 krad by a [60Co] source; and the study showed that effective immunisation was not dependent on the presence of a mature worm infection or on cercarial penetration of the skin by the immunising infection, as artificially transformed schistosomula were as immunogenic when injected into sheep as cercariae that penetrated the skin. The results opened up the possibility of making a live vaccine against ovine schistosomiasis, with the caveats that the problem of live parasite storage needed to be overcome and that a more efficient immunising schedule was needed. Other reports described highly effective immunisation of sheep with irradiated *S. bovis* cercariae [14] and irradiated schistosomula [15].

The first attempts at immunising cattle (zebu calves) were against *S. bovis* in Sudan and involved vaccination with 3 krad-irradiated homologous larval parasites first under experimental laboratory challenge using irradiated schistosomula or cercariae [16], and then in the field, under natural challenge when the calves (50% immunised with irradiated schistosomula) were allowed to graze in a *S. bovis*-endemic area for 10 months [17]. In both trials, vaccination was safe and, compared with control animals, the vaccinated animals had higher growth rates and significantly fewer adult worms and tissue and faecal eggs, indicating that zebu cattle could be protected effectively against *S. bovis* by vaccination with irradiated parasites.

An inherent problem in the production of a potential live radiation-attenuated vaccine at this time was the limited shelf-life of the attenuated parasites but new techniques to successfully cryopreserve schistosomula, including vitrification (solidifying a liquid without crystal formation) [18], were developed by Eric James and his team, which enabled their indefinite storage. In 1985, a cryopreserved homologous radiation-attenuated schistosomula vaccine evoked a good level of protection in sheep against *S. bovis* challenge [19].

At about the same time, effective irradiated vaccines were also being developed in China against *S. japonicum* infections, first in mice, and then in domestic pigs, sheep, cattle and buffaloes. These livestock animals, particularly water buffalo (*Bubalus bubalis*), represent important reservoirs of *S. japonicum*, so their vaccination provides a highly suitable approach to control schistosomiasis by zoonotic transmission interruption. The initial experiments were undertaken by Hsü and his team and were reported in 1983 [20] and 1984 [21]. The first study [20] used experimental infections with cattle calves receiving a vaccine of approximately 10,000 irradiated schistosomula followed by a challenge with 500 normal cercariae; the best results, in terms of reduced worm counts, involved three injections (partly given intramuscularly and partly intradermal) of larvae irradiated with 36 krad. The second study [21] was essentially a repeat with calves being perfused later (54–57 days as opposed to one month in the earlier experiment), thereby allowing the infection to mature to egg production, although the reduction in worm numbers was similar. The efficacy of this irradiated vaccine was field tested in vaccinated yearling cattle that were naturally challenged in an area in China highly endemic for schistosomiasis [21]; at perfusion, significant reductions in worm burden and liver eggs were recorded in the vaccinees compared with controls.

Although the work was undertaken in 1979 and 1980, Xu et al. [22] reported in 1993 on trials in bovines of vaccinations with single or double doses of 10,000 or 20,000 cryopreserved irradiated (CI) (20 krad) *S. japonicum* schistosomula together with 1 mL bacille Calmett-Guérin (BCG); worm numbers were reduced by 55–65% in vaccinated water buffalo (*Bubalus bubalis*) and cattle calves after being challenged with 500–1000 cercariae. A field test of the vaccine (10,000 CI schistosomula) resulted in a worm reduction of 53% in vaccinated water buffalo (*Bubalus bubalis*) calves [22]. Intradermal vaccination with 30,000 freeze-thaw (FT) schistosomula and BCG by the same group provided 57% protection in cattle. Similar levels of protection were obtained in sheep immunised with CI and FT schistosomula following challenge with 500 cercariae [23].

Cercariae have also been used as the irradiated vaccine source. Shi et al., in a report published in 1990 [24], vaccinated water buffaloes three times with 10,000 *S. japonicum* cercariae irradiated with a cheap, simple and portable UV light source at a dose of 400 μW min/cm^2. A challenge infection of 1000 untreated cercariae was given to vaccinated and naive control animals; the experiment was terminated six weeks post-challenge and, compared with controls, the vaccinated animals developed 89% resistance to infection with S. japonicum. Using a similar vaccination regimen, the same group undertook a study in pigs with a challenge infection of 1000 untreated cercariae given 2.5 or 6 months after the last immunization, with age-matched naïve pigs challenged as controls; immunized animals developed 90% resistance against the challenge [25].

The use of live schistosomula or cercariae vaccines attenuated by ionizing radiation or by biochemical means [26] potentially provides a method to protect domestic livestock against infection with schistosomes, but they have generally not found favour as a practical means of vaccinating domestic animals in the field (or humans) and they have never been used on a large scale. The reasons for this include: (1) the high production costs and labour-intensive efforts necessary to obtain the large numbers of cercariae required from infected snails; (2) the difficulties in standardizing the dose of ionizing radiation in order to induce larval attenuation and to ensure irradiated parasites do not retain some level of infectivity, thereby causing a breakthrough infection if insufficiently irradiated; (3) the requirement for cryo-preservation in order to store and then transport attenuated parasites over long distances; and (4) the safety issues associated with potential toxicity of administering a live vaccine and local inflammatory responses at the site of vaccination.

Thus, although in general the initial successes with irradiated schistosome vaccines were encouraging, with the research benefitting from substantial funding support during the 1970–1990s, progress stalled thereafter. This was mainly due to a change in research emphasis when the new advances in recombinant DNA technology were applied for the development of schistosome vaccines. Consequently, limited work has been undertaken on livestock animals with live attenuated schistosome vaccines in the past 25 years. In one approach protocols were established to compare the level of protection induced by recombinant and naked plasmid DNA formulations with the gold standard gamma or UV-irradiated cercarial vaccines in pigs [27,28]. Another avenue involved systematically investigating cellular and humoral immune responses generated by the protective UV-attenuated S. japonicum cercarial vaccine in pigs in order to identify key molecules involved in the process leading to resistance, thereby providing a paradigm for the development of an optimal vaccine formulation for both veterinary and clinical application [25,29–33].

3. The Impact of Recombinant DNA Technology on the Development of Animal Vaccines for Schistosomiasis

As indicated, in efforts to circumvent the perceived problems of using live, attenuated S. japonicum schistosomula or cercariae as vaccines to prevent infection in domestic livestock, and with the new techniques in genetic manipulation fast making ground, the research focus changed. Many groups attempted to reproduce or even improve on the protection afforded by substituting native antigens or chemically-defined schistosomal antigens genetically engineered in bacteria or yeast as recombinant proteins, or as plasmid DNA vaccines. The three most tested molecules tested in livestock have been glutathione S-transferases, paramyosin and triose-phosphate isomerase, details for which now follow.

3.1. The Glutathione S-Transferases

Two of the first schistosome molecules to be cloned and expressed (first in E. coli and then yeast) were the 28 kDa glutathione-S-transferase from S. mansoni (28 GST, P28 or Sm28) [34] and the 26 kDa GST homologue (termed Sj26) from S. japonicum [35]. The molecular cloning of the genes encoding the 28 GSTs of S. bovis, S. japonicum and S. haematobium soon followed [36]. The GSTs are enzyme isoforms that catalyse the detoxification of lipophilic molecules by thiol-conjugation.

They were considered attractive vaccine candidates in ruminants and other mammals because it was hypothesised that antibody-mediated neutralization of this detoxification function could render the schistosome vulnerable to toxic products generated by immune attack at the tegument or in the gut [37]. Accordingly, it was shown that native GST and GP38, which shares protective epitopes with keyhole limpet haemocyanin (KLH), exhibited vaccine potential against *S. mansoni* in small animal experiments [34]. Subsequently, native forms of *S. bovis* GST and KLH were tested for vaccine efficacy against *S. bovis* in Zebu cattle, and this resulted in specific antibodies being generated against both molecules and, depending on the vaccination schedule, significant reductions in faecal and tissue eggs also resulted; notably, however, vaccination did not reduce adult worm numbers [38]. In contrast, whereas vaccination of goats [39] and sheep [40] with recombinant *S. bovis*-derived 28GST (recombinant *S. bovis* 28GST), followed by experimental challenge with *S. bovis* cercariae, resulted in reduced worm burden, there was no impairment of fecundity. In a further report, immunization of calves with recombinant *S. bovis* 28GST induced significant reductions in female worm numbers, faecal eggs counts, and the number of viable eggs (determined by miracidial counts), in animals exposed to natural *S. mattheei* infection in the field [41]. In contrast, the same immunization schedule generated no protective effect against a massive (10,000 cercariae) single experimental challenge with *S. mattheei*. Being highly susceptible to *S. mattheei* infection, calves produce high parasite recovery rates, and the effect of vaccination and the generated immune response may have been insufficient to protect the animals, raising questions of the biological relevance of massive experimental challenges in the evaluation of protective immunity to schistosomiasis [41,42].

Subsequently, although considerable work on the schistosome GST vaccines focused on *S. mansoni* and then *S. haematobium*, it was clear that the very significant inhibition of female worm fecundity and egg viability was the most evident host protective effect generated against the GSTs of all schistosome species, including *S. japonicum*, by homologous vaccination [43]. The exact mechanism whereby anti-GST antibodies affected egg production and viability remained unanswered, but the phenomenon appeared to be associated with their inhibition of the enzymatic activity of GST, the consequent impairment in prostaglandin biosynthesis (prostaglandin D2 orchestrates various stages of the host immune response), and the resultant effect on schistosome biology, including a reduction in female worm fecundity [44].

Following on from the work with *S. mansoni* GSTs, partial protection was recorded in Chinese sheep and bovines vaccinated with *S. japonicum* 28 kDa GST (Sj28GST), either as a recombinant protein or plasmid DNA vaccine [45–47], but most reports were of the vaccine potential of the 26 kDa GST isoform (Sj26GST) in different mammalian hosts [48,49] (Table 1). Recombinant (r) Sj26GST induced a prominent anti-fecundity effect, as well as a significant, albeit moderate, level of protection in terms of reduced worm burdens in sheep, cattle and pigs, following challenge infection with *S. japonicum* [48–52]. Similar levels of vaccine efficacy were obtained in water buffaloes vaccinated with purified rSj26GST [50,52]. Anti-Sj26GST antibodies were generated in the immunized water buffaloes and, following challenge with *S. japonicum*, the typical anti-fecundity effect was observed with decreased numbers (circa 50%) of faecal eggs and eggs deposited in host livers and intestines [52]. As well, the rSjc26GST vaccine reduced the egg-hatching capacity of *S. japonicum* eggs into viable miracidia by nearly 40% [52]. Encouragingly, field trials demonstrated that the protective effect of rSj26GST against *S. japonicum* could be maintained in cattle and water buffaloes for at least 12 months post-vaccination [53,54], but whereas research to improve efficacy has continued using the murine model of schistosomiasis japonica (e.g., [55]), it is disappointing that there have been no further trials of the vaccine in livestock animals. The picture is somewhat brighter in regards to paramyosin, with some of the early work and recent progress on this vaccine candidate now being described.

Table 1. *S. japonicum* vaccines tested in domestic livestock.

Host	Antigen	Method of Immunization Regimen	Vaccine Efficacy			Ref
			Worm Burden Reduction %	Liver Egg Burden Reduction %	Fecal Egg Reduction %	
Pig	UV-attenuated cercariae	Single/three immunizations	59–78	89	86–99.7	[31]
	Irradiated cercariae		>95	>95	>95	[28]
	SjC23-pcDNA3.1 DNA	Conjunction with/without IL-12	29–58	48–56		[56]
	SjTPI-pcDNA3.1 DNA	Conjunction with/without IL-12	46–48	49–66		[57]
	Paramyosin	Conjugated with alum or TiterMax	32–34			[27]
	Paramyosin	Montanide ISA 206	52–58			[58]
	SjCTPI DNA	Fused to bovine heat shock protein 70	41–51	42–62	33–52 (miracidial hatching)	
	SjC23DNA	(Hsp70) and boosted with a plasmid DNA encoding IL-12	45–51	43–54	47–52 (miracidial hatching)	[10]
Water buffalo	Sjc26GST (field study)	Twenty months after vaccination, the infection rate in buffaloes was reduced by 60–68%				[53]
	Sjc26GST		22	50	50	[52]
	Sj28GST (field study)	Injected with Freund's adjuvants	37	33	62 (miracidial hatching)	[46]
	Cryopreserved-irradiated and freeze-thaw schistosomula	Single/twice intradermal vaccination	62–65			[22]
	Cercariae UV irradiated	Six immunizations	89			[24]
Goat	Sj31 and Sj32	DNA priming-protein boosting	21–32	47–52	48–54 (miracidial hatching)	[59]
	Sj26GST		30	60		[54]
Cattle	Sj28GST-DNA	Three immunizations	44	19	77	[47]
	Sj23-DNA		33	34	66	
	Sj28GST + Sj23-DNA		38	48	68	
Sheep	Sj26GST	Injected with Freund's adjuvants	54–62	42–55	11–38	[45,46]
	Sj28GST		61–69	59–69	43–60	
	Sj23		58–66	56–66	40–58	
	Native Paramyosin			68	43	
	Paramyosin			56	16	

3.2. Paramyosin

Paramyosin is a large (97 kDa) coiled-coil myofibrillar protein restricted to invertebrates. In schistosomes it is found on the tegumental surface of lung stage schistosomula, in the cercarial secretory glands, and in the muscles of adult worms and larvae [60]. This molecule first generated interest as a vaccine candidate based on results of experiments in mice targeting *S. mansoni* [60]. Trials in sheep with native and an expressed and purified recombinant fragment of Chinese strain *S. japonicum* paramyosin (Sj-97) resulted in significant partial protection being obtained [45]. Subsequently, vaccine experiments in pigs [27] and water buffaloes [61], using full length Chinese *S. japonicum* paramyosin, yielded further encouraging protective efficacy against challenge infection, although the protection was again only partial. At this time (the early 2000s) the limitations to wide-spread use of recombinant (r) Sj-97 as a vaccine were the size of the protein, the inadequate expression levels obtained, resulting in low yields of the recombinant protein, its insolubility in yeast and bacterial expression systems, the inevitable costs of its up-scaled production and purification, and the funds required for large-scale buffalo vaccine trials in the field; this resulted in a halting in its progression as a priority vaccine candidate.

In 2008, however, Jiz et al. [62] published a new robust method for the pilot-scale expression and purification of rSj-97 by its extraction from *E. coli* inclusion bodies and purification with sequential anion-exchange, hydroxyapatite, and size exclusion chromatography. The purified protein was greater than 95% pure, free of significant endotoxin contamination, adopted an alpha-helical coiled-coil tertiary structure, bound immunoglobulin and collagen, and represented a significant step forward towards preclinical evaluation of paramyosin as a vaccine for schistosomiasis [63]. The same team showed that the rSj-97 vaccine, adjuvanted with Montanide ISA 206, was safe, well tolerated and robustly immunogenic among water buffaloes resident in four villages in Leyte, the Philippines, an area highly endemic for schistosomiasis japonica [64]. They conducted three vaccine trials (in 2008, in 2013 and in 2016) to assess the level of protection generated in water buffaloes with the rSj-97 vaccine; animals received and tolerated well three doses (250 μg/dose or 500 μg/dose) of rSj97 plus Montanide ISA 206 at 4 weekly intervals before a challenge infection with 1000 *S. japonicum* cercariae [58]. The 3 × 250 μg/dose of rSj97 (2008 and 2013 trials) did not result in a significant reduction in worm burden in vaccinated animals compared with controls injected with ISA 206 emulsified with lyophilisation buffer, but the increased dosage (3 × 500 μg/dose of rSj97) in the 2013 and 2016 trials resulted in a significantly lower worm burden (by 57.8% in both trials) in vaccinated water buffaloes compared with controls [58]. The trialled rSj97/ISA206 vaccine resulted in a mixed immune response with induction of both IgG1 and IgG2 anti-paramyosin antibodies, but no conclusive correlation was found between isotype distribution and protection [58]. The group also reported undertaking a trial in buffaloes with the rSj97-ISA206 vaccine followed by six months of community-based field exposure after vaccination [58], but the results have not yet been released.

3.3. Triose-Phosphate Isomerase (TPI)

Another leading anti-schistosome vaccine candidate is triose-phosphate isomerase (TPI). Following its uptake in schistosomes, glucose is metabolised via glycolysis to provide critical energy in the form of ATP to ensure parasite survival; TPI is a highly efficient enzyme and pivotal in this process, converting glyceraldehyde-3-phosphate to dihydroxyacetone phosphate. It is located in most cells of the adult schistosome and on the surface membranes of newly transformed schistosomula, the stage in the mammalian host that is considered the most likely target of an anti-schistosome vaccine [50]; a plasmid DNA vaccine encoding *S. japonicum* Chinese strain TPI (SjCTPI) was shown to reduce worm burdens in mice and pigs [57,65]. Subsequently, the efficacy of SjCTPI and the 23 kDa integral membrane protein tetraspanin (SjC23), independently, and as fusions with bovine heat-shock protein 70 (Hsp70), co-administered with an interleukin-12-expressing plasmid as adjuvant, were assessed as DNA vaccines in China in water buffaloes against experimental *S. japonicum* challenge [10]. The most encouraging vaccine was the SjCTPI-Hsp70 construct, which reduced worm burdens by

51.2%, reduced liver eggs by 61.5%, reduced faecal eggs by 52.1% and resulted in a 52.1% reduction in hatching of faecal miracidia [10]. The SjCTPI-Hsp70 vaccine has subsequently undergone field testing in bovines against natural *S. japonicum* challenge in China. The trial comprised a four-year double-blind cluster randomised intervention in 12 administrative villages around the schistosomiasis-endemic Dongting Lake in Hunan Province, designed to assess the impact of a multi-component integrated control strategy, including bovine vaccination using a heterologous 'prime-boost' delivery of the SjCTPI vaccine, on schistosome transmission. The study design and baseline results have been published [66]. In brief, the integrated control strategies included: (a) Combined human mass chemotherapy and the bovine SjCTPI vaccine or placebo vaccine; (b) Combined mollusciciding of snails and bovine SjCTPI vaccine or placebo vaccine; (c) No other intervention (treatment of infected individuals only) and bovine SjCTPI vaccine or placebo vaccine. The primary end-point for the study is human infection rate, with secondary endpoints including bovine infection rate, snail infection prevalence and the density of infected snails.

4. Challenges and Opportunities for the Future

In summary, many of the *S. japonicum* vaccines tested in domestic livestock include enzymes, muscle components and membrane proteins (Table 1) [67,68]. DNA vaccines have found particular appeal as they generate both T-cell and B-cell (or antibody-mediated) immune responses, their preparation and production are convenient and cost-effective, and they can even be used in the field without a cold chain. Another advantage of applying DNA vaccines compared with other approaches is the possibility of targeting the in vivo expressed recombinant antigen to different cell compartments. Furthermore, methods such as prime-boost regimens and the use of adjuvants (such as IL-12) in combination with a DNA vaccine can enhance its protective efficacy.

Other than some proteomic analyses of *S. bovis* and the *S. bovis*-host interface, aimed at identifying potential new vaccine and drug targets [69], it is surprising that no recent research has been reported in the development and testing of different vaccines targeting schistosomiasis infections caused by *S. bovis* and *S. mattheei* in livestock, despite the early encouraging successes. This may be somewhat short-sighted as it has been recently argued that animal schistosomiasis likely causes a considerable drain, both directly and indirectly, on the local economy of many poor communities in sub-Saharan Africa [70]. Further, the zoonotic component of schistosomiasis transmission in Africa appears to be far more significant and important than previously thought [6], and this may impact on the current WHO vision to eliminate schistosomiasis as a public health issue by 2025. Consequently, it has been considered that extending treatment to include animal hosts in a One Health approach, as has been successfully undertaken in China, would be both of economic and public health benefit. The positioning of an animal-based transmission blocking vaccine as part of an integrated control package fits well into this scenario, as was recognised as an outcome of two workshops co-sponsored by the Bill and Melinda Gates Foundation and the National Institute of Allergy and Infectious Diseases on schistosomiasis elimination strategies and the potential role of a vaccine [71,72]. Some proposed Preferred Product Characteristics for a clinical versus a veterinary vaccine against schistosomiasis were formulated at one of these workshops, indicating that the safety profile of the latter is more straightforward and less rigorous [71]. Whereas this characteristic could potentially reduce the costs of deploying a schistosomiasis vaccine for use in livestock as opposed to one for human application, an evaluation of the economics and benefits of applying the two different types of vaccine needs to be undertaken.

One significant challenge impacting on the future development of veterinary-targeted vaccines to aid in the control of schistosomiasis continues to be our rather scanty knowledge of the immunology of schistosome infections in natural livestock hosts, especially bovines, compared with experimental model animals, such as mice. This is due, in part, to the high cost of purchasing and maintaining large animals for immunobiological studies and the scarcity and high price of immunological reagents for studying the relevant immune responses. Nevertheless, some recent research has provided new insights on immunity against schistosomiasis japonica in field-exposed natural hosts such as cattle and water buffalo, particularly the immune response generated against migrating schistosome larvae, the likely targets of an anti-schistosome vaccine. In an important study, McWilliam et al. [73] investigated the immune response evoked in the lungs and skin, the major sites of larval migration, in previously *S. japonicum*-exposed and re-challenged water buffaloes. A powerful allergic-type response was generated in the skin with IL-5 transcript levels being elevated, with IL-10 levels decreased. In addition, a Th1 type immune profile was demonstrated in stimulated cells from the lung-draining lymph node, whereas a predominant Th2 type immune response was apparent in stimulated cells from the skin-draining lymph node; these immune responses reflected the timing of parasite migration and occurred consecutively. The intense Th2 type profile generated at the cercarial penetration site differs markedly from that evident in mice, suggesting a possible mechanism of immunity. Furthermore, the study suggested that a reduced/delayed immune response occurred in buffaloes challenged with high numbers of cercariae compared with lower numbers, particularly in the skin.

In tandem with studies comparing immune responses in buffalo (in which age-related resistance likely occurs) and yellow cattle (in which it does not) against schistosomiasis [74,75], and further immunological exploration of the self-cure effect in older buffalo and other livestock hosts such as pigs against schistosomes [76], the investigation by McWilliam et al. [73] provides a unique, in-depth appreciation of the immunobiology of schistosomiasis in a natural host. Such studies can aid in the design and delivery of more effective anti-schistosome vaccines that will complement current control options so as to achieve and sustain future elimination goals.

Author Contributions: D.P.M. conducted the literature review, and drafted and revised the manuscript. H.Y., B.M.T., L.Y. and P.C. revised the manuscript and provided intellectual content. All authors read and approved the final manuscript.

Acknowledgments: The authors would like to thank the National Health and Medical Research Council of Australia (NHMRC) for providing financial support for their research on schistosomiasis through Project (APP1002245, APP1098244) and Program (APP1037304, APP1132975) grants. DPM is a NHMRC Senior Principal Research Fellow (APP1102926).

References

1. De Bont, J.; Vercruysse, J. Schistosomiasis in cattle. *Adv. Parasitol.* **1998**, *41*, 285–364. [PubMed]
2. Charlier, J.; van der Voort, M.; Kenyon, F.; Skuce, P.; Vercruysse, J. Chasing helminths and their economic impact on farmed ruminants. *Trends Parasitol.* **2014**, *30*, 361–367. [CrossRef] [PubMed]
3. Webster, B.L.; Diaw, O.T.; Seye, M.M.; Webster, J.P.; Rollinson, D. Introgressive hybridization of *Schistosoma haematobium* group species in Senegal: Species barrier break down between ruminant and human schistosomes. *PLoS Negl. Trop. Dis.* **2013**, *7*, e2110. [CrossRef] [PubMed]
4. Boissier, J.; Grech-Angelini, S.; Webster, B.L.; Allienne, J.F.; Huyse, T.; Mas-Coma, S.; Toulza, E.; Barre-Cardi, H.; Rollinson, D.; Kincaid-Smith, J.; et al. Outbreak of urogenital schistosomiasis in Corsica (France): An epidemiological case study. *Lancet Infect. Dis.* **2016**, *16*, 971–979. [CrossRef]
5. King, K.C.; Stelkens, R.B.; Webster, J.P.; Smith, D.F.; Brockhurst, M.A. Hybridization in parasites: Consequences for adaptive evolution, pathogenesis, and public health in a changing world. *PLoS Pathog.* **2015**, *11*, e1005098. [CrossRef] [PubMed]
6. Leger, E.; Webster, J.P. Hybridizations within the genus *Schistosoma*: Implications for evolution, epidemiology and control. *Parasitology* **2017**, *144*, 65–80. [CrossRef] [PubMed]
7. Bergquist, R.; Utzinger, J.; McManus, D.P. Trick or treat: The role of vaccines in integrated schistosomiasis control. *PLoS Negl. Trop. Dis.* **2008**, *2*, e244. [CrossRef] [PubMed]
8. Bergquist, R.M.; Donald, M. Schistosomiasis vaccine development: The missing link. In *Schistosoma Biology, Pathology, Control*; Jamieson, B.G.M., Ed.; CRC Press: Boca Raton, FL, USA, 2017; pp. 462–478.

9. Williams, G.M.; Sleigh, A.C.; Li, Y.; Feng, Z.; Davis, G.M.; Chen, H.; Ross, A.G.; Bergquist, R.; McManus, D.P. Mathematical modelling of schistosomiasis japonica: Comparison of control strategies in the People's Republic of China. *Acta Trop.* **2002**, *82*, 253–262. [CrossRef]

10. Da'dara, A.A.; Li, Y.S.; Xiong, T.; Zhou, J.; Williams, G.M.; McManus, D.P.; Feng, Z.; Yu, X.L.; Gray, D.J.; Harn, D.A. DNA-based vaccines protect against zoonotic schistosomiasis in water buffalo. *Vaccine* **2008**, *26*, 3617–3625. [CrossRef] [PubMed]

11. Gray, D.J.; Williams, G.M.; Li, Y.; Chen, H.; Li, R.S.; Forsyth, S.J.; Barnett, A.G.; Guo, J.; Feng, Z.; McManus, D.P. A cluster-randomized bovine intervention trial against *Schistosoma japonicum* in the People's Republic of China: Design and baseline results. *Am. J. Trop. Med. Hyg.* **2007**, *77*, 866–874. [PubMed]

12. Gordon, C.A.; Acosta, L.P.; Gray, D.J.; Olveda, R.M.; Jarilla, B.; Gobert, G.N.; Ross, A.G.; McManus, D.P. High prevalence of *Schistosoma japonicum* infection in Carabao from Samar Province, the Philippines: Implications for transmission and control. *PLoS Negl. Trop. Dis.* **2012**, *6*, e1778. [CrossRef] [PubMed]

13. Taylor, M.G.; James, E.R.; Nelson, G.S.; Bickle, Q.; Dunne, D.W.; Webbe, G. Immunisation of sheep against *Schistosoma mattheei* using either irradiated cercariae or irradiated schistosomula. *J. Helminthol.* **1976**, *50*, 1–9. [CrossRef] [PubMed]

14. Hussein, M.F.; Bushara, H.O. Investigations on the development of an irradiated vaccine for animal schistosomiasis. In *Nuclear Techniques in Animal Production and Health*; International Atomic Energy Agency: Vienna, Austria, 1976; pp. 421–431.

15. Taylor, M.G.; James, E.R.; Bickle, Q.; Hussein, M.F.; Andrews, B.J.; Dobinson, A.R.; Nelson, G.S. Immunization of sheep against *Schistosoma bovis* using an irradiated schistosomular vaccine. *J. Helminthol.* **1979**, *53*, 1–5. [CrossRef] [PubMed]

16. Bushara, H.O.; Hussein, M.F.; Saad, A.M.; Taylor, M.G.; Dargie, J.D.; Marshall, T.F.; Nelson, G.S. Immunization of calves against *Schistosoma bovis* using irradiated cercariae of schistosomula of *S. bovis*. *Parasitology* **1978**, *77*, 303–311. [CrossRef] [PubMed]

17. Majid, A.A.; Bushara, H.O.; Saad, A.M.; Hussein, M.F.; Taylor, M.G.; Dargie, J.D.; Marshall, T.F.; Nelson, G.S. Observations on cattle schistosomiasis in the Sudan, a study in comparative medicine. III. Field testing of an irradiated *Schistosoma bovis* vaccine. *Am. J. Trop. Med. Hyg.* **1980**, *29*, 452–455. [CrossRef] [PubMed]

18. James, E.R. Cryopreservation of helminths. *Parasitol. Today* **1985**, *1*, 134–139. [CrossRef]

19. James, E.R.; Dobinson, A.R.; Lucas, S.B.; Andrews, B.J.; Bickle, Q.D.; Taylor, M.G.; Ham, P.J. Protection of sheep against *Schistosoma bovis* using cryopreserved radiation-attenuated schistosomula. *J. Helminthol.* **1985**, *59*, 51–55. [CrossRef] [PubMed]

20. Hsu, S.Y.; Hsu, H.F.; Xu, S.T.; Shi, F.H.; He, Y.X.; Clarke, W.R.; Johnson, S.C. Vaccination against bovine schistosomiasis japonica with highly X-irradiated schistosomula. *Am. J. Trop. Med. Hyg.* **1983**, *32*, 367–370. [CrossRef] [PubMed]

21. Hsu, S.Y.; Xu, S.T.; He, Y.X.; Shi, F.H.; Shen, W.; Hsu, H.F.; Osborne, J.W.; Clarke, W.R. Vaccination of bovines against schistosomiasis japonica with highly irradiated schistosomula in China. *Am. J. Trop. Med. Hyg.* **1984**, *33*, 891–898. [CrossRef] [PubMed]

22. Xu, S.; Shi, F.; Shen, W.; Lin, J.; Wang, Y.; Lin, B.; Qian, C.; Ye, P.; Fu, L.; Shi, Y.; et al. Vaccination of bovines against schistosomiasis japonica with cryopreserved-irradiated and freeze-thaw schistosomula. *Vet. Parasitol.* **1993**, *47*, 37–50. [PubMed]

23. Xu, S.; Wu, H.; Fu, L.; Tzian, T.; Lin, B.; Tzian, T.; Chu, H. Tests to immunize sheep by freezing *Schistosoma japonicum* larva vaccines. *China J. Vet. Sci. Technol.* **1990**, *2*, 19–20.

24. Shi, Y.E.; Jiang, C.F.; Han, J.J.; Li, Y.L.; Ruppel, A. *Schistosoma japonicum*: An ultraviolet-attenuated cercarial vaccine applicable in the field for water buffaloes. *Exp. Parasitol.* **1990**, *71*, 100–106. [CrossRef]

25. Shi, Y.E.; Jiang, C.F.; Han, J.J.; Li, Y.L.; Ruppel, A. Immunization of pigs against infection with *Schistosoma japonicum* using ultraviolet-attenuated cercariae. *Parasitology* **1993**, *106*, 459–462. [CrossRef] [PubMed]

26. Chi, L.W.; Andreus, J.; Yates, R.A.; Kiley, L.A.; Liu, S.X. Worm burden and lymphocyte response in mice immunized with N-methyl-N'-nitro-N-nitrosoguanidine attenuated cercariae of *Schistosoma japonicum*. *Chin. Med. J.* **1988**, *101*, 181–186. [PubMed]

27. Chen, H.; Nara, T.; Zeng, X.; Satoh, M.; Wu, G.; Jiang, W.; Yi, F.; Kojima, S.; Zhang, S.; Hirayama, K. Vaccination of domestic pig with recombinant paramyosin against *Schistosoma japonicum* in China. *Vaccine* **2000**, *18*, 2142–2146. [CrossRef]

28. Bickle, Q.D.; Bogh, H.O.; Johansen, M.V.; Zhang, Y. Comparison of the vaccine efficacy of gamma-irradiated *Schistosoma japonicum* cercariae with the defined antigen Sj62(IrV-5) in pigs. *Vet. Parasitol.* **2001**, *100*, 51–62. [CrossRef]

29. Abdel-Hafeez, E.H.; Kikuchi, M.; Watanabe, K.; Ito, T.; Yu, C.; Chen, H.; Nara, T.; Arakawa, T.; Aoki, Y.; Hirayama, K. Proteome approach for identification of schistosomiasis japonica vaccine candidate antigen. *Parasitol. Int.* **2009**, *58*, 36–44. [CrossRef] [PubMed]

30. Tian, F.; Lin, D.; Wu, J.; Gao, Y.; Zhang, D.; Ji, M.; Wu, G. Immune events associated with high level protection against *Schistosoma japonicum* infection in pigs immunized with UV-attenuated cercariae. *PLoS ONE* **2010**, *5*, e13408. [CrossRef] [PubMed]

31. Lin, D.; Tian, F.; Wu, H.; Gao, Y.; Wu, J.; Zhang, D.; Ji, M.; McManus, D.P.; Driguez, P.; Wu, G. Multiple vaccinations with UV-attenuated cercariae in pig enhance protective immunity against *Schistosoma japonicum* infection as compared to single vaccination. *Parasites Vectors* **2011**, *4*. [CrossRef] [PubMed]

32. Tian, F.; Hou, M.; Chen, L.; Gao, Y.; Zhang, X.; Ji, M.; Wu, G. Proteomic analysis of schistosomiasis japonica vaccine candidate antigens recognized by UV-attenuated cercariae-immunized porcine serum IgG2. *Parasitol. Res.* **2013**, *112*, 2791–2803. [CrossRef] [PubMed]

33. Abdel-Hafeez, E.H.; Watanabe, K.; Kamei, K.; Kikuchi, M.; Chen, H.; Daniel, B.; Yu, C.; Hirayama, K. Pilot study on interferon-gamma-producing T cell subsets after the protective vaccination with radiation-attenuated cercaria of *Schistosoma japonicum* in the miniature pig model. *Trop. Med. Health* **2014**, *42*, 155–162. [CrossRef] [PubMed]

34. Balloul, J.M.; Sondermeyer, P.; Dreyer, D.; Capron, M.; Grzych, J.M.; Pierce, R.J.; Carvallo, D.; Lecocq, J.P.; Capron, A. Molecular cloning of a protective antigen of schistosomes. *Nature* **1987**, *326*, 149–153. [CrossRef] [PubMed]

35. Saint, R.B.; Beall, J.A.; Grumont, R.J.; Mitchell, G.F.; Garcia, E.G. Expression of *Schistosoma japonicum* antigens in *Escherichia coli*. *Mol. Biochem. Parasitol.* **1986**, *18*, 333–342. [CrossRef]

36. Trottein, F.; Godin, C.; Pierce, R.J.; Sellin, B.; Taylor, M.G.; Gorillot, I.; Silva, M.S.; Lecocq, J.P.; Capron, A. Inter-species variation of schistosome 28-kDa glutathione S-transferases. *Mol. Biochem. Parasitol.* **1992**, *54*, 63–72. [CrossRef]

37. Mitchell, G.F. Glutathione *S*-transferases—Potential components of anti-schistosome vaccines? *Parasitol. Today* **1989**, *5*, 34–37. [CrossRef]

38. Bushara, H.O.; Bashir, M.E.; Malik, K.H.; Mukhtar, M.M.; Trottein, F.; Capron, A.; Taylor, M.G. Suppression of *Schistosoma bovis* egg production in cattle by vaccination with either glutathione S-transferase or keyhole limpet haemocyanin. *Parasite Immunol.* **1993**, *15*, 383–390. [CrossRef] [PubMed]

39. Boulanger, D.; Trottein, F.; Mauny, F.; Bremond, P.; Couret, D.; Pierce, R.J.; Kadri, S.; Godin, C.; Sellin, E.; Lecocq, J.P.; et al. Vaccination of goats against the trematode *Schistosoma bovis* with a recombinant homologous schistosome-derived glutathione S-transferase. *Parasite Immunol.* **1994**, *16*, 399–406. [CrossRef] [PubMed]

40. Boulanger, D.; Schneider, D.; Chippaux, J.P.; Sellin, B.; Capron, A. *Schistosoma bovis*: Vaccine effects of a recombinant homologous glutathione S-transferase in sheep. *Int. J. Parasitol.* **1999**, *29*, 415–418. [CrossRef]

41. De Bont, J.; Vercruysse, J.; Grzych, J.M.; Meeus, P.F.; Capron, A. Potential of a recombinant *Schistosoma bovis*-derived glutathione S-transferase to protect cattle against experimental and natural *S. mattheei* infection. *Parasitology* **1997**, *115*, 249–255. [CrossRef] [PubMed]

42. Grzych, J.M.; De Bont, J.; Liu, J.; Neyrinck, J.L.; Fontaine, J.; Vercruysse, J.; Capron, A. Relationship of impairment of schistosome 28-kilodalton glutathione S-transferase (GST) activity to expression of immunity to *Schistosoma mattheei* in calves vaccinated with recombinant *Schistosoma bovis* 28-kilodalton GST. *Infect. Immun.* **1998**, *66*, 1142–1148. [PubMed]

43. Capron, A. Schistosomiasis: Forty years' war on the worm. *Parasitol. Today* **1998**, *14*, 379–384. [CrossRef]

44. Herve, M.; Angeli, V.; Pinzar, E.; Wintjens, R.; Faveeuw, C.; Narumiya, S.; Capron, A.; Urade, Y.; Capron, M.; Riveau, G.; et al. Pivotal roles of the parasite PGD2 synthase and of the host D prostanoid receptor 1 in schistosome immune evasion. *Eur. J. Immunol.* **2003**, *33*, 2764–2772. [CrossRef] [PubMed]

45. Taylor, M.G.; Huggins, M.C.; Shi, F.; Lin, J.; Tian, E.; Ye, P.; Shen, W.; Qian, C.G.; Lin, B.F.; Bickle, Q.D. Production and testing of *Schistosoma japonicum* candidate vaccine antigens in the natural ovine host. *Vaccine* **1998**, *16*, 1290–1298. [CrossRef]

46. Shi, F.; Zhang, Y.; Ye, P.; Lin, J.; Cai, Y.; Shen, W.; Bickle, Q.D.; Taylor, M.G. Laboratory and field evaluation of *Schistosoma japonicum* DNA vaccines in sheep and water buffalo in China. *Vaccine* **2001**, *20*, 462–467. [CrossRef]

47. Shi, F.; Zhang, Y.; Lin, J.; Zuo, X.; Shen, W.; Cai, Y.; Ye, P.; Bickle, Q.D.; Taylor, M.G. Field testing of *Schistosoma japonicum* DNA vaccines in cattle in China. *Vaccine* **2002**, *20*, 3629–3631. [CrossRef]

48. McManus, D.P. Prospects for development of a transmission blocking vaccine against *Schistosoma japonicum*. *Parasite Immunol.* **2005**, *27*, 297–308. [CrossRef] [PubMed]

49. Wu, Z.D.; Lu, Z.Y.; Yu, X.B. Development of a vaccine against *Schistosoma japonicum* in China: A review. *Acta Trop.* **2005**, *96*, 106–116. [CrossRef] [PubMed]

50. McManus, D.P.; Loukas, A. Current status of vaccines for schistosomiasis. *Clin. Microbiol. Rev.* **2008**, *21*, 225–242. [CrossRef] [PubMed]

51. Liu, S.X.; Song, G.C.; Xu, Y.X.; Yang, W.; McManus, D.P. Anti-fecundity immunity induced in pigs vaccinated with recombinant *Schistosoma japonicum* 26 kDa glutathione-*S*-transferase. *Parasite Immunol.* **1995**, *17*, 335–340. [CrossRef] [PubMed]

52. Shuxian, L.; Yongkang, H.; Guangchen, S.; Xing-song, L.; Yuxin, X.; McManus, D.P. Anti-fecundity immunity to *Schistosoma japonicum* induced in Chinese water buffaloes (*Bos buffelus*) after vaccination with recombinant 26 kDa glutathione-S-transferase (reSjc26GST). *Vet. Parasitol.* **1997**, *69*, 39–47. [CrossRef]

53. He, Y.K.; Liu, S.X.; Zhang, X.Y.; Chen, G.C.; Luo, X.S.; Li, Y.S.; Xu, Y.X.; Yu, X.L.; Yang, R.Q.; Chen, Y.; et al. Field assessment of recombinant *Schistosoma japonicum* 26 kDa glutathione S-transferase in Chinese water buffaloes. *Southeast Asian J. Trop. Med. Hyg.* **2003**, *34*, 473–479.

54. Wu, Z.; Liu, S.; Zhang, S.; Tong, H.; Gao, Z.; Liu, Y.; Lin, D.; Liu, Z.; Wu, G.; Yi, H.; et al. Persistence of the protective immunity to *Schistosoma japonicum* in Chinese yellow cattle induced by recombinant 26 kDa glutathione-S-transferase (reSjc26GST). *Vet. Parasitol.* **2004**, *123*, 167–177. [CrossRef] [PubMed]

55. Cheng, P.C.; Lin, C.N.; Peng, S.Y.; Kang, T.F.; Lee, K.M. Combined IL-12 Plasmid and recombinant SjGST enhance the protective and anti-pathology effect of SjGST DNA vaccine against *Schistosoma japonicum*. *PLoS Negl. Trop. Dis.* **2016**, *10*. [CrossRef] [PubMed]

56. Zhu, Y.; Ren, J.; Da'dara, A.; Harn, D.; Xu, M.; Si, J.; Yu, C.; Liang, Y.; Ye, P.; Yin, X.; et al. The protective effect of a *Schistosoma japonicum* Chinese strain 23 kDa plasmid DNA vaccine in pigs is enhanced with IL-12. *Vaccine* **2004**, *23*, 78–83. [CrossRef] [PubMed]

57. Zhu, Y.; Si, J.; Harn, D.A.; Xu, M.; Ren, J.; Yu, C.; Liang, Y.; Yin, X.; He, W.; Cao, G. *Schistosoma japonicum* triose-phosphate isomerase plasmid DNA vaccine protects pigs against challenge infection. *Parasitology* **2006**, *132*, 67–71. [CrossRef] [PubMed]

58. Wu, H.W.; Fu, Z.Q.; Lu, K.; Pond-Tor, S.; Meng, R.; Hong, Y.; Chu, K.; Li, H.; Jiz, M.; Liu, J.M.; et al. Vaccination with recombinant paramyosin in Montanide ISA206 protects against *Schistosoma japonicum* infection in water buffalo. *Vaccine* **2017**, *35*, 3409–3415. [CrossRef] [PubMed]

59. Tang, L.; Zhou, Z.; Chen, Y.; Luo, Y.; Wang, L.; Chen, L.; Huang, F.; Zeng, X.; Yi, X. Vaccination of goats with 31 kDa and 32 kDa *Schistosoma japonicum* antigens by DNA priming and protein boosting. *Cell. Mol. Immunol.* **2007**, *4*, 153–156. [PubMed]

60. Gobert, G.N.; Stenzel, D.J.; Jones, M.K.; Allen, D.E.; McManus, D.P. *Schistosoma japonicum*: Immunolocalization of paramyosin during development. *Parasitology* **1997**, *114*, 45–52. [CrossRef] [PubMed]

61. McManus, D.P.; Wong, J.Y.; Zhou, J.; Cai, C.; Zeng, Q.; Smyth, D.; Li, Y.; Kalinna, B.H.; Duke, M.J.; Yi, X. Recombinant paramyosin (rec-Sj-97) tested for immunogenicity and vaccine efficacy against *Schistosoma japonicum* in mice and water buffaloes. *Vaccine* **2001**, *20*, 870–878. [CrossRef]

62. Jiz, M.; Wu, H.W.; Meng, R.; Pond-Tor, S.; Reynolds, M.; Friedman, J.F.; Olveda, R.; Acosta, L.; Kurtis, J.D. Pilot-scale production and characterization of paramyosin, a vaccine candidate for schistosomiasis japonica. *Infect. Immun.* **2008**, *76*, 3164–3169. [CrossRef] [PubMed]

63. Jiz, M.A.; Wu, H.; Olveda, R.; Jarilla, B.; Kurtis, J.D. Development of paramyosin as a vaccine candidate for schistosomiasis. *Front. Immunol.* **2015**, *6*. [CrossRef] [PubMed]

64. Jiz, I.M.; Mingala, C.N.; Lopez, I.F.M.; Chua, M.; Gabonada, F.G., Jr.; Acosta, L.P.; Wu, H.; Kurtis, J.D. A field trial of recombinant *Schistosoma japonicum* paramyosin as a potential vaccine in naturally-infected water buffaloes. *Ann. Parasitol.* **2016**, *62*, 295–299.

65. Zhu, Y.; Si, J.; Ham, D.A.; Yu, C.; He, W.; Hua, W.; Yin, X.; Liang, Y.; Xu, M.; Xu, R. The protective immunity produced in infected C57BL/6 mice of a DNA vaccine encoding *Schistosoma japonicum* Chinese strain

triose-phosphate isomerase. *Southeast Asian J. Trop. Med. Public Health* **2002**, *33*, 207–213. [PubMed]

66. Gray, D.J.; Li, Y.S.; Williams, G.M.; Zhao, Z.Y.; Harn, D.A.; Li, S.M.; Ren, M.Y.; Feng, Z.; Guo, F.Y.; Guo, J.G.; et al. A multi-component integrated approach for the elimination of schistosomiasis in the People's Republic of China: Design and baseline results of a 4-year cluster-randomised intervention trial. *Int. J. Parasitol.* **2014**, *44*, 659–668. [CrossRef] [PubMed]

67. Tebeje, B.M.; Harvie, M.; You, H.; Loukas, A.; McManus, D.P. Schistosomiasis vaccines: Where do we stand? *Parasites Vectors* **2016**, *9*. [CrossRef] [PubMed]

68. You, H.; McManus, D.P. Vaccines and diagnostics for zoonotic schistosomiasis japonica. *Parasitology* **2015**, *142*, 271–289. [CrossRef] [PubMed]

69. De la Torre-Escudero, E.; Perez-Sanchez, R.; Manzano-Roman, R.; Oleaga, A. *Schistosoma bovis*-host interplay: Proteomics for knowing and acting. *Mol. Biochem. Parasitol.* **2017**, *215*, 30–39. [CrossRef] [PubMed]

70. Gower, C.M.; Vince, L.; Webster, J.P. Should we be treating animal schistosomiasis in Africa? The need for a One Health economic evaluation of schistosomiasis control in people and their livestock. *Trans. R. Soc. Trop. Med. Hyg.* **2017**, *111*, 244–247. [CrossRef] [PubMed]

71. Mo, A.X.; Colley, D.G. Workshop report: Schistosomiasis vaccine clinical development and product characteristics. *Vaccine* **2016**, *34*, 995–1001. [CrossRef] [PubMed]

72. Mo, A.X.; Agosti, J.M.; Walson, J.L.; Hall, B.F.; Gordon, L. Schistosomiasis elimination strategies and potential role of a vaccine in achieving global health goals. *Am. J. Trop. Med. Hyg.* **2014**, *90*, 54–60. [CrossRef] [PubMed]

73. McWilliam, H.E.; Piedrafita, D.; Li, Y.; Zheng, M.; He, Y.; Yu, X.; McManus, D.P.; Meeusen, E.N. Local immune responses of the Chinese water buffalo, *Bubalus bubalis*, against *Schistosoma japonicum* larvae: Crucial insights for vaccine design. *PLoS Negl. Trop. Dis.* **2013**, *7*, e2460. [CrossRef] [PubMed]

74. Wang, T.; Zhang, S.; Wu, W.; Zhang, G.; Lu, D.; Ornbjerg, N.; Johansen, M.V. Treatment and reinfection of water buffaloes and cattle infected with *Schistosoma japonicum* in Yangtze River Valley, Anhui province, China. *J. Parasitol.* **2006**, *92*, 1088–1091. [CrossRef] [PubMed]

75. Yang, J.; Fu, Z.; Feng, X.; Shi, Y.; Yuan, C.; Liu, J.; Hong, Y.; Li, H.; Lu, K.; Lin, J. Comparison of worm development and host immune responses in natural hosts of *Schistosoma japonicum*, yellow cattle and water buffalo. *BMC Vet. Res.* **2012**, *8*. [CrossRef] [PubMed]

76. Li, Y.S.; McManus, D.P.; Lin, D.D.; Williams, G.M.; Harn, D.A.; Ross, A.G.; Feng, Z.; Gray, D.J. The *Schistosoma japonicum* self-cure phenomenon in water buffaloes: Potential impact on the control and elimination of schistosomiasis in China. *Int. J. Parasitol.* **2014**, *44*, 167–171. [CrossRef] [PubMed]

11

Field Evaluation of a Loop-Mediated Isothermal Amplification (LAMP) Platform for the Detection of *Schistosoma japonicum* Infection in *Oncomelania hupensis* Snails

Zhi-Qiang Qin [1], Jing Xu [1], Ting Feng [1], Shan Lv [1], Ying-Jun Qian [1], Li-Juan Zhang [1], Yin-Long Li [1], Chao Lv [1], Robert Bergquist [2], Shi-Zhu Li [1] and Xiao-Nong Zhou [1,*]

[1] Key Laboratory of Parasite and Vector Biology, Ministry of Health; National Institute of Parasitic Diseases, Chinese Center for Disease Control and Prevention, Shanghai 200025, China; qinzq1008@hotmail.com (Z.-Q.Q.); xujing@nipd.chinacdc.cn (J.X.); fengting@nipd.chinacdc.cn (T.F.); lvshan@nipd.chinacdc.cn (S.L.); yjqiancn@163.com (Y.-J.Q.); zhanglj@nipd.chinacdc.cn (L.-J.Z.); liyl@nipd.chinacdc.cn (Y.-L.L.); lvchao@nipd.chinacdc.cn (C.L.); lisz@chinacdc.cn (S.-Z.L.)

[2] Ingerod, SE-454 94 Brastad, Sweden; robert.bergquist@outlook.com

* Correspondence: zhouxn1@chinacdc.cn

Abstract: *Schistosoma* infection in snails can be monitored by microscopy or indirectly by sentinel mice. As both these approaches can miss infections, more sensitive tests are needed, particularly in low-level transmission settings. In this study, loop-mediated isothermal amplification (LAMP) technique, designed to detect a specific 28S ribosomal *Schistosoma japonicum* (Sj28S) gene with high sensitivity, was compared to microscopy using snail samples from 51 areas endemic for schistosomiasis in five Chinese provinces. In addition, the results were compared with those from polymerase chain reaction (PCR) by adding DNA sequencing as a reference. The testing of pooled snail samples with the LAMP assay showed that a dilution factor of 1/50, i.e., one infected snail plus 49 non-infected ones, would still result in a positive reaction after the recommended number of amplification cycles. Testing a total of 232 pooled samples, emanating from 4006 snail specimens, showed a rate of infection of 6.5%, while traditional microscopy found only 0.4% positive samples in the same materials. Parallel PCR analysis confirmed the diagnostic accuracy of the LAMP assay, with DNA sequencing even giving LAMP a slight lead. Microscopy and the LAMP test were carried out at local schistosomiasis-control stations, demonstrating that the potential of the latter assay to serve as a point-of-care (POC) test with results available within 60–90 min, while the more complicated PCR test had to be carried out at the National Institute of Parasitic Diseases (NIPD) in Shanghai, China. In conclusion, LAMP was found to be clearly superior to microscopy and as good as, or better than, PCR. As it can be used under field conditions and requires less time than other techniques, LAMP testing would improve and accelerate schistosomiasis control.

Keywords: *Schistosoma japonicum*; *Oncomelania hupensis*; snail; 28S ribosomal DNA; PCR; loop-mediated isothermal amplification (LAMP); pooled samples; China

1. Introduction

Schistosomiasis, one of the neglected tropical diseases (NTDs), is a public health problem caused by one of six species of the *Schistosoma* parasite that affects >200 million people in Africa, South America and Southeast Asia. However, the prevalence of schistosomiasis, based on stool examination and urine filtration, strongly understates the presumed real figure, as indicated by more sensitive techniques [1,2]. In China, the Philippines and three small pockets of the Indonesian island Sulawesi, the disease is a zoonosis caused by *Schistosoma japonicum* [1–3]. In China, the required intermediate snail host, *Oncomelania hupensis*, is widely distributed in the country's endemic areas, ranging from the Yangtze River Valley and the southern plains, to the mountainous regions of Sichuan and Yunnan in the west [4]. In 2004, a new integrated control strategy was introduced [5,6] involving reduction of infection sources by fencing off transmission sites, the replacement of water buffaloes (an important reservoir) with tractors for agricultural work and improved sanitation via access to clean water and latrines. These approaches have markedly reduced the infection rate in humans, domestic animals and the intermediate snail host [7]. The changes accomplished are so profound that it has become difficult to monitor the remaining transmission sites by only testing humans and domestic animals [8]. Conversely, snail diagnosis by microscopy or the use of the sentinel mice approach [9] are not only labor-intensive and time-consuming, but are also not sufficiently sensitive. To sustain the success achieved with regard to schistosomiasis elimination in China, highly sensitive snail-monitoring systems capable of assessing residual transmission in real time are now needed.

Due to its high sensitivity, molecular diagnosis has emerged as a promising approach for the detection of a suspected, low-level presence of pathogens [10–13]. However, a lack of the resources essential for this kind of diagnostics—such as bio-safety cabinets, a stable supply of electricity and well-experienced technicians, which are rare in peripheral laboratories in developing countries—limits the implementation of sophisticated technology.

The loop-mediated isothermal amplification (LAMP) technology employs a polymerase that amplifies the target DNA gene sequence with high specificity and rapidity under isothermal conditions [14]. Hamburger and colleagues investigated the use of this technique for the detection of infections due to *S. mansoni* and *S. haematobium,* showing excellent results, not only confirming that the LAMP technique works in the laboratory, but also in the field in Africa [15]. The usefulness and high sensitivity of LAMP-assisted snail diagnosis was later confirmed in Brazil by Gandasegui et al. [16] and in China by Kumagai et al. [17]. The latter research group developed a diagnostic platform based on a target 28S ribosomal DNA (rDNA) specific for *S. japonicum* (not reacting with *S. mansoni*) and showed that snails experimentally infected with only one miracidium could be detected less than 24 h after infection. As part of this study, we explored the application of LAMP using pooled snail samples, i.e., instead of testing each snail separately, we combined snails, however never in numbers exceeding 50 snails per pooled sample, based on preliminary dilution tests (see Results). The protocol used was derived from a visual LAMP-detection method developed by Tomita et al. [18], where the amplification of the pyrophosphate ion by-product combines with a divalent metal ion to form an insoluble salt. Adding calcein, a bivalent fluorescein/manganese complex, to the reaction solution results in a strong fluorescent signal from positive reactions, enabling visual discrimination by the naked eye without specialized equipment. We compared the results of the LAMP assay with the outcome using a polymerase chain reaction (PCR), applying DNA sequencing to determine the identity of the amplified product.

The purpose of the present study was not only to confirm the sensitivity of the LAMP method when used for the detection of *S. japonicum* DNA in infected snails in known endemic settings, but also to investigate and validate its application under field conditions soon after snail collection. An added aim was to determine if the LAMP procedure could be speeded up by testing pooled DNA samples in place of testing the snails individually.

2. Materials and Methods

This study constitutes an evaluation of LAMP-based snail diagnosis with the eventual aim of being part of a platform integrating different kinds of data and, thereby, enabling improved surveillance of schistosomiasis transmission. *O. hupensis* snails were collected during the spring over a period of three years (2013–2015) from all endemic regions in China, covering five provinces. The LAMP approach used is shown schematically in the form of a flow chart (Figure 1). As we were interested to see if the field work could be accelerated by testing samples consisting of pooled snails, DNA from various numbers of snails was investigated before the main study was undertaken.

Figure 1. Flow chart of loop-mediated isothermal amplification (LAMP) and PCR for detecting *S. japonicum*-infected snails.

2.1. Ethical Statement

Although this study did not include human sera or experimental animal data, an ethical statement is required to initiate any research project. Thus, we hereby state that all procedures performed within this study were conducted following animal husbandry guidelines of the Chinese Academy of Medical Sciences and with permission from the Experimental Animal Committee (National Institute of Parasitic Diseases (NIPD), Chinese Center for Diseases Control and Prevention, (China CDC) with ethical clearance number IPD-2012-5.

2.2. Snail Sampling Procedure

O. hupensis snails were collected from areas with known human schistosomiasis infection rates varying between 0.9% and 2.8% [19]. We used snails collected in April/May each year from 51 villages in 15 counties in Hunan, Hubei, Jiangxi, Anhui and Yunnan provinces. Most collection spots were in marshlands, except in Yunnan Province, where the snails were found in irrigation and drainage ditches. Systematic sampling was applied for snail investigation using survey frames of 250 m^2 in the marshlands and smaller areas spaced 50 m apart along the ditches [20,21]. All live snails found, together numbering 4006 specimens, were kept and transferred to the laboratory for testing.

2.3. Microscopy Testing and DNA Extraction

After having been crushed by pressure between clean glass plates and the pieces of shell removed, the snails were examined individually under the microscope at low magnification (generally 10×) to certify whether cercariae and/or sporocysts were present. After microscopy testing, 232 pooled snail samples from the 4006 single snails, were collected for further genomic DNA extraction. The snail soft tissues were pooled in clean 2.0 or 10.0 mL tubes (not exceeding 50 snail bodies in each) with 400–1000 μL of DNA lysis buffer (Qiagen, Valencia, CA, USA) added into each tube and the tissue collections homogenized. Subsequently, 20–50 μL of ProteinK (Qiagen, Valencia, CA, USA) was added to the snail homogenates with the tubes kept in a water bath at 56 °C, for 2–3 h, after which the supernatant of snail homogenates was saved and passed through a DNA binding column (Qiagen, Valencia, CA, USA). Finally, the dedicated DNA binding column was washed by the washing buffer

(Qiagen, Valencia, CA, USA) and the genomic DNA recovered by eluting the DNA-binding column with nuclease-free water. The recovered DNA samples were used for further testing by the LAMP assay and conventional PCR.

2.4. PCR Assay

A conventional PCR assay (PCR kit purchased from Takara Biotech, Dalian, China) was carried out in parallel with the LAMP assay (see below). Paired primer strands, i.e., 5′-GGTTTGACTATTAT TGTTGAGC-3′ and 5′-CTCACCTTAGTTCGGACTGA-3′ targeting the *S. japonicum* 28S (Sj28S) rDNA (Accession:EU835689.1) were used [17]. The ingredients were 1 μL of each primer (10 pmol/L each), 3 μL DNA template, 0.2 mM deoxynucleotide (dNTP) solution, 1.25 units of highly thermostable DNA polymerase from the thermophilic bacterium *Thermus aquaticus* (Taq DNA) and 2.5 μL $10\times$ buffer (pH 8.8 Tris-HCl, KCl and $MgCl_2$). The initial activation (cycle 1) was set for 3 min at 94 °C followed by 33 cycles of 30 s at 94 °C, 56 °C for 50 s and 72 °C for 1 min. The final extension step was carried out for 7 min at 72 °C. The amplified product was visualized by agarose gel electrophoresis (1.5%) with ethidium bromide staining.

2.5. DNA Sequencing

In order to make sure that the PCR product of all 14 positive samples exactly matched the target sequence, the 330 bp band of each PCR product was separated by gel electrophoresis, cloned into the Pmd19-T vector (Takara Biotech, Dalian, China), transferred into *E. coli* cells, strain DH5α, and then cultured in Luria-Bertani (LB) medium with ampicillin (100 μg/mL) at 37 °C in a 5.0 mL tube. After 12–16 h of culture, plasmid DNA was extracted from the bacterial colonies using a DNA extraction kit. The purified plasmid DNA was sent to a commercial company (Sangon Biotech, Co., Ltd., Shanghai, China) for sequence analysis, confirming the sample to be a complete match to Sj28S rDNA when compared with the National Center for Biotechnology Information (NCBI) database. One sample found to be positive by LAMP but negative by PCR, was subjected to an additional agarose gel analysis, thus we isolated the target band and sent the purified product for DNA sequence analysis to Sangon Biotech.

2.6. LAMP Assay

(A)   Reagent stock solution set-up and primer sequence

    a.   The $2\times$ reaction mixture: pH 8.8 Tris buffer (40 mM), KCl (20 M), $MgSO_4$ (16 mM), $(NH_4)_2SO_4$ (20 mM), Tween 20 (0.2%), betaine (1.6 M), dNTPs (2.8 mM each).

    b.   Calcein working solution ($2\times$ composition): Calcein (50 μM), $MnCl_2$ (1 mM).

    c.   Sj28S gene primers [17], (5′-3′, Sangon; HPLC purification): F3 (GCTTTGTCCTTCGGG CATTA), B3 (GGTTTCGTAACGCCCAATGA), FIP (ACGCAACTGCCAACGTGACATACT GGTCGGCTTGTTACTAGC), BIP (TGGTAGACGATCCACCTGACCCCTCGCGCACATGT TAAACTC)

(B)   Amplification (60–90 min)

We produced a reaction mixture of 7.5 μL nuclease-free water, 12.5 μL of $2\times$ reaction buffer, 1.0 μL of $25\times$ primer mixture, 1.0 μL (8 μ/μL) of Bst, a *Bacillus stearothermophilus* DNA polymerase homologue used for DNA strand displacement and 1.0 μL calcein. We used 0.2 mL reaction tubes dispensing 23 μL of the reaction mixture together with 2.0 μL of the sample to be tested into each tube. In addition, 23 μL of the reaction mixture was added to the Sj28S rDNA target in a second tube (the positive control) and also to the nuclease-free water in second tube (the negative control). All reaction tubes were incubated at 65 °C for 60~90 min, followed by the inactivation of the enzyme by the incubation of the tubes at 85 °C for 5 min. The tubes were then observed by the unaided eye to observe the color of the reaction changing from orange to yellow-green in the presence of LAMP (see Results).

2.6.1. Testing Samples with Life Cycle Stages of *S. japonicum*

Laboratory-bred *O. hupensis* snails were challenged with *S. japonicum* miracidia and the next life cycle stages of *S. japonicum* were thus transferred to the *O. hupensis* snails. To confirm whether DNA from different developing stage of *S. japonicum* could be detected by the LAMP assay, we performed the test with DNA collected from a mother sporocyst, a daughter sporocyst and a mature cercaria from these laboratory-based snails (infected and non-infected). Furthermore, to study whether DNA from other *Schistosoma* species would cross-react in the LAMP assay *Trichobilharzia* cercariae, emanating from a common bird-specific *Schistosoma* species, was also subjected to testing using the same procedure as described above under 2.5 and 2.6.

2.6.2. Pooled Snail Samples

To evaluate the detection limit of the LAMP method before the main study, we performed a preliminary test in which one schistosome-positive snail was mixed with different numbers of schistosome-negative snails at the following ratios: 1/4, 1/9, 1/19, 1/49, 1/99 and 1/199. For practical reasons, each snail pool in the main study came from the same area (though the different pools investigated contained different sets of snails). Depending on availability, the number of snails in the pools could not be standardized but it was always kept at ≤50. The result of this exercise was 232 snail pools made out of the total number of snails collected (4006). Depending on how many snails were pooled, the pools were kept in 2.0 mL or 10 mL centrifuge tubes together with 400 µL or 1.0 mL, of a lysis buffer from a DNeasy blood and tissue kit, (Qiagen, Valencia, CA, USA).

2.7. Validation

To assess the quality of the LAMP assay, a panel of nucleic acid extracts and test kits were dispatched to 28 separate testing health agency laboratories in the endemic areas at the provincial and county levels, where laboratory personnel were well-trained to operate the LAMP assay. Each nucleic acid sample was thawed, divided into 100 µL aliquots, coded and refrozen. The next day, all samples were packaged and sent by overnight shipment to the 28 separate laboratories. Each laboratory tested each sample 5 times using a standard LAMP protocol provided by National Institute of Parasitic Diseases (NIPD) at China CDC, based in Shanghai. The samples were validated against the true results, kept at the NIPD, which were unknown to the staff carrying out the testing in the health agency laboratories. The outcomes were scored according to a 0–100 scale, where 5 equal results were given a score of 100, 4 equal results were given a score of 80, and so on. To make sure that the LAMP test had the required specificity, it was applied (in parallel with the PCR assay) to 20 pools produced from a total of 1000 individual snails that had previously also been investigated by microscopy.

3. Results

As seen in Figure 2, the preliminary test of the snail pools in different ratios showed that large-scale testing could be carried out based on 50 snails without the risk of missing a positive result.

The ready-to-use LAMP test kit evaluated here detected 7.5 times more infected snails than microscopy, while the PCR results were consistent with those of the LAMP assay, except with respect to a single snail pool that was found to be positive by LAMP and negative by PCR. Out of the 232 pooled snail samples tested, 217 were found to be negative and 14 positive by both assays (Table 1), while the remaining single sample, found positive by LAMP but negative by PCR, was found to be positive by DNA sequence analysis, underlining LAMP's superiority. As can be seen in Table 2, none of the diagnostic approaches produced false positive results when applied to snail samples from non-endemic areas. The results further demonstrated that the schistosome DNA included in a single miracidium is sufficient to be amplified by the LAMP assay, making it possible to detect the schistosome infection already at the sporocyst stages in the snail, as well as when mature cercariae are ready for release.

The *Trichobilharzia* cercariae used to test the specificity were negative, confirming the specificity of the test (Figure 3).

Figure 2. Investigation of the LAMP diagnostic capability by testing serial dilutions of the Sj28S gene component. The following dilutions of infected and uninfected snails are shown: 1/4 (tube no. 1); 1/9 (tube no. 2); 1/19 (tube no. 3); 1/49 (tube no. 4); 1/99 (tube no. 5) and 1/199 (tube no. 6).

Table 1. Comparison between microscopy, LAMP and PCR in screening snail samples.

Province	No. of Counties Included	No. of Villages Included	No. of Snails Tested	No. of Pooled Samples	Microscopy		LAMP		PCR	
					Pos. *	%	Pos. *	%	Pos. *	%
Hubei	2	5	599	38	1	0.5	3	7. 9	3	7.9
Hunan	2	6	716	80	0	0	2	2.5	2	2.5
Jiangxi	6	25	1183	34	0	0	5	14.7	4	11.8
Anhui	2	6	698	43	0	0	1	2.3	1	2.3
Yunnan	3	9	810	37	0	0	4	10.8	4	10.8
Total	15	51	4006	232	1	0.4	15	6.5	14	6.0

* Positive.

Table 2. Screening snail samples in three non-endemic areas: comparison between microscopy, LAMP and PCR.

Province	No. of Counties Included	No. of Villages Included	No. of Snails Tested	No. of Pooled Samples	Microscopy		LAMP		PCR	
					Pos. *	%	Pos. *	%	Pos. *	%
Shanghai	2	2	200	4	0	0	0	0	0	0
Zhejiang	2	2	500	10	0	0	0	0	0	0
Guangxi	2	2	300	6	0	0	0	0	0	0
Total	6	6	1000	20	0	0	0	0	0	0

* Positive.

Figure 3. Detection of the Sj28S gene component in the different parasite developmental stages of *S. japonicum* in *O. hupensis* by the LAMP method. 1. Negative control (nuclease-free water); 2. Positive control (Sj28 plasmid DNA); 3. Cercariae; 4. Specificity control (*Trichobilharzia* cercariae); 5. Negative control (pooled snail DNA from a non-endemic area); 6. Mother sporocyst; 7. Daughter sporocyst.

The 28 different laboratories at the provincial and county health agency levels, belonging to the inter-laboratory panel, demonstrated an almost total agreement with respect to the results over the three reported years. Only four laboratories showed slightly lower scores, one with a score of 80 in

2013, two with a score of 60 in 2014, and one with a score of 80 in 2014 and a score of 90 in 2015 (Table 3). Importantly, with the exception of one laboratory, those with scores lower than 100 in one year did not have the same score in other years.

Table 3. Inter-laboratory comparison using LAMP for the detection of intermediate snail hosts infected by *S. japonicum.*

Province	Laboratory	Score 2013	Score 2014	Score 2015
Hunan	IPD	100	100	100
	Hanshou	-	100	100
	Yuanjiang	-	100	100
	Yueyang	-	100	100
Hubei	CDC	100	100	100
	Gongan	-	100	100
	Hanchuan	-	100	100
	Jiangling	-	100	100
Anhui	IPD	100	100	100
	Wuhu	-	100	100
	Anqin	-	100	100
	Guichi	-	100	100
Jiangxi	IPD	100	100	100
	Poyang	-	60	100
	Duchang	-	60	100
Jiangsu	IPD	100	100	100
	Qixia	-	100	100
Sichuan	CDC	100	100	100
	Renshou	-	100	100
	Guanghan	-	100	100
Yunnan	CDC	100	100	100
	Dali	-	80	90
	Eryuan	-	100	100
Shanghai	CDC	100	100	100
Guangdong	CDC	100	100	100
Fujian	CDC	100	100	100
Zhejiang	IPD	100	100	100
Guangxi	CDC	80	100	100

CDC = Center for Disease Control and Prevention; IPD= Provincial Institute of Parasitic Diseases; Scores are the levels of agreement between five tests. The number of samples from 2013 was not sufficient to be tested in all laboratories (signified with a dash in the table).

4. Discussion

Estimates of the prevalence of *S. japonicum* infection in its obligatory vector snail can be used as a proxy for areas at risk of schistosomiasis. As already pointed out by Hamburger et al. [12] and reiterated by Abbasi et al. [13], the snail infection rate provides a measure of the transmission from humans (and other definitive reservoir hosts) to the snail and can, therefore, serve as a marker of residual infection in an area. However, traditional snail diagnosis depends on the labor-intensive, time-consuming individual dissection of thousands of collected snails from the field and the results are not sufficiently sensitive to support this statement, but with the advent of molecular diagnostics this has changed. The successful use of the LAMP technique shown here promises to revolutionize snail surveillance, not only in the laboratory but also in field [13–17]. The reported results are timely, as the use of snail control as a complementary approach along with chemotherapy is again being proposed as a potentially necessary means to achieve the elimination of schistosomiasis [22].

PCR-based assays have been around since the mid-1970s [10], but were not used for schistosomiasis diagnosis until the end of the 1990s and the early 2000s, first for snails [12] and later also for human infections [23,24]. However, the instability and variability inherent in enzymatic processes, as well as the need for advanced equipment, limit PCR applications in the field. In this regard, the LAMP approach is superior, as it can be adapted for application in field laboratories [25] by using ready-mixed reagents suitable for shipment at ambient temperature, together with sample storage under minimal refrigeration [13–16]. The development of a surveillance platform based on molecular diagnostic techniques and characterized by simplicity and reliability, yet with high throughput, requires an approach that is adaptable to county-level laboratories with limited resources. The manganese/calcein method of Tomita et al. [18] is an important contribution in this regard as it enables the recognition of small quantities of DNA by means of a fluorescent signal emitted from the sample solution after amplification, and has been successfully used in China by Kumagai et al. [17]. Other attempts to increase readability and sensitivity include the use of various dyes, e.g., SYBR green (Singh et al., 2017) or hydroxyl napthol blue (Ali et al., 2017) which have also produced good results [26,27]. Dyes have the advantage of being independent of refrigeration.

Any increase of the dilution factor would considerably accelerate the area needed to be tested. We found a dilution ratio of 1/50 to be useful (Figure 2), but if the number of infected snails decreases, as it is supposed to do with the elimination program in force, the risk of mistakenly declaring an area free of transmission increases if the snail pool contains too few snails. This could be counteracted by using a higher number of snails in the pool and increasing the time of amplification for the test, however, the risk for false positives would then rise.

The strength of the present study is not only that it further improves the potential of the LAMP test that has already proved successful for snail diagnosis [16,17], but also that it targets a gene specific for *S. japonicum* and provides validation leading to the reliable use of the pooled-snail approach piloted by Hamburger et al. for *S. mansoni* [15] and Tong et al. for *S. japonicum* [20]. A further advantage of the LAMP technique is that although it is highly technical, it is easy to perform in basic laboratory settings common in rural areas. It is also easy to learn, as shown by the excellent agreement over three years in the many places included in this study. In addition, while sporocysts and parasite germ balls are easily missed by traditional microscopic methods, the snails containing mother or daughter sporocysts were both positive the day after infection. Therefore, the LAMP assay is an appropriate method for the detection of pre-patent infections. As seen in Table 1, the outcome of testing with PCR and the LAMP approach largely agreed, indicating that the sensitivity of the two techniques is the same in practice. However, theoretically the latter has an advantage since the one sample reacting negatively by PCR was positive when tested with the LAMP test. Comparison with microscopy, on the other hand, clearly showed that molecular testing is superior and should be used in the future. The excellent agreement between all 28 field laboratories (Table 3) shows that we are now ready to change from microscopy to molecular testing, preferably using LAMP, as it lends itself to use in the field. It is suggested that this kind of snail testing be included together with the diagnostic testing of humans and domestic animals in a joint surveillance and response platform based on only high-resolution techniques.

The risk of schistosomiasis still exists in China and snail control remains a significant challenge in the field [28]. In the present study, the LAMP results indicate that Hunan, Hubei, Jiangxi, Anhui, and Yunnan Provinces contain infected snails, underlining the risk of schistosomiasis transmission. The results can be used to guide further local investigations and snail control activities.

5. Conclusions

The LAMP platform is an effective method for monitoring snails in endemic field sites. Despite expensive reagents and the risk of contamination that requires specific training of the staff in charge, we recommend that the LAMP-based test replace microscopy for snail diagnosis due to its greater accuracy and reduced delay in delivering results.

Author Contributions: S.-Z.L. and X-N.Z. conceived and designed the project, and supervised the study. Z.-Q.Q. performed most of the experiments and analyzed the data and wrote the original draft. J.X. helped analyze the data, R.B. helped organize and write the article. T.F., C.L., Y.-L.L. and Y.-J.Q. helped with DNA extraction, PCR and LAMP experiments. S.L. and L.-J.Z. helped with snail samples collection in field. All authors reviewed and approved the manuscript.

References

1.   McManus, D.P.; Dunne, D.W.; Sacko, M.; Utzinger, J.; Vennervald, B.J.; Zhou, X.N. Schistosomiasis. *Nat. Rev. Dis. Primers* **2018**, *4*, 13. [CrossRef]

2.   Assaré, R.K.; Tra, M.B.I.; Ouattara, M.; Hürlimann, E.; Coulibaly, J.T.; N'Goran, E.K.; Utzinger, J. Sensitivity of the point-of-care circulating cathodic antigen urine cassette test for diagnosis of *Schistosoma mansoni* in low-endemicity settings in Côte d'Ivoire. *Am. J. Trop. Med. Hyg.* **2018**. [CrossRef]

3.   Hadidjaja, P. Clinical study of Indonesian schistosomiasis at Lindu lake area, Central Sulawesi. *Southeast Asian J. Trop. Med. Public Health* **1984**, *15*, 507–514. [PubMed]

4.   Zhu, G.; Fan, J.; Peterson, A.T. *Schistosoma japonicum* transmission risk maps at present and under climate change in mainland China. *PLoS Negl. Trop. Dis.* **2017**, *11*, e0006021. [CrossRef] [PubMed]

5.   Wang, L.D.; Chen, H.G.; Guo, J.G.; Zeng, X.J.; Hong, X.L.; Xiong, J.J.; Wu, X.H.; Wang, X.H.; Wang, L.Y.; Xia, G.; et al. A strategy to control transmission of *Schistosoma japonicum* in China. *N. Engl. J. Med.* **2009**, *360*, 121–128. [CrossRef] [PubMed]

6.   Wang, L.D.; Guo, J.G.; Wu, X.H.; Chen, H.G.; Wang, T.P.; Zhu, S.P.; Zhang, Z.H.; Steinmann, P.; Yang, G.J.; Wang, S.P.; et al. China's new strategy to block *Schistosoma japonicum* transmission: Experiences and impact beyond schistosomiasis. *Trop. Med. Int. Health* **2009**, *14*, 1475–1483. [CrossRef] [PubMed]

7.   Sun, L.P.; Wang, W.; Hong, Q.B.; Li, S.Z.; Liang, Y.S.; Yang, H.T.; Zhou, X.N. Approaches being used in the national schistosomiasis elimination programme in China: A review. *Infect. Dis. Poverty* **2017**, *6*, 55. [CrossRef]

8.   Spear, R.C.; Seto, E.Y.; Carlton, E.J.; Liang, S.; Remais, J.V.; Zhong, B.; Qiu, D. The challenge of effective surveillance in moving from low transmission to elimination of schistosomiasis in China. *Int. J. Parasitol.* **2011**, *41*, 1243–1247. [CrossRef]

9.   Yang, K.; Sun, L.P.; Liang, Y.S.; Wu, F.; Li, W.; Zhang, J.F.; Huang, Y.X.; Hang, D.R.; Liang, S.; Bergquist, R.; et al. *Schistosoma japonicum* risk in Jiangsu province, People's Republic of China: Identification of a spatio-temporal risk pattern along the Yangtze River. *Geospat. Health* **2013**, *8*, 133–142. [CrossRef]

10. Erlich, H.A. Polymerase chain reaction. *J. Clin. Immunol.* **1989**, *9*, 437–447. [CrossRef]

11. Notomi, T.; Okayama, H.; Masubuchi, H.; Yonekawa, T.; Watanabe, K.; Amino, N.; Hase, T. Loop-mediated isothermal amplification of DNA. *Nucleic Acids Res.* **2000**, *28*, E63. [CrossRef] [PubMed]

12. Hamburger, J.; He-Na; Xin, X.Y.; Ramzy, R.M.; Jourdane, J.; Ruppel, A. A polymerase chain reaction assay for detecting snails infected with bilharzia parasites (*Schistosoma mansoni*) from very early prepatency. *Am. J. Trop. Med. Hyg.* **1998**, *59*, 872–876. [CrossRef] [PubMed]

13. Abbasi, I.; King, C.H.; Muchiri, E.M.; Hamburger, J. Detection of *Schistosoma mansoni* and *Schistosoma haematobium* DNA by loop-mediated isothermal amplification: Identification of infected snails from early prepatency. *Am. J. Trop. Med. Hyg.* **2010**, *83*, 427–432. [CrossRef] [PubMed]

14. Notomi, T.; Mori, Y.; Tomita, N.; Kanda, H. Loop-mediated isothermal amplification (LAMP): Principle, features, and future prospects. *J. Microbiol.* **2015**, *53*, 1–5. [CrossRef] [PubMed]

15. Hamburger, J.; Abbasi, I.; Kariuki, C.; Wanjala, A.; Mzungu, E.; Mungai, P.; Muchiri, E.; King, C.H. Evaluation of loop-mediated isothermal amplification suitable for molecular monitoring of schistosome-infected snails in field laboratories. *Am. J. Trop. Med. Hyg.* **2013**, *88*, 344–351. [CrossRef]

16. Gandasegui, J.; Fernández-Soto, P.; Muro, A.; Simões Barbosa, C.; Lopes de Melo, F.; Loyo, R.; de Souza Gomes, E.C. A field survey using LAMP assay for detection of *Schistosoma mansoni* in a low-transmission area of schistosomiasis in Umbuzeiro, Brazil: Assessment in human and snail samples. *PLoS Negl. Trop. Dis.* **2018**, *12*, e0006314. [CrossRef] [PubMed]

17. Kumagai, T.; Furushima-Shimogawara, R.; Ohmae, H.; Wang, T.P.; Lu, S.; Chen, R.; Wen, L.; Ohta, N. Detection of early and single infections of *Schistosoma japonicum* in the intermediate host snail, *Oncomelania hupensis*, by PCR and loop-mediated isothermal amplification (LAMP) assay. *Am. J. Trop. Med. Hyg.* **2010**, *83*, 542–548. [CrossRef]

18. Tomita, N.; Mori, Y.; Kanda, H.; Notomi, T. Loop-mediated isothermal amplification (LAMP) of gene sequences and simple visual detection of products. *Nat. Protoc.* **2008**, *3*, 877–882. [CrossRef]

19. Lei, Z.L.; Zhang, L.J.; Xu, Z.M.; Dang, H.; Xu, J.; Lv, S.; Cao, C.L.; Li, S.Z.; Zhou, X.N. Endemic status of schistosomiasis in People's Republic of China in 2014. *Zhongguo Xue Xi Chong Bing Fang Zhi Za Zhi* **2015**, *27*, 563–569. (In Chinese)

20. Tong, Q.B.; Chen, R.; Zhang, Y.; Yang, G.J.; Kumagai, T.; Furushima-Shimogawara, R.; Lou, D.; Yang, K.; Wen, L.Y.; Lu, S.H.; et al. A new surveillance and response tool: Risk map of infected *Oncomelania hupensis* detected by loop-mediated isothermal amplification (LAMP) from pooled samples. *Acta Trop.* **2015**, *141 Pt B*, 170–177. [CrossRef]

21. Xun-Ping, W.; An, Z. Study of spatial stratified sampling strategy of *Oncomelania hupensis* snail survey based on plant abundance. *Zhongguo Xue Xi Chong Bing Fang Zhi Za Zhi* **2017**, *29*, 420–425. (In Chinese) [PubMed]

22. Lo, N.C.; Gurarie, D.; Yoon, N.; Coulibaly, J.T.; Bendavid, E.; Andrews, J.R.; King, C.H. Impact and cost-effectiveness of snail control to achieve disease control targets for schistosomiasis. *Proc. Natl. Acad. Sci. USA* **2018**, *115*, E584–E591. [CrossRef] [PubMed]

23. Pontes, L.A.; Dias-Neto, E.; Rabello, A. Detection by polymerase chain reaction of *Schistosoma mansoni* DNA in human serum and feces. *Am. J. Trop. Med. Hyg.* **2002**, *66*, 157–162. [CrossRef] [PubMed]

24. He, P.; Gordon, C.A.; Williams, G.M.; Li, Y.; Wang, Y.; Hu, J.; Gray, D.J.; Ross, A.G.; Harn, D.; McManus, D.P. Real-time PCR diagnosis of *Schistosoma japonicum* in low transmission areas of China. *Infect. Dis. Poverty* **2018**, *7*, 8. [CrossRef] [PubMed]

25. Wilisiani, F.; Tomiyama, A.; Katoh, H.; Hartono, S.; Neriya, Y.; Nishigawa, H.; Natsuaki, T. Development of a LAMP assay with a portable device for real-time detection of begomoviruses under field conditions. *J. Virol. Methods* **2018**. [CrossRef] [PubMed]

26. Singh, R.; Singh, D.P.; Savargaonkar, D.; Singh, O.P.; Bhatt, R.M.; Valecha, N. Evaluation of SYBR green I based visual loop-mediated isothermal amplification (LAMP) assay for genus and species-specific diagnosis of malaria in *P. vivax* and *P. falciparum* endemic regions. *J. Vector Borne Dis.* **2017**, *54*, 54–60. [PubMed]

27. Ali, S.A.; Kaur, G.; Boby, N.; Sabarinath, T.; Solanki, K.; Pal, D.; Chaudhuri, P. Rapid and visual detection of leptospira in urine by LigB-LAMP assay with pre-addition of dye. *Mol. Cell. Probes* **2017**, *36*, 29–35. [CrossRef]

28. Yang, Y.; Zheng, S.B.; Yang, Y.; Cheng, W.T.; Pan, X.; Dai, Q.Q.; Chen, Y.; Zhu, L.; Jiang, Q.W.; Zhou, Y.B. The Three Gorges Dam: Does the flooding time determine the distribution of schistosome-transmitting snails in the middle and lower reaches of the Yangtze River, China? *Int. J. Environ. Res. Public Health* **2018**, *15*, 1304. [CrossRef]

12

Potential Impact of Climate Change on Schistosomiasis: A Global Assessment Attempt

Guo-Jing Yang [1,2,*] and Robert Bergquist [3]

[1]   Department of Epidemiology and Public Health, Swiss Tropical and Public Health Institute, Socinstrasse 57, CH-4002 Basel, Switzerland
[2]   University of Basel, CH-4002 Basel, Switzerland
[3]   Ingerod, SE-454 94 Brastad, Sweden; robert.bergquist@outlook.com
*   Correspondence: guojingyang@hotmail.com

Abstract: Based on an ensemble of global circulation models (GCMs), four representative concentration pathways (RCPs) and several ongoing and planned Coupled Model Intercomparison Projects (CMIPs), the Intergovernmental Panel on Climate Change (IPCC) predicts that global, average temperatures will increase by at least 1.5 °C in the near future and more by the end of the century if greenhouse gases (GHGs) emissions are not genuinely tempered. While the RCPs are indicative of various amounts of GHGs in the atmosphere the CMIPs are designed to improve the workings of the GCMs. We chose RCP4.5 which represented a medium GHG emission increase and CMIP5, the most recently completed CMIP phase. Combining this meteorological model with a biological counterpart model accounted for replication and survival of the snail intermediate host as well as maturation of the parasite stage inside the snail at different ambient temperatures. The potential geographical distribution of the three main schistosome species: *Schistosoma japonicum*, *S. mansoni* and *S. haematobium* was investigated with reference to their different transmission capabilities at the monthly mean temperature, the maximum temperature of the warmest month(s) and the minimum temperature of the coldest month(s). The set of six maps representing the predicted situations in 2021–2050 and 2071–2100 for each species mainly showed increased transmission areas for all three species but they also left room for potential shrinkages in certain areas.

Keywords: climate change; schistosomiasis; distribution; intermediate snail host; transmission; modelling

1. Introduction

Schistosomiasis, caused by trematode parasites with a predilection for intestinal and urogenital venous circulation in the human definitive host, is one of the neglected tropical diseases (NTDs) selected for increased attention by the World Health Organization (WHO) [1]. Six different species of *Schistosoma* are capable of infecting humans, each depending on a certain snail species as an intermediate host. Humans infect snails by depositing parasite eggs (excreted in feces or urine) in waterlogged areas and humans are infected or reinfected when in contact with water containing schistosome cercariae released from infected snails. The disease is generally chronic, although schistosomiasis is often a contributing factor to premature death, direct mortality is comparatively low. Transmission of schistosomiasis has been reported in 78 countries and more than 800 million people in Africa, Latin America, the Middle East and Southeast Asia live in areas endemic to schistosomiasis [2], with up to 250 million actually infected [3]. Chemotherapy in amounts sufficient for more than 100 million school age children per year has been pledged by the private sector and development partners, but there is still a large discrepancy between the number of people requiring preventive treatment and those actually receiving it [4]. In addition, the number of people suffering from this infection continues to rise as a reflection of ongoing population growth, which is particularly high in endemic areas.

Schistosomiasis is not as neglected as many other tropical diseases since it has a large research focus and still remains one of the most prevalent infections in the world, estimated to correspond to 4.5 million disability-adjusted life years (DALYs) by the WHO Expert Committee in 2002 [5]. However, this estimate was based on a wider range of pathologies than that used in the global burden of disease (GBD) study of 1990 [6]. It was also higher than the updated GBD in 2010 [7] that put the burden of schistosomiasis at 3.3 million DALYs. Importantly, however, the GBD figure of 2010 was high enough to put this disease as no. 3 after malaria and tuberculosis on the NTD list [3]. This increase was due to the inclusion of diarrhea, dysuria and anemia in the DALY score which was not counted before. While later updates [8] show a sharply lower DALY score for schistosomiasis, other authors [9–11] hold that the true impact of this disease is several-fold higher because of the low weight given by the GBD estimates to subtle symptoms and pathology in individuals with infections too light to be revealed by diagnostics based on parasite egg-detection. Indeed, high-definition circulating antigen tests, such as the point-of-care circulating cathodic antigen (POC-CCA) assay indicates that the current number of infections may be at least 10 times higher than that shown by egg-detection [12].

The epidemiology of schistosomiasis (and that of all other organisms) must be seen in the light of the perceived ongoing climate change. The latest half century has seen signs of global warming, mainly thought to be due to the burning of coal and oil at an increasingly large scale. From 1990, reports relevant for our understanding of climate change, including options for its mitigation, are regularly produced by the Intergovernmental Panel on Climate Change (IPCC) [13] for the United Nations Framework Convention on Climate Change (UNFCCC). IPCC bases its assessments on the published, scientific literature and opinions of invited independent researchers. An important part of its work is to do with global circulation models (GCMs), which are currently used to predict the climate for the next 80 years based on complex mathematical representations of the Earth's energy balance between atmosphere, total land mass, sea and ice cover. These components interact as a coupled system, whose status emerges from equations based on the dynamic values of various climate variables, e.g., temperature, winds, etc., at each point on the globe. Climate modelling uses current and historic data to attempt the prediction of future climate scenarios from the present time to the end of the 21st century.

The projections of the GCMs disagree due to various forms of natural variability included in the models. Fortuitously, this variability can be reduced by averaging an ensemble of simulations, resulting in universal agreement. Generally, such averaged model ensembles produce simulations of current and past large-scale climates that agree with observation. Further confidence comes from the fact that converging GCMs also produce an accurate 'hindcast' of previous climate change that took place in the 1900s. Evidence is already available in the form of a rising average global temperature and amplified warming of air and oceans, particularly in the Arctic, leading to rising sea levels, dry places becoming dryer and wet places wetter.

The fact, temperature changes impact snail distributions in general as well as the maturation of the intermediate stages of the parasite inside this intermediate host, makes a discussion of future changes in the distribution of schistosomiasis complex. However, it is useful to know that water temperature below freezing puts an absolute limit to snail survival. Indeed, the climate-dependent, long-term (as opposed to seasonal) movements of the 'frost line' at northern latitudes indicates a diffuse zone north of which schistosomiasis transmission cannot occur. Immediately south of this zone, transmission is governed by the prevailing temperature and the time it stays above a certain limit, a fact rooted in the relationship between the development of plants and the ambient temperature first mentioned in the 1700s by Réaumur who coined the 'degree-day unit' and used it as a measure of crop maturation [14]. This unit, now called the growing degree-day (GDD), is defined as the amount of heat an organism needs to accumulate to achieve full development. Although its main application remains in agriculture, the GDD concept has also been used for predicting the development of parasites [15], monitoring snail replication as well as the maturation of the schistosome sporocyst stages inside the snail [16,17].

The effect of temperature alterations with regard to the potential distribution of schistosomiasis has been addressed in China [17–19] and Africa [20,21], but a global picture of potential long-term transmission alterations ascribed to climate change is still missing. To address this question, we felt that it was warranted to theorize about the intermediate- and long-term global distribution possibilities of this disease considering possible future dispersion of the intermediate snail host into non-endemic areas. The IPCC focuses a lot on temperature predictions and this variable has a strong influence on snail survival. Importantly, even minor temperature increases play a role if they cover a sufficiently long period of the annual cycle. For these reasons, we used GDD as the key parameter to evaluate the potential, future transmission risk of schistosomiasis.

2. Materials and Methods

When preparing the risk maps, we only considered the predicted temperature increase in relation to two required needs. These were the needs of the snail (three species) and that of the parasite stages inside the snail (mother sporocyst, daughter sporocyst and cercaria). Naturally, this approach was highly theoretical as many parameters other than temperature govern the potential distribution of schistosomiasis. However, it represents a first step in an investigation that can be developed further.

2.1. Study Area

Aiming to give a global overview of potential risk areas, a digital map of the world with country boundaries was downloaded from ArcGIS (ESRI, Redlands, CA, USA). Areas of particular risk for the change in schistosomiasis transmission were the current northern limits of the infection and slopes bordering high-altitude mountains. The southern limit was the southernmost tip of Africa and Chile and Brazil in South America as the sea rather than temperature limiting transmission at all other longitudes.

2.2. Meteorological Model

Modelling future temperatures builds on four representative concentration pathways (RCPs) representing four greenhouse gas concentration (not emission) trajectories, which were adopted by the IPCC for its 5th assessment report (AR5) in 2014 [22]. These RCPs superseded the Special Report on Emissions Scenarios (SRES) projections published in 2000 and were previously used for this purpose. Unlike simpler models which make mixing assumptions regarding processes internal to a presumed cell, while other functions govern the interface between such cells, the GCMs describe four possible climate futures, which are all considered possible depending on how much greenhouse gases (GHGs) are emitted in the years to come (see Figure 1). The four RCPs, i.e., RCP2.6, RCP4.5, RCP6 and RCP8.5 are named after a possible range of 'radiative' forcing relative to pre-industrial values (+2.6, +4.5, +6.0, and +8.5 W/m^2, respectively) [23].

The IPCC relies also on Coupled Model Intercomparison Project (CMIP) experiments, a collaborative series of experiments designed to improve our knowledge of the GCMs and their interactions. The most recently completed phase of the project is CMIP5, which includes more metadata describing model simulations than previous phases. The findings are summarized in AR5 (https://cmip.llnl.gov/cmip5/index.html). In this study, all models were based on CMIP5 with RCP4.5, which represented a medium GHG emission increase. The temperature prediction data used were derived from GCMs created in a grid format of 0.5 × 0.5 degrees latitude and longitude by five well-known research centers representing the most generally accepted view of the world's major climate systems (Table 1). The datasets we used consisted of a baseline temperature based on the 1961–1990 period and predicted periods 2021–2050 and 2071–2100. These were based on an ensemble of the five predicted climate scenarios between 2006 and 2100 with special reference to the monthly mean temperature (T_{mean}), the maximum temperature of the warmest months (T_{max}) and the minimum temperature of the coldest months (T_{min}), which are reminiscent of the BIO$_1$, BIO$_5$ and BIO$_6$ variables of the 'WorldClim' dataset [24]. Thirty years of averaged monthly temperatures (T_{mean}, T_{max} and T_{min}) spanning the periods 2021–2050 and 2071–2100 were extracted.

Table 1. The five global circulation models used in this study.

GCM [a]	Characteristics	Developing Centre
ACCE-SS1-0	Based on the UK MetOffice UM atmosphere model, the GFDL MOM4p1 ocean model, the LANL CICE4.1 sea-ice model and the MOSES2 land surface model.	The Australian Community Climate and Earth-System Simulator (ACCESS) weather models
IPSL-CM5A_LR	An atmosphere-land-ocean-sea ice model with representations of the carbon cycle; the stratospheric chemistry and the tropospheric aerosol chemistry	Institut Pierre Simon Laplace Climate Modelling Centre (IPSL-CMC) of Centre National de la Recherche Scientifique (CNRS); Paris; France
HadGEM2-AO	A configuration of the HadGEM2 model which is an atmosphere-only simulation with other component interfaces replaced with ancillary file input.	UK Met Office Hadley Centre
CanESM2	The second generation Canadian Earth System Model (CanESM2) consists of the physical coupled atmosphere-ocean model CanCM4 coupled to a terrestrial carbon model (CTEM) and an ocean carbon model (CMOC).	Canadian Centre for Climate Modelling and Analysis
GISS-E2-H-CC	Based on Earth system models that include interactive atmospheric chemistry, aerosols, carbon cycle and other tracers, as well as the standard atmosphere, ocean, sea ice and land surface components.	National Aeronautics and Space Administration (NASA) Goddard Institute for Space Studies

[a] Global Circulation Model.

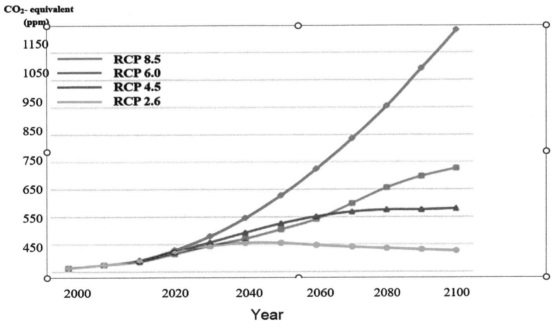

Figure 1. Estimated future equivalent atmospheric CO_2 concentrations including all 'forcing' agents according to the four representative concentration pathways (RCPs).

2.3. Biological Model

The GDD, being the temperature above a critical threshold multiplied by the duration needed, can be articulated as $T_{ave} - T_{base}$, where the former is the average daily temperature and the latter the base temperature or the lowest temperature at which development of an organism can occur. The annual sum of GDD, termed AGDD, determines fairly well the potential for the spatial distribution of living organisms. As the level of the GDD required to complete the development of an organism is fairly constant, organisms with high heat unit requirements are more likely to develop into mature stages in areas where AGDD is high. We found this unit useful for use as a means to define the geographical limits of schistosomiasis transmission, mainly based on the climate impact on the snail intermediate host but also on its effect on the development of the sporocyst inside the snail.

With the aim of assessing the effect of temperature on schistosomiasis development, we created biological models with reference to the parasites by calculating potential transmission indices (PTIs) derived from GDD and AGDD. The GDDs for *S. japonicum*, *S. mansoni* and *S. haematobium* were 853, 268 and 298 degree-days, respectively [17,25,26] and the efficient temperature ranges (T_{low} and T_{high}) for the development of *S. japonicum*, *S. mansoni* and *S. haematobium* were 18–35 °C, 16–35 °C and 18–32 °C, respectively [16,25,26]. The AGDD for each grid was calculated by summing up the difference between the mean monthly temperature (T_{ij}) at location i and month j and the efficient temperature range for parasite development:

$$AGDD_i = \sum_{j=1}^{12} (T_{ij} - T_{low}) \times day_j \times 1(T_{low} < T_{ij} < T_{high}), \tag{1}$$

where day_j indicates the number of days in month j, $1(\dots)$ is the indicator function, giving the value of 1 if the condition within the parenthesis is true, otherwise 0.

The PTI_i was calculated for each pixel grid i in the periods 1961–1990, 2021–2050 and 2071–2100, according to Equation (2). Only PTI values above 1 were considered to be of relevance (i.e., areas where schistosomiasis transmission could potentially occur).

$$PTI_i = (AGDD_i/GDD_s) \times 1(AGDD_i/GDD_s > 1), \tag{2}$$

Oncomelania, the intermediate snail host of *S. japonicum*, can only survive if the January mean temperature is higher than 0 °C [17,18], while the most common *S. mansoni* snail host exists in areas where the yearly T_{max} is between 20–33 °C [27]. The corresponding optimal temperature range of the intermediate snail host for *S. haematobium* is 15.5–31 °C [28]. The vector survival threshold masks were overlapped on the PTI maps for the three different *Schistosoma* species investigated.

2.4. Geographical Information System (GIS) and Risk Assessment

We created a GIS database using ArcGIS, version 10.5 (ESRI; Redlands, CA, USA) for the investigation of baseline and change of transmission regions.

2.4.1. Baseline, Predicted Transmission Region and PTI

The PTI of the three main different schistosomiasis species for the periods 1961–1990, 2021–2050 and 2071–2100 were imported and presented as map overlays. On top of the PTI layer, we overlapped the thresholds for the intermediate hosts for the three species: 0 °C of the January T_{mean} for *Oncomelania* (*S. japonicum*), yearly T_{max} between 20 °C and 33 °C for the *Biomphalaria* snail species (*S. mansoni*) and a T_{max} between 15.5 °C and 31 °C for the *Bulinus* species (*S. haematobium*).

2.4.2. Change of Transmission Region, PTI due to Predicted Climate Change

We compared the spatial extent of the sensitive potential transmission region at two time periods: 2021–2050 vs. baseline 1961–1990 and 2071–2100 vs. baseline. We highlighted the change of PTI between the two time periods to present the transmission intensity difference due to the predicted climate change.

2.5. Model Validation by Ground Truth Data

S. japonicum was selected to evaluate the model prediction. All prediction results by pixel grids were compared with the same format data derived from the historic schistosomiasis transmission data provided by National Institute of Parasitic Diseases (NIPD), China Centers for Disease Control (CDC).

The model sensitivity and specificity of the prediction results were evaluated by the following three equations:

$$SE = \frac{Pe}{Pte},\tag{3}$$

$$SP = \frac{Pn}{Ptn},\tag{4}$$

$$TM = \frac{Pen}{Pa},\tag{5}$$

where SE is sensitivity, SP is specificity, TM is the total agreement rate, Pe is the correctly predicted endemic pixels, Pte is all endemic pixels, Pn is the correctly predicted endemic pixels, Ptn is all non-endemic pixels, Pen is correctly predicted endemic and non-endemic pixels and Pa are all pixels.

3. Results

3.1. Change of Transmission Region and PTI for Schistosomiasis due to Climate Change

The average temperatures predicted by the IPCC for the two time periods 2021–2050 and 2071–2100, based on the average of the five GCM results, seemed increasingly likely in the event that efforts to curb the GHG emissions were not stepped up more than they were so far. Figures 2–4 use IPCC'S predicted temperatures for the two future time periods 2021–2050 and 2071–2100 but rather than comparing with a preindustrial average, we used the 1961–1990 period for which we had available PTI data as a baseline. The blue color shown in the figures designated the ocean, while the background of each plot was based on the PTI baseline.

For *S. japonicum*, we only applied the low temperature constraints. The global warming displayed heterogeneous patterns with respect to snail survival. For example, the current areas endemic for *S. japonicum* in the Sichuan Province were predicted to become unsuitable for snail habitats. On the other hand, the downstream regions between the Sichuan and Hunan/Hubei provinces corresponding to the area above the Three Gorges Dam, which is currently non-endemic, might well present a potential endemic risk in the future. The predicted potential transmission areas of *S. japonicum* moving northward was not so obvious in 2021–2050 as it might have become in the 2071–2100 period.

For *S. mansoni* and *S. haematobium*, in both timeframes forecast, the potential transmission areas could retreat from the Saharan areas as the desert might encroach on this part of the continent due to diminishing or discontinued rainfall. The future transmission areas of *S. mansoni* might shrink more than those of *S. haematobium*, while schistosomiasis in Ethiopia and other highlands in Africa could reach higher with warmer temperatures.

(a) between 2021–2050   (b) between 2071–2100

Figure 2. Change of risk area for *S. japonicum* vs. the baseline. (a) 2021–2050 vs. the baseline, (b) 2071–2050 vs. the baseline.

Figure 3. Change of risk area for *S. mansoni* vs. the baseline. (**a**) 2021–2050 vs. the baseline, (**b**) 2071–2050 vs. the baseline.

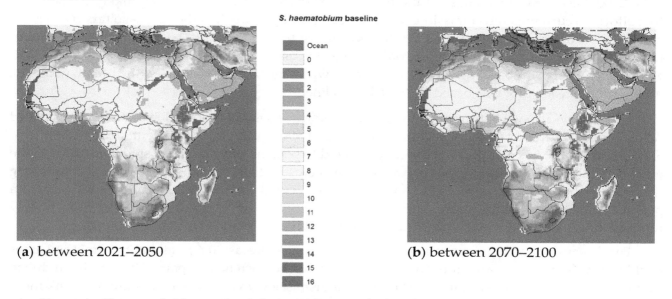

Figure 4. Change of risk area for *S. haematobium* vs. the baseline. (**a**) 2021–2050 vs. the baseline, (**b**) 2071–2050 vs. the baseline.

Suitability varies from 0 over the spectrum to the most likely (red). Grey areas signify areas that might potentially shrink as the temperature would become less suited to the specific snails for the different schistosomal species.

3.2. Model Validation by Ground Truth Data

The model prediction results were validated by the ground truth data in China. The sensitivity and specificity of model prediction were 0.78 and 0.89, respectively. The total prediction match rate was 0.88.

4. Discussion

Three schistosome species pose the main infection risk for humans. *S. japonicum* is the single schistosome species in China, the Philippines and three closely situated small foci in Celebes, Indonesia. It is transmitted by *Oncomelania* snails, whose latitudinal movements over land during most of the last million years may have been prevented by the development of the Himalaya plateau serving as a barrier. The endemic areas for *S. mansoni* and *S. haematobium* overlap to a great extent on the

African continent and in the Middle East, but not everywhere. The former, the most abundant of the schistosome species, has also found an exclusive niche in the Northeast part of South America and on some of the Caribbean islands but are now disappearing from the latter, however this is not due to climate change [29]. Its distribution is supported by the broad geographic range of *Biomphalaria* spp. snails that serve as obligatory hosts for its larval stages. Recently, however, *Bi. straminea* has been identified in the Hong Kong Special Administrative Region and Shenzhen City in the Guangdong Province of China and has remained there since the 1970s [30], a fact that could eventually result in transmission of *S. mansoni* in parallel with *S. japonicum* in China. *S. haematobium* is confined to Africa and the Middle East due to its reliance on *Bulinus* spp. intermediate snail hosts [31]. Although this schistosome species must also have been brought from Africa to Latin America during the slave trade of the 16th and 17th century, only *S. mansoni* became established there because of the absence of *Bulinus* snails. Although this information indicates that schistosome species and their specific snails can spread into various new areas, this is not of a magnitude that requires it to be considered when discussing the risk for schistosomiasis due to temperature augmentation.

To assess the potential impact of climate change on the transmission of schistosomiasis in the world we developed a biological model using available data from the literature. Compared to *S. japonicum*, both *S. mansoni* and *S. haematobium* required less total heat energy to complete one generation [17,25,26]. Therefore, the transmission intensity of the two latter species is generally somewhat stronger than that of *S. japonicum*. However, the three different intermediate snail hosts had different temperature thresholds for survival that came into play in certain geographical areas. For example, the distribution of the *Oncomelania* snail, utilized by *S. japonicum*, was constrained by the temperature in January (when below 0 °C), which effectively limited its progress northwards, while *Biomphalaria* (*S. mansoni*) and *Bulinus* (*S. haematobium*) had thermal requirements that included an annual T_{max} of 15.5–31 °C and 20–33 °C respectively [27], which is one of the factors (so far) keeping these snails from entering Europe and other northern territories. Interestingly, *S. haematobium* appears to have a better chance of a foothold in Europe than *S. mansoni*, at least in the middle part of the century (Figure 3).

With respect to snail survival, the GDD approach in 2008 predicted an extension of 662,373 and 783,883 km^2 potentially endemic areas for schistosomiasis japonica in China in 2030 and 2050, respectively [17]. Yang et al. noted that the 0–1 °C January isotherm of 1971–2000 had already shifted from 33°15′ N to 33°41′ N compared to the 1961–1990 baseline, expanding the area by 41,335 km^2, resulting in an additional 20.7 million people at risk of schistosomiasis in China [32]. For *S. japonicum*, the predicted temperature increases based on our biological model and the average ensemble of the five GCM models would result in transmission starting to extend northward by 2050 (Figure 2a) adding a considerably larger margin by 2100 (Figure 2b). It is also conceivable that the transmission intensity will increase in areas already endemic for schistosomiasis.

It is important for the existence or absence of the parasite and vital for prediction model validation that more information is made available also for *S. mansoni* and *S. haematobium*. However, the change in the geographic transmission region for these two species due to climate change is more complex than in China. With temperatures increasing above T_{max}, the historic transmission areas surrounding the Sahara region would retreat from the equator reducing the transmission regions of both species. However, the current risk areas would extend further into the northern or southern current marginal transmission areas, including the Mediterranean countries. Indeed, schistosomiasis hematobia has recently been identified in Corsica, France [33]. Although it is questionable whether this extension into Europe is due to climate change, rather large areas of southern Europe will become habitable for the snail hosts in the future (Figures 3 and 4). Overall, however, the total transmission areas should be reduced. The changing transmission patterns in terms of region and intensity are heterogeneous and new populations at risk will probably appear. Further research is warranted to work out the geographical probabilities.

A limitation of our current modelling approach is that it emphasizes the role of temperature but does not take into account the role of rainfall and the potential interaction between temperature and rainfall. It is difficult to say whether our model is conservative or whether these additional effects might further amplify the extent of changes predicted on the basis of temperature alone. Thus, recent improvements in modelling global trends in precipitation and water availability should become an integral part of present and future predictions of climate change and variability on infectious disease dynamics, including schistosomiasis. Recent years have seen widespread massive flooding, which can lead to snail dispersal and an epidemic outbreak of schistosomiasis if occurring in or close to endemic areas. In addition, the issue of altitude, that has been neglected so far, might under-evaluate changing transmission patterns in mountainous regions, which would have major implications for parts of China and many African countries. Additionally, most climate studies, including the current one, discuss large geographical scales, i.e., national, regional and global levels. To capture localized climate changes, regional climate models are needed that can assign meteorological parameters at relatively small scales also. Such climate models can provide information with useful local detail including realistic extreme events and generate detailed projections of the future climate. Any discussion of the future distribution of schistosomiasis, presumed to be induced by climate change would be futile without exact information of the prevailing distribution of the infection, both in humans and in the intermediate snail host. It is therefore critical that the diagnostic techniques applied are sensitive enough to find even the lightest infection.

This work is based on the best possible models available today on the future climate for the rest of the century. Without a doubt, however, future increased computing power will permit more comprehensive simulations, better represented parameterized processes and more accurate projections at all levels, which might well result in slightly different projections. In addition, natural phenomena, such as cataclysmic volcanic eruptions like that which occurred in Krakatoa in 1883, major meteoric hits, etc., that would completely upend any prediction of the kind discussed here cannot be completely ruled out. Even without such events, we still expect further changes in the forthcoming 6th assessment report (AR6) scheduled for release in 2022.

Author Contributions: Conceptualization, G.Y.; Formal analysis, G.Y.; Investigation, R.B.; Writing—original draft, G.Y.; Writing—review & editing, R.B.

References

1. WHO. 2012. Available online: http://www.who.int/neglected_diseases/NTD_RoadMap_2012_Fullversion. pdf (accessed on 15 October 2018).
2. Steinmann, P.; Keiser, J.; Bos, R.; Tanner, M.; Utzinger, J. Schistosomiasis and water resources development: Systematic review, meta-analysis, and estimates of people at risk. *Lancet Infect. Dis.* **2006**, *6*, 411–425. [CrossRef]
3. Hotez, P.; Alvarado, M.; Basáñez, M.; Bolliger, I.; Bourne, R.; Boussinesq, M.; Brooker, S.; Brown, A.; Buckle, G.; Budke, C.; et al. (DALYs and HALE Collaborators). The gobal burden of disease study 2010: Interpretation and implications for the neglected tropical diseases. *PLoS Negl. Trop. Dis.* **2014**, *8*, e2865. [CrossRef] [PubMed]
4. WHO. Schistosomiasis Fact Sheet of 20 February 2018. Available online: http://www.who.int/news-room/fact-sheets/detail/schistosomiasis (accessed on 20 August 2018).
5. WHO (World Health Organization). *Prevention and Control of Schistosomiasis and Soil-Transmitted Helminthiasis: Report of a WHO Expert Committee*; World Health Organization: Geneva, Switzerland, 2002.
6. Murray, C.J.; Lopez, A.D.; Jamison, D.T. The global burden of disease in 1990: Summary results, sensitivity analysis and future directions. *Bull. World Health Organ.* **1994**, *723*, 495–509.
7. Murray, C.J.L.; Vos, T.; Lozano, R.; Naghavi, M.; Flaxman, A.D.; Michaud, C.; Ezzati, M.; Shibuya, K.; Salomon, J.A.; Abdalla, S.; et al. Disability-adjusted life years (DALYs) for 291 diseases and injuries in 21 regions, 1990–2010: A systematic analysis for the Global Burden of Disease Study 2010. *Lancet* **2012**, *380*, 2197–2223. [CrossRef]

8. Hay, S.I.; Abajobir, A.A.; Abate, K.H.; Abbafati, C.; Abbas, K.M.; Abd-Allah, F.; Abdulkader, R.S.; Abdulle, A.M.; Abebo, T.A.; Abera, S.F.; et al. Global, regional, and national disability-adjusted life-years (DALYs) for 333 diseases and injuries and healthy life expectancy (HALE) for 195 countries and territories, 1990–2016: A systematic analysis for the Global Burden of Disease Study 2016. *Lancet* **2017**, *39010100*, 1260–1344. [CrossRef]

9. King, C.H. Health metrics for helminth infections. *Acta Trop.* **2015**, *141 Pt B*, 150–160. [CrossRef]

10. King, C.H. It's Time to Dispel the Myth of "Asymptomatic" Schistosomiasis. *PLoS Negl. Trop. Dis.* **2015**, *92*, e0003504. [CrossRef] [PubMed]

11. King, C.H.; Galvani, A.P. Underestimation of the global burden of schistosomiasis. *Lancet* **2018**, *39110118*, 307–308. [CrossRef]

12. Bergquist, R.; van Dam, G.J.; Xu, J. Diagnostic tests for schistosomiasis. In *Schistosoma: Biology, Pathology and Control*; Jamieson, B.G.M., Ed.; CRC Press: Boca Raton, FL, USA, 2016; pp. 401–439.

13. IPCC. Principles Governing IPCC Work, Approved 1–3 October 1998, Last Amended 14–18 October 2013. Available online: https://ipcc.ch/pdf/ipcc-principles/ipcc-principles.pdf (accessed on 5 september 2018).

14. Bonhomme, R. Bases and limits to using 'degree.day' units. *Eur. J. Agron.* **2000**, *13*, 1–10. [CrossRef]

15. Bernal, J.; Gonzalez, D. Experimental assessment of a degree-day model for predicting the development of parasites in the field. *J. Appl. Entiron.* **1993**, *116*, 459–466. [CrossRef]

16. Yang, G.J.; Utzinger, J.; Sun, L.P.; Hong, Q.B.; Vounatsou, P.; Tanner, M.; Zhou, X.N. Effect of temperature on the development of *Schistosoma japonicum* within *Oncomelania hupensis*, and hibernation of *O. hupensis*. *Parasitol. Res.* **2007**, *100*, 695–700. [CrossRef] [PubMed]

17. Zhou, X.N.; Yang, G.J.; Yang, K.; Wang, X.H.; Hong, Q.B.; Sun, L.P.; Malone, J.B.; Kristensen, T.K.; Bergquist, N.R.; Utzinger, J. Potential Impact of Climate Change on Schistosomiasis Transmission in China. *Am. J. Trop. Med. Hyg.* **2008**, *78*, 188–194. [CrossRef] [PubMed]

18. Yang, G.J.; Vounatsou, P.; Zhou, X.N.; Tanner, M.; Utzinger, J.E. Electrophoretic detection of genetic variability among Schistosoma japonicum isolates by sequence-related amplified polymorphism. *Parasitologia* **2005**, *47*, 127–134.

19. Zhu, G.; Fan, J.; Peterson, A. Schistosoma japonicum transmission risk maps at present and under climate change in mainland China. *PLoS Negl. Trop. Dis.* **2017**, *1110*, e0006021. [CrossRef] [PubMed]

20. McCreesh, N.; Nikulin, G.; Booth, M. Predicting the effects of climate change on *Schistosoma mansoni* transmission in eastern Africa. *Parasit. Vectors* **2015**, *8*, 4. [CrossRef] [PubMed]

21. Stensgaard, A.S.; Booth, M.; Nikulin, G.; McCreesh, N. Combining process-based and correlative models improves predictions of climate change effects on *Schistosoma mansoni* transmission in eastern Africa. *Geosp. Health* **2016**, *11* (Suppl. 1), 406. [CrossRef] [PubMed]

22. Moss, R.; Babiker, M.; Brinkman, S.; Calvo, E.; Carter, T.; Edmonds, J.; Elgizouli, I.; Emori, S.; Erda, L.; Hibbard, K.; et al. *Towards New Scenarios for Analysis of Emissions: Climate Change, Impacts and Response Strategies*; Intergovernmental Panel on Climate Change: Geneva, Switzerland, 2008; Volume 132.

23. IPPC Working Group I. The Scientific Basis. Available online: https://www.ipcc.ch/ipccreports/tar/wg1/029.htm (accessed on 5 September 2018).

24. Hijmans, R.J.; Cameron, S.E.; Parra, J.L.; Jones, P.G.; Jarvis, A. Very high resolution interpolated climate surfaces for global land areas. *Int. J. Clim.* **2005**, *25*, 1965–1978. [CrossRef]

25. Pflüger, W. Experimental epidemiology of schistosomiasis. I. The prepatent period and cercarial production of *Schistosoma mansoni* in *Biomphalaria* snails at various constant temperatures. *Parasitol. Res.* **1980**, *63*, 159–169.

26. Pflüger, W.; Roushdy, M.Z.; El-Emam, M. Prepatency of *Schistosoma haematobium* in snails at different constant temperatures. *J. Egypt. Soc. Parasitol.* **1983**, *13*, 513–519. [PubMed]

27. Malone, J.B.; Yilma, J.M.; McCarroll, J.C.; Erko, B.; Mukaratirwa, S.; Zhou, X. Satellite climatology and the environmental risk of Schistosoma mansoni in Ethiopia and east Africa. *Acta Trop.* **2001**, *79*, 59–72. [CrossRef]

28. Kalinda, C.; Chimbari, M.J.; Mukaratirwa, S. Schistosomiasis in Zambia: A systematic review of past and present experiences. *Infect. Dis. Poverty* **2018**, *71*, 41. [CrossRef] [PubMed]

29. Hewitt, R.; Willingham, A.L. Elimination of Schistosomiasis in the Caribbean. *TropicalMed* **2018**, in press.

30. Habib, M.R.; Guo, Y.H.; Lv, S.; Gu, W.B.; Li, X.H.; Zhou, X.N. Predicting the spatial distribution of *Biomphalaria straminea*; a potential intermediate host for *Schistosoma mansoni* in China. *Geosp. Health* **2016**, *113*, 453. [CrossRef] [PubMed]

31.   Mandahl-Barth, G. The species of the genus Bulinus: Intermediate hosts of Schistosoma. *Bull. World Health Organ.* **1965**, *331*, 33–44.

32.   Yang, G.; Vounatsou, P.; Zhou, X.N.; Tanner, M.; Utzinger, J. A potential impact of climate change and water resource development on the transmission of *Schistosoma japonicum* in China. *Parassitologia* **2005**, *47*, 127–134. [PubMed]

33.   Berry, A.; Moné, H.; Iriart, X.; Mouahid, G.; Aboo, O.; Boissier, J.; Fillaux, J.; Cassaing, S.; Debuisson, C.; Valentin, A.; et al. *Schistosomiasis haematobium*, Corsica, France. *Emerg. Infect. Dis.* **2014**, *209*, 1595–1597. [CrossRef] [PubMed]

13

A Call for Systems Epidemiology to Tackle the Complexity of Schistosomiasis, its Control and its Elimination

Stefanie J. Krauth [1,*], Julie Balen [2], Geoffrey N. Gobert [3] and Poppy H. L. Lamberton [1,4,*]

[1] Institute for Biodiversity, Animal Health and Comparative Medicine, University of Glasgow, Glasgow G12 8QQ, UK
[2] School of Health and Related Research, University of Sheffield, Sheffield S1 4DA, UK; j.balen@sheffield.ac.uk
[3] School of Biological Sciences, Queen's University Belfast, Belfast BT9 7BL, UK; G.Gobert@qub.ac.uk
[4] Wellcome Centre for Molecular Parasitology, University of Glasgow, Glasgow G12 8QQ, UK
[*] Correspondence: Stefanie.Krauth@glasgow.ac.uk (S.J.K.); Poppy.Lamberton@glasgow.ac.uk (P.H.L.L.)

Abstract: Ever since the first known written report of schistosomiasis in the mid-19th century, researchers have aimed to increase knowledge of the parasites, their hosts, and the mechanisms contributing to infection and disease. This knowledge generation has been paramount for the development of improved intervention strategies. Yet, despite a broad knowledge base of direct risk factors for schistosomiasis, there remains a paucity of information related to more complex, interconnected, and often hidden drivers of transmission that hamper intervention successes and sustainability. Such complex, multidirectional, non-linear, and synergistic interdependencies are best understood by looking at the integrated system as a whole. A research approach able to address this complexity and find previously neglected causal mechanisms for transmission, which include a wide variety of influencing factors, is needed. Systems epidemiology, as a holistic research approach, can integrate knowledge from classical epidemiology, with that of biology, ecology, social sciences, and other disciplines, and link this with informal, tacit knowledge from experts and affected populations. It can help to uncover wider-reaching but difficult-to-identify processes that directly or indirectly influence exposure, infection, transmission, and disease development, as well as how these interrelate and impact one another. Drawing on systems epidemiology to address persisting disease hotspots, failed intervention programmes, and systematically neglected population groups in mass drug administration programmes and research studies, can help overcome barriers in the progress towards schistosomiasis elimination. Generating a comprehensive view of the schistosomiasis system as a whole should thus be a priority research agenda towards the strategic goal of morbidity control and transmission elimination.

Keywords: schistosomiasis; systems epidemiology; systems thinking; complexity; neglected tropical diseases; interdisciplinarity

1. A Brief History of the Discovery, Research, and Control of Schistosomiasis

The parasites now classified as *Schistosoma* spp. were first described in 1851 in Egypt by Theodor Bilharz [1]. Within a year, the involvement of these pathogens in the then-termed "endemic haematuria of warm climates" and the "dysenterische Veränderung des Dickdarms" (dysenteric pathology of the colon) became evident [1,2]. With estimated local prevalence ranging from 50–90% [3,4], and deaths from infections not uncommon, the disease initially named Bilharzia was recognised as a serious public health concern [3,4]. The parasite Bilharz first described as *Distomum haematobium* [1] was later renamed *Bilharzia haematobium* [3] and finally re-classified as *Schistosoma haematobium* [5].

Ever since Bilharz's description, researchers have worked to understand the parasite's developmental biology and identify strategies to help prevent infection, interrupt transmission, and reduce disease burden worldwide.

Bilharzia parasites were described in 1882 as "without question, the most dangerous [of human] parasite[s]" [3]. It was argued that, although other, more serious parasites existed, these were less common and therefore schistosomiasis should be considered the "schlimmerer Feind der Menschheit" ("worse enemy of humankind") [4]. Attempts to control the disease were rolled out soon after its discovery and efforts have increased over the last two decades [6]. For example, one of the first schistosomiasis health education interventions was implemented in 1882. After recognising that infection takes place at water points, a printed memorandum was sent to employees of the British Eastern Telegraph company stationed in Egypt, and later made public [3]. In seeking to prevent human infection, a comprehensive understanding of the life cycle and mode of infection became important research priorities. Observations and experiments in the late 19th century led to hypotheses on how the parasite enters the human body, a point of biology debated in the literature of the time [3,4,7,8]. The most popular theory at the time suggested that ingestion of unclean water was the mode of infection [3,4], but skin penetration was also hypothesised early on and, although at first discounted, led to the policy of forbidding people to bathe in open waters [7,8]. Concurrently, efforts searching for an insect or mollusc intermediate host were ongoing due to analogies drawn from *Distoma* species [4].

Much progress has been made in the understanding of schistosomiasis since these early days. The biology of the parasites is now well described, intermediate host snails identified, and an effective antischistosomal drug—praziquantel—was developed in the 1970s, capable of treating infections caused by all species [9–13]. Nevertheless, Fritsch's 1887 quote, "Even when we understand the life history [of Bilharzia] completely, we might not be able to sufficiently protect ourselves against this malicious foe" (translated from German) [4], remains true today, with over 200 million people still infected and over half of those demonstrating detectable symptoms [14].

Current international strategic goals, as outlined by the World Health Organisation (WHO), aim for morbidity control, and once this is reached for the elimination of schistosomiasis as a public health problem "where appropriate" by 2020 [6,15,16]. With such ambitious goals, it is important to consider how severe historical levels of schistosomiasis once were. If existing interventions were to be discontinued, interrupted, or otherwise unsuccessful, schistosomiasis prevalence, intensity, and associated morbidity could be at risk of returning to former historical levels [17,18].

Despite major research advances, many aspects of the biological, ecological, socio-cultural, economic, and political drivers of schistosomiasis are yet to be elucidated. To identify improved control measures, reduce disease transmission, and achieve elimination in the future, it is key to understand which factors and/or processes directly and indirectly influence exposure, infection, transmission, and disease development, as well as how these are interrelated. One priority area for research should therefore be to better understand, and engage with, the schistosomiasis "system" as a whole.

2. Systems Epidemiology: Systems Thinking for Epidemiology

To overcome current shortcomings of control efforts and move towards schistosomiasis elimination, there is a need to improve intervention strategies. It is well understood that health and disease are affected by multiple, diverse, and complex influences ranging from host immunology and parasite biology through to exposure, social environment, ecology, climate, and access to preventative and curative services [19–23]. Control strategies need to be designed around an improved understanding of the comprehensive range of broader factors influencing disease transmission and intervention successes. Their complex interrelationships, emergent properties, and non-linear feedback-loops all need to be considered. Such interdependencies in a system cannot be identified by considering each of the factors individually. These relationships are best understood by looking at the system as a whole [20,23,24]. Traditional epidemiological approaches, largely reductionist in nature, deal with a limited number of directly related factors, narrowing down causal mechanisms to smaller components that enable us to draw generalisable conclusions [25,26]. This approach has been paramount to uncover many risk factors of *Schistosoma* transmission. However, the direct and indirect interrelated causal mechanisms of the disease are hard to integrate using standard epidemiological approaches. In contrast to reductionist approaches, systems sciences address system-wide behaviours and collective effects. In systems thinking, a system is understood as consisting of many components that, through their interactions with each other, form a complex whole with system-wide properties that can give rise to emergent behaviour, adaptations, and feedback loops [27].

The application of general systems thinking to epidemiology and health research as a tool to integrate knowledge from different areas of research has long been proposed for several diseases [19,28–30]. However, to our knowledge this is the first time it has been proposed specifically for schistosomiasis or any neglected tropical disease (NTD). Systems thinking has well-defined advantages over reductionist approaches. A good example of a health issue of which we now have a system-wide understanding is obesity [24,28,29]. A system influence diagram created by Shiftn (2008) illustrates the complex interrelationships of multiple factors influencing obesity [28]. Such "influence models" can be used to formulate appropriate research hypotheses and address the multiple factors across levels of influence and across disciplines [23,26,29]. With influence diagrams, the whole-disease system can be effectively visualised and analysed for underlying causal mechanisms driving changes in infections and intervention successes/failures. This type of analysis can provide the starting point for more in-depth studies on the dynamics of human–parasite systems as well as for more contextually-relevant intervention/implementation research. Co-creating and discussing influence diagrams can, in turn, enhance stakeholders' understanding of underlying behaviours of a specific system [24].

In their thematic series, "Advancing the application of systems thinking in health" Adam (2014) and colleagues discussed how the application of various systems methods has helped authors uncover reasons for poor health outcomes, such as systems-wide impacts on neonatal health in Uganda and has gone on to identify high leverage points [30]. Other authors linked a range of factors including government opposition, alternative medicine, and strong media coverage to changes in vaccination rates [31]. Adam (2014) emphasised the importance of including evidence beyond traditional epidemiology and economic analysis into the design and evaluation of public health interventions and discussed the usefulness of visual representations for the analysis and interpretation of a system [30]. We build on these ideas by proposing the integration of systems science tools and systems modelling into the field of epidemiology for schistosomiasis and other NTDs. This approach, described as "systems epidemiology", will more effectively integrate knowledge to better understand and control schistosomiasis, as well as focus on contextually relevant factors.

The central goal of a systems epidemiologist would be to uncover principles governing the behaviour and outputs of the entire system, not limited to the behaviour of its individual parts. Working together in a trans-disciplinary manner, researchers, policymakers, health providers, and the affected population could generate much-needed insights into the drivers of persisting *Schistosoma* transmission.

3. Systems Epidemiology as Described in Broader Existing Literatures

Systems epidemiology has, to the best of our knowledge, not yet been applied in the form we propose here. However, the term has been used several times in recent publications across a range of scopes and other topics [19,32–34]. In the majority of these studies, systems epidemiology refers to integrating systems biology tools, such as high-throughput molecular analysis of biomarkers, with epidemiological research questions. For example, the integration of genomics, transcriptomics, proteomics, and metabolomics with epidemiological research was conducted to clarify underlying mechanisms of the effects of food on human health [32]. In addition, a multi-omic approach was employed to understand human pathophysiology in cardiovascular disease and cancer [33,34]. Including multi-omic measurements to analyse complex biological data is an important strategy to uncover the exact mechanisms involved in exposure through to disease development. However, systems biology comprises only the micro-system that influences disease development; i.e., mechanisms only taking place after host exposure to the parasite. In contrast, systems epidemiology can be defined in a wider context, whereby mechanisms related to environmental, social, and demographic aspects of disease are needed to complement the systems biology data, as previously proposed for the control of tuberculosis [19].

We therefore argue that systems epidemiology needs to move beyond the application of systems biology, towards a more holistic understanding of health. Systems epidemiology should combine classical epidemiology with social sciences, natural sciences (including systems biology), ecology, economics, health policy and systems research, and other relevant disciplines and sub-disciplines. This would more effectively characterise the relevant physical and socio-political environments of endemic regions, and access (or lack of) to relevant services, as well as the biology and the co-evolution of the hosts and the pathogen. We argue that applying a systems epidemiology approach to schistosomiasis research is imperative for assessing factors that contribute to persistent disease hotspots, failed intervention programmes, and systematically missed population groups in mass drug administration (MDA) campaigns and/or research studies. Findings from such an approach, we believe, can help overcome current barriers in the progress towards schistosomiasis elimination.

4. The Call for Systems Epidemiology Approaches in Schistosomiasis Control

Over the last two decades, the global agendas outlined in the Millennium and Sustainable Development Goals (MDGs and SDGs, respectively) have raised the profile of schistosomiasis and other poverty-related diseases which had, in the post-colonial era, received reduced attention by international and national governmental agencies [35]. The WHO recommends repeated MDA with praziquantel to reduce schistosomiasis intensity and associated morbidity [14]. In certain areas where the elimination of schistosomiasis as a public health problem, or the interruption of schistosomiasis transmission, are deemed possible, the WHO recommends MDA plus complementary public health interventions [14]. MDA reduces the number of Schistosoma eggs released into the environment, thus reducing human to snail transmission and potentially lowering transmission back into humans [14,36,37]. MDA campaigns have made substantial reductions in morbidity rates and have improved public health overall [37]. These successes sparked an increased push towards disease elimination [6,15,16]. However, MDA success varies considerably, with greater reductions in infection intensities and prevalence in areas which were initially classified as low endemicity (<10% of school-aged children infected), but with often disappointing effects in many moderate and high endemicity areas [21,38]. Despite increased funding, extensive praziquantel donations and national control programmes running for over a decade in several countries, hotspots of high transmission and severe morbidity remain [21,38,39].

While the benefits of MDA to schistosomiasis morbidity reductions are well established, it is now evident that MDA alone is unlikely to achieve elimination [21,36,37,40,41]. Many authors have discussed reasons for MDA programme failures, including treatment compliance, inadequate coverage, treatment efficacy, open defecation/urination behaviours, water contact behaviours, snail density, available infrastructure, and many more [21,36,40,42–47]. Because schistosomiasis is so deeply embedded in broader physical, social, political, and economic systems, the factors influencing intervention successes (or failures) also span these systems [40,42,45]. Several integrated control measures have been proposed to overcome currently identified shortcomings of MDA-only strategies. These propose the inclusion of health education, agricultural policy interventions, sanitation improvements, water supply improvements, engineering interventions, snail control, and behavioural interventions, etc. [48–53]. Extending control measures in this way aims to target both the transmission of schistosomiasis from snails to humans and from humans to snails. Most of these measures aim to increase treatment compliance, provide physical barriers around urine or faeces, and/or decrease snail density. The proposed measures in these studies are based on factors known to contribute to transmission and disease burden. However, a comprehensive summary of all prevailing factors influencing the disease and its transmission in specific settings, and how changing one aspect impacts another aspect as well as the overall system, has, to date, not been generated. Due to the complexity of the issues, it is unfeasible to identify, measure, and include all factors in a single study and researchers often need to focus on a subset of relevant factors that are measurable and feasible for analysis. A research approach and associated toolkit able to deal with this complexity, including a variety of influencing factors, is urgently needed if WHO goals are to be met.

5. How to Apply Systems Epidemiology Approaches to Schistosomiasis Control

To exemplify the complexity of the schistosomiasis system, Figures 1 and 2 illustrate a preliminary interrelationship diagram of empirically tested or hypothesised interactions from a large body of literature and expert knowledge. These figures represent a first "brainstormed" draft of the broader interaction network for schistosomiasis that could be created using systems epidemiology tools. Detailing the complete nature and direction of these interactions would take considerable future research. Nevertheless, already from this crude diagram, interesting observations emerge. For example, factors from the social environment are especially well-connected to other factors in the system (Figure 3). While social environment factors rarely directly interact with infection mechanisms, they are connected with other factors which, in turn, influence exposure and/or treatment coverage and thereby infection rates of a community. These factors affect, e.g., the likelihood of having high-risk water contact, access to treatment, and treatment compliance—which are all well-documented MDA programmatic issues [21,47,54]. Social environment factors vary between communities and settings, since social and cultural norms vary between groups [55–57]. Additionally, social environment factors are not easily quantifiable and often need qualitative research approaches to elucidate them. However qualitative research remains neglected and still occasionally overlooked or misunderstood. This is perhaps best exemplified in the 2016 systematic review on treatment compliance in NTD control programmes, in which qualitative findings were discussed in half a sentence noting: "Other studies provided only qualitative or anecdotal data or reasons for low or non-compliance" [47]. Qualitative research is especially valuable and urgently needed when assessing treatment uptake in order to find missing factors to explain low compliance. Complete whole-system diagrams could further be compared with other, more commonly used methods, such as Bayesian networks [58], to compare combined qualitative and quantitative approaches.

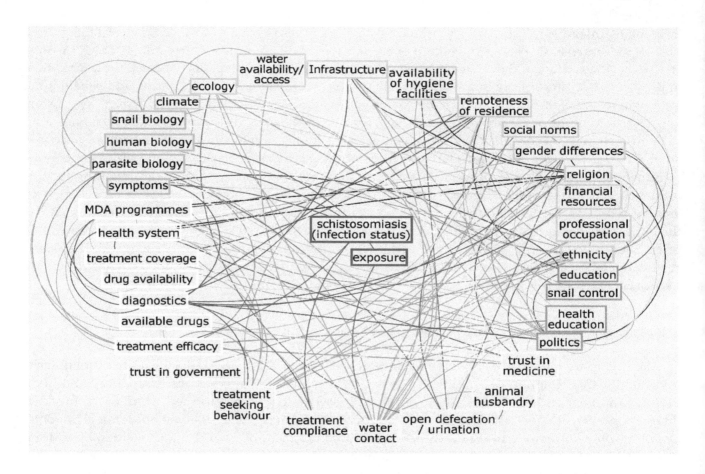

Figure 1. Potential network of factors influencing schistosomiasis infection and disease created with Vensim [59] and GIMP [60]. Connections are a collection of empirically tested or hypothesised relationships. Colours are for illustrative purposes only. This diagram resulted from ongoing brainstorming of connections from a large body of literature and expert knowledge. The diagram aims to exemplify the complexity of the schistosomiasis system without claims of completeness and without detailing the exact nature and direction of interactions. It is meant solely for the purpose of an example of what a systems diagram for schistosomiasis could provide. The full diagram(s) would need to be developed through extensive empirical and theoretical research.

Understanding schistosomiasis control as a systems issue requires a strong interdisciplinary and transdisciplinary approach. Strategies are needed to enable researchers and programme managers to adequately assess and integrate issues across disciplines and in different settings. Creating an empirically based system for understanding interrelationships between relevant issues in schistosomiasis transmission and intervention successes/failures is needed. A comprehensive interrelationship diagram, detailing the nature and direction of the system-wide connections would need to be based on the integration of published knowledge from researchers, with informal knowledge from experts and local populations. Methods to collect and analyse data would include repeated modelling sessions and participatory workshops with stakeholders from a range of backgrounds. This would be the first step towards establishing a systems epidemiology research approach for the control and elimination of schistosomiasis and other NTDs.

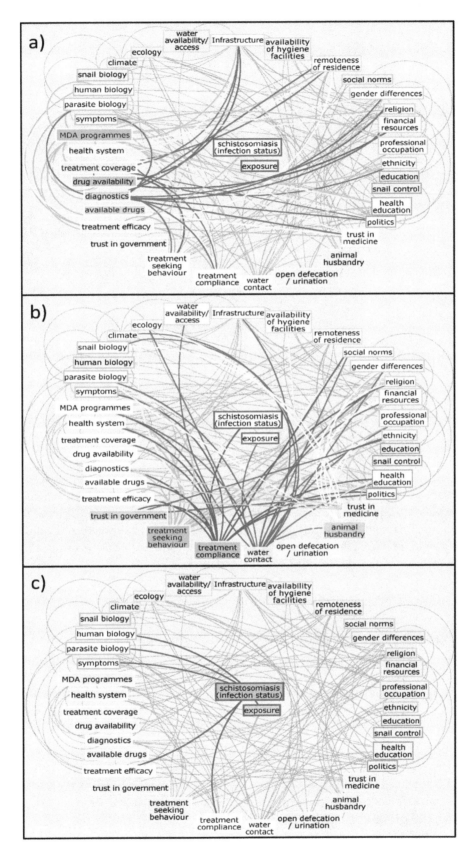

Figure 2. Potential network of factors influencing schistosomiasis infection and disease with individual connections highlighted for (**a**) clinical, (**b**) behavioural, and (**c**) exposure and infection aspects. Colours are for illustrative purposes only; white boxes indicate where the highlighted variables connect to. Different clusters are highlighted by coloured outlines: green: biological aspects; white: clinical aspects; yellow: behavioural aspects; orange: social aspects; purple: politics, policy, and services aspects; turquoise: physical environment; red: exposure and infection.

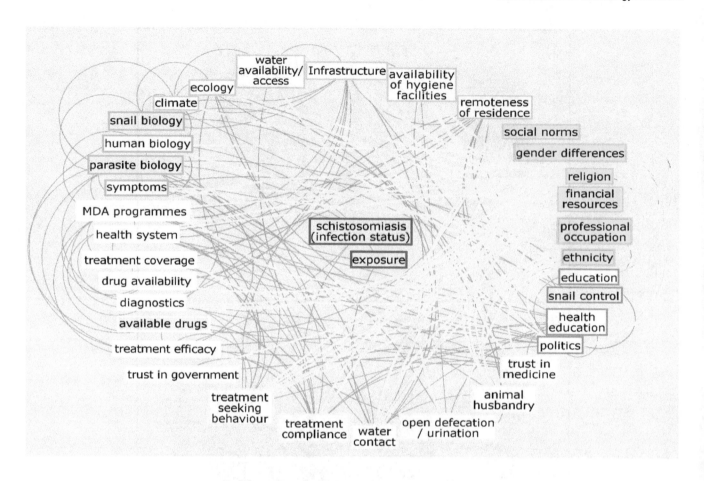

Figure 3. Interconnectedness of social factors with other aspects of the schistosomiasis. White boxes indicate where the highlighted variables connect to. Social aspects illustrated: social norms, gender differences, religion, financial resources, professional occupation, and ethnicity. Although they do not interact directly with infection status or exposure, social aspects underlie and influence many other factors that are, in turn, connected to exposure and infection.

6. Conclusions

Understanding the broader systems-relations and influences of a disease, as well as how best to address these factors with limited resources, is an important challenge. The overall goal is to establish sustainable, contextually relevant, and cost-effective approaches to tackle persistent hotspots of disease transmission. Moving beyond current research and implementation practice, towards complex system analyses and interventions for a disease such as schistosomiasis will help research and policy communities identify how best to achieve WHO goals along the road to elimination. Using a systems thinking toolset, we can connect and integrate knowledge from across a range of disciplines including classical epidemiology, molecular parasitology, ecology, medical anthropology, social and political sciences, and health policy and systems research to identify multiple target points for future schistosomiasis control programmes. This would remove or minimise elusive barriers to success, enabling the global health community to move a step closer towards the elimination of schistosomiasis worldwide.

Author Contributions: Conceptualization, S.J.K. and P.H.L.L.; literature review, S.J.K.; writing—original draft preparation, S.J.K.; writing—review and editing, P.H.L., J.B., G.N.G. visualization, S.J.K.

Acknowledgments: We would like to thank Axel Hochstetter for his help with the extensive figure editing.

References

1. Bilharz, T.; Siebold, C.T.E. Ein beitrag zur helminthographia humana. *Z. Wiss. Zool. Abt. A* **1852**, *4*, 53–76.
2. Bilharz, T. Fernere mittheilungen über *Distomum haematobium*. *Z. Wiss. Zool. Abt. A* **1852**, *4*, 454–456.
3. Cobbold, T.S. Remarks on injurious parasites of Egypt in relation to water-drinking. *Br. Med. J.* **1882**, *2*, 503–504. [CrossRef]
4. Fritsch, G. Zur anatomie der *Bilharzia haematobia* (cobbold). *Arch. Mikrosk. Anat.* **1887**, *31*, 192–223. [CrossRef]
5. Hemming, F. Opinions and declarations rendered by the international commission on zoological nomenclature. Opinion 147. *Bull. Zool. Nomencl.* **1943**, *2*, 123–132.
6. Rollinson, D.; Knopp, S.; Levitz, S.; Stothard, J.R.; Tchuem Tchuente, L.A.; Garba, A.; Mohammed, K.A.; Schur, N.; Person, B.; Colley, D.G.; et al. Time to set the agenda for schistosomiasis elimination. *Acta Trop.* **2013**, *128*, 423–440. [CrossRef] [PubMed]
7. Kartulis, S. Weitere beiträge zur pathologischen anatomie der bilharzia (*Distomum haematobium*, cobbold). *Arch. Pathol. Anat. Physiol. Klin. Med.* **1898**, *152*, 474–486. [CrossRef]
8. Looss, A. Zur anatomie und histologie der *Bilharzia haematobia* (cobbold). *Arch. Mikrosk. Anat.* **1895**, *46*, 1–108. [CrossRef]
9. Gordon, R.M.; Davey, T.H.; Peaston, H. The transmission of human bilharziasis in Sierra Leone, with an account of the life-cycle of the schistosomes concerned, *S. mansoni* and *S. haematobium*. *Ann. Trop. Med. Parasitol.* **1934**, *28*, 323–418. [CrossRef]
10. King, C.H. The evolving schistosomiasis agenda 2007–2017—Why we are moving beyond morbidity control toward elimination of transmission. *PLoS Negl. Trop. Dis.* **2017**, *11*, e0005517. [CrossRef]
11. Lampe, P. The development of *Schistosoma mansoni*. *Proc. R. Soc. Med.* **1927**, *1510*, 56–62.
12. Leiper, R.T.; Atkinson, E.L. Observations on the spread of Asiatic schistosomiasis. *Br. Med. J.* **1915**, *1*, 201–203. [CrossRef]
13. Machemer, L.; Lorke, D. Mutagenicity studies with praziquantel, a new anthelmintic drug, in mammalian systems. *Arch. Toxicol.* **1978**, *39*, 187–197. [CrossRef] [PubMed]
14. World Health Organization. *Schistosomiasis, W. Progress Report 2001–2011 and Strategic Plan 2012–2020*; World Health Organization: Geneva, Switzerland, 2013.
15. World Health Organization. *Elimination of Schistosomiasis. 65th World Health Assembly, Resolution WHA65*; World Health Organization: Geneva, Switzerland, 2012.
16. Toor, J.; Alsallaq, R.; Truscott, J.E.; Turner, H.C.; Werkman, M.; Gurarie, D.; King, C.H.; Anderson, R.M. Are we on our way to achieving the 2020 goals for schistosomiasis morbidity control using current world health organization guidelines? *Clin. Infect. Dis.* **2018**, *66*, S245–S252.
17. Gurarie, D.; Yoon, N.; Li, E.; Ndeffo-Mbah, M.; Durham, D.; Phillips, A.E.; Aurelio, H.O.; Ferro, J.; Galvani, A.P.; King, C.H. Modelling control of Schistosoma haematobium infection: Predictions of the long-term impact of mass drug administration in Africa. *Parasites Vectors* **2015**, *8*, 529. [CrossRef]
18. Mitchell, K.M.; Mutapi, F.; Mduluza, T.; Midzi, N.; Savill, N.J.; Woolhouse, M.E.J. Predicted impact of mass drug administration on the development of protective immunity against *Schistosoma haematobium*. *PLoS Negl. Tropl. Dis.* **2014**, *8*, e3059. [CrossRef]
19. Comas, I.; Gagneux, S. The past and future of tuberculosis research. *PLoS Pathog.* **2009**, *5*, e1000600. [CrossRef]
20. El-Sayed, A.M.; Galea, S. *Systems Science and Population Health*; Oxford University Press: Oxford, UK, 2017.
21. Kittur, N.; Binder, S.; Campbell, C.H.; King, C.H.; Kinung'hi, S.; Olsen, A.; Magnussen, P.; Colley, D.G. Defining persistent hotspots: Areas that fail to decrease meaningfully in prevalence after multiple years of mass drug administration with praziquantel for control of schistosomiasis. *Am. J. Trop. Med. Hyg.* **2017**, *97*, 1810–1817. [CrossRef]
22. Nithiuthai, S.; Anantaphruti, M.T.; Waikagul, J.; Gajadhar, A. Waterborne zoonotic helminthiases. *Vet. Parasitol.* **2004**, *126*, 167–193. [CrossRef]
23. Sturmberg, J.P. *The Value of Systems and Complexity Sciences for Healthcare*; Springer Publishing: Berlin, Germany, 2016.
24. Newell, B.; Proust, K.; Dyball, R.; McManus, P. Seeing obesity as a systems problem. *N. S. W. Public Health Bull.* **2008**, *18*, 214–218. [CrossRef]

25. Epstein, P.R.; Ferber, D. *Changing Planet, Changing Health: How the Climate Crisis Threatens Our Health and What We Can Do about It*; University of California Press: Berkeley, CA, USA, 2011.

26. Joffe, M.; Gambhir, M.; Chadeau-Hyam, M.; Vineis, P. Causal diagrams in systems epidemiology. *Emerg. Themes Epidemiol.* **2012**, *9*, 1. [CrossRef] [PubMed]

27. Bar-Yam, Y. *General Features of Complex Systems*; Encyclopedia of Life Support Systems (EOLSS), UNESCO, EOLSS Publishers: Oxford, UK, 2002.

28. Shift cvba. Shift Obesity System Influence Diagram. Available online: http://www.shiftn.com/obesity/Full-Map.html (accessed on 6 December 2018).

29. Huang, T.T.; Drewnowski, A.; Kumanyika, S.K.; Glass, T.A. A systems-oriented multilevel framework for addressing obesity in the 21st century. *Prev. Chronic Dis.* **2009**, *6*, A82. [PubMed]

30. Adam, T. Advancing the application of systems thinking in health. *Health Res. Policy Syst.* **2014**, *12*, 50. [CrossRef] [PubMed]

31. Varghese, J.; Kutty, V.R.; Paina, L.; Adam, T. Advancing the application of systems thinking in health: Understanding the growing complexity governing immunization services in Kerala, India. *Health Res. Policy Syst.* **2014**, *12*, 47. [CrossRef]

32. Cornelis, M.C.; Hu, F.B. Systems epidemiology: A new direction in nutrition and metabolic disease research. *Curr. Nutr. Rep.* **2013**, *2*, 225–235. [CrossRef] [PubMed]

33. Haring, R.; Wallaschofski, H. Diving through the "-omics": The case for deep phenotyping and systems epidemiology. *OMICS* **2012**, *16*, 231–234. [CrossRef] [PubMed]

34. Lund, E.; Dumeaux, V. Systems epidemiology in cancer. *Cancer Epidemiol. Biomarkers Prev.* **2008**, *17*, 2954–2957. [CrossRef]

35. Israelian, N. A brief history of neglected tropical diseases. *Immpress Magazine*, 17 October 2016. Available online: http://www.immpressmagazine.com/a-brief-history-of-neglected-tropical-diseases/ (accessed on 6 December 2018).

36. Gurarie, D.; Lo, N.C.; Ndeffo-Mbah, M.L.; Durham, D.P.; King, C.H. The human-snail transmission environment shapes long term schistosomiasis control outcomes: Implications for improving the accuracy of predictive modeling. *PLoS Negl. Trop. Dis.* **2018**, *12*, e0006514. [CrossRef]

37. Webster, J.P.; Molyneux, D.H.; Hotez, P.J.; Fenwick, A. The contribution of mass drug administration to global health: Past, present and future. *Philos. Trans. R. Soc. Lond. Ser. B Biol. Sci.* **2014**, *369*, 20130434. [CrossRef]

38. Crellen, T.; Walker, M.; Lamberton, P.H.L.; Kabatereine, N.B.; Tukahebwa, E.M.; Cotton, J.A.; Webster, J.P. Reduced efficacy of praziquantel against *Schistosoma mansoni* is associated with multiple rounds of mass drug administration. *Clin. Infect. Dis.* **2016**, *63*, 1151–1159.

39. Lo, N.C.; Addiss, D.G.; Hotez, P.J.; King, C.H.; Stothard, J.R.; Evans, D.S.; Colley, D.G.; Lin, W.; Coulibaly, J.T.; Bustinduy, A.L.; et al. A call to strengthen the global strategy against schistosomiasis and soil-transmitted helminthiasis: The time is now. *Lancet Infect. Dis.* **2017**, *17*, E64–E69. [CrossRef]

40. Allen, T.; Parker, M. Deworming delusions? Mass drug administration in east African schools. *J. Biosoc. Sci.* **2016**, *48* (Suppl. 1), S116–S147. [CrossRef] [PubMed]

41. Sokolow, S.H.; Wood, C.L.; Jones, I.J.; Swartz, S.J.; Lopez, M.; Hsieh, M.H.; Lafferty, K.D.; Kuris, A.M.; Rickards, C.; De Leo, G.A. Global assessment of schistosomiasis control over the past century shows targeting the snail intermediate host works best. *PLoS Negl. Trop. Dis.* **2016**, *10*, e0004794. [CrossRef] [PubMed]

42. Chami, G.F.; Kontoleon, A.A.; Bulte, E.; Fenwick, A.; Kabatereine, N.B.; Tukahebwa, E.M.; Dunne, D.W. Profiling nonrecipients of mass drug administration for schistosomiasis and hookworm infections: A comprehensive analysis of praziquantel and albendazole coverage in community-directed treatment in Uganda. *Clin. Infect. Dis.* **2016**, *62*, 200–207. [CrossRef] [PubMed]

43. Dyson, L.; Stolk, W.A.; Farrell, S.H.; Hollingsworth, T.D. Measuring and modelling the effects of systematic non-adherence to mass drug administration. *Epidemics* **2017**, *18*, 56–66. [CrossRef]

44. Hastings, J. Rumours, riots and the rejection of mass drug administration for the treatment of schistosomiasis in Morogoro, Tanzania. *J. Biosoc. Sci.* **2016**, *48*, S16–S39. [CrossRef] [PubMed]

45. Person, B.; Knopp, S.; Ali, S.M.; A'Kadir, F.M.; Khamis, A.N.; Ali, J.N.; Lymo, J.H.; Mohammed, K.A.; Rollinson, D. Community co-designed schistosomiasis control interventions for school-aged children in Zanzibar. *J. Biosoc. Sci.* **2016**, *48* (Suppl. 1), S56–S73. [CrossRef] [PubMed]

46.   Riccardi, N.; Nosenzo, F.; Peraldo, F.; Sarocchi, F.; Taramasso, L.; Traverso, P.; Viscoli, C.; Di Biagio, A.; Derchi, L.E.; De Maria, A. Increasing prevalence of genitourinary schistosomiasis in Europe in the migrant era: Neglected no more? *PLoS Negl. Trop. Dis.* **2017**, *11*, e0005237. [CrossRef]

47.   Shuford, K.V.; Turner, H.C.; Anderson, R.M. Compliance with anthelmintic treatment in the neglected tropical diseases control programmes: A systematic review. *Parasites Vectors.* **2016**, *9*, 29. [CrossRef]

48.   Knopp, S.; Mohammed, K.A.; Ali, S.M.; Khamis, I.S.; Ame, S.M.; Albonico, M.; Gouvras, A.; Fenwick, A.; Savioli, L.; Colley, D.G.; et al. Study and implementation of urogenital schistosomiasis elimination in Zanzibar (Unguja and Pemba islands) using an integrated multidisciplinary approach. *BMC Public Health* **2012**, *12*, 930. [CrossRef]

49.   Lee, Y.H.; Jeong, H.G.; Kong, W.H.; Lee, S.H.; Cho, H.I.; Nam, H.S.; Ismail, H.A.H.A.; Alla, G.N.A.; Oh, C.H.; Hong, S.T. Reduction of urogenital schistosomiasis with an integrated control project in Sudan. *PLoS Negl. Trop. Dis.* **2015**, *9*, e3423. [CrossRef] [PubMed]

50.   Raso, G.; Esse, C.; Dongo, K.; Ouattara, M.; Zouzou, F.; Hurlimann, E.; Koffi, V.A.; Coulibaly, G.; Mahan, V.; Yapi, R.B.; et al. An integrated approach to control soil-transmitted helminthiasis, schistosomiasis, intestinal protozoa infection, and diarrhea: Protocol for a cluster randomized trial. *JMIR Res. Protoc.* **2018**, *7*, e145. [CrossRef] [PubMed]

51.   Tian-Bi, Y.N.T.; Ouattara, M.; Knopp, S.; Coulibaly, J.T.; Hurlimann, E.; Webster, B.; Allan, F.; Rollinson, D.; Meite, A.; Diakite, N.R.; et al. Interrupting seasonal transmission of *Schistosoma haematobium* and control of soil-transmitted helminthiasis in northern and central Côte d'Iivoire: A score study protocol. *BMC Public Health* **2018**, *18*, 186. [CrossRef] [PubMed]

52.   Xu, J.; Xu, J.F.; Li, S.Z.; Zhang, L.J.; Wang, Q.; Zhu, H.H.; Zhou, X.N. Integrated control programmes for schistosomiasis and other helminth infections in P.R. China. *Acta Trop.* **2015**, *141*, 332–341. [CrossRef] [PubMed]

53.   Yang, Y.; Zhou, Y.B.; Song, X.X.; Li, S.Z.; Zhong, B.; Wang, T.P.; Bergquist, R.; Zhou, X.N.; Jiang, Q.W. Integrated control strategy of schistosomiasis in the People's Republic of China: Projects involving agriculture, water conservancy, forestry, sanitation and environmental modification. *Adv. Parasitol.* **2016**, *92*, 237–268. [PubMed]

54.   Ross, A.G.P.; Chau, T.N.; Inobaya, M.T.; Olveda, R.M.; Li, Y.S.; Harn, D.A. A new global strategy for the elimination of schistosomiasis. *Int. J. Infect. Dis.* **2017**, *54*, 130–137. [CrossRef]

55.   Henrich, J.; Boyd, R. The evolution of conformist transmission and the emergence of between-group differences. *Evol. Hum. Behav.* **1998**, *19*, 215–241. [CrossRef]

56.   Schultz, P.W.; Nolan, J.M.; Cialdini, R.B.; Goldstein, N.J.; Griskevicius, V. The constructive, destructive, and reconstructive power of social norms. *Psychol. Sci.* **2007**, *18*, 429–434. [CrossRef] [PubMed]

57.   Sherif, M. *The Psychology of Social Norms*; Harper and Brothers Publishing: New York, NY, USA, 1936.

58.   Ghahramani, Z. Learning dynamic Bayesian networks. In *Adaptive Processing of Sequences and DATA Structures*; Giles, C.L., Gori, M., Eds.; Springer: New York, NY, USA, 1998; pp. 168–197.

59.   Ventana Systems Inc. *Vensim*; Ventana Systems Inc.: Harvard, MA, USA, 2015.

60.   GIMP.org. Available online: https://www.gimp.org/ (accessed on 29 January 2019).

14

Treading the Path towards Genetic Control of Snail Resistance to Schistosome Infection

Damilare O. Famakinde

Department of Medical Microbiology and Parasitology, College of Medicine, University of Lagos, Idi-Araba, Surulere, Lagos 100254, Nigeria; damfam.joe@gmail.com

Abstract: Schistosomiasis remains the most important tropical snail-borne trematodiasis that threatens many millions of human lives. In achieving schistosomiasis elimination targets, sustainable control of the snail vectors represents a logical approach. Nonetheless, the ineffectiveness of the present snail control interventions emphasizes the need to develop new complementary strategies to ensure more effective control outcomes. Accordingly, the use of genetic techniques aimed at driving resistance traits into natural vector populations has been put forward as a promising tool for integrated snail control. Leveraging the *Biomphalaria-Schistosoma* model system, studies unraveling the complexities of the vector biology and those exploring the molecular basis of snail resistance to schistosome infection have been expanding in various breadths, generating many significant discoveries, and raising the hope for future breakthroughs. This review provides a compendium of relevant findings, and without neglecting the current existing gaps and potential future challenges, discusses how a transgenic snail approach may be adapted and harnessed to control human schistosomiasis.

Keywords: schistosomiasis; vector control; snail resistance; gene drive; transgenic snail

1. Introduction

It is presently more than a century since malacological discoveries established that various genera of freshwater snails (Mollusca: Gastropoda) serve as biological vectors of human diseases caused by parasitic trematodes. These findings have made the study of snail biology an important aspect of infectious disease research, particularly in tropical helminthology. Among these human snail-borne trematodiases, schistosomiasis (bilharziasis) ranks as the most important disease, afflicting more than 206 million humans [1], and being responsible for over 3.51 million disability-adjusted life years (DALYs) [2], most prominently in the tropics. Most cases of human schistosomiasis are caused by three parasitic schistosomes (blood flukes): *Schistosoma haematobium*, *S. mansoni*, and *S. japonicum* [3]. Both *S. haematobium* and *S. mansoni* are found in Africa and the Middle East; only *S. mansoni* occurs in the Americas, and *S. japonicum* is a major disease-causing species in China, Indonesia, and the Philippines [3]. However, the geographical distribution of these flukes is synchronous to, and importantly determined by, the local distribution of their snail vectors. *S. haematobium* is transmitted by *Bulinus* snails, *S. mansoni* by *Biomphalaria* snails, and *S. japonicum* by *Oncomelania* snails [4].

The human-to-snail-to-human transmission of *Schistsosoma* occurs when adult male and female living in copula within the human host mate and produce fertilized eggs. Some of the eggs are voided with urine (in *S. haematobium*) or feces (in *S. mansoni* and *S. japonicum*) into the environment. The eggs that reach the vectors' freshwater habitats hatch and release the enclosed miracidia larvae, which swim actively to locate and infect their snail vectors. A miracidium that successfully infects a susceptible vector undergoes intramolluscan polyembryonic development to produce thousands of actively-swimming tailed cercariae larvae that emerge continuously from the snail host for the rest of the its lifetime (spanning months) [3–6]. Human infection with schistosomes is acquired through skin contact with, and subsequent penetration by, the cercariae during recreational, domestic, or occupational activities with contaminated water [5]. Following penetration, the worms transform into immature schistosomes (schistosomulae) and are carried in body circulation, from where they enter the portal veins and mature in about 5–7 weeks [3,5]. Mature worm pairs migrate to their preferred host sites—*S. mansoni* and *S. japonicum* to the mesenteric venules of the bowel or rectum, and *S. haematobium* to the venous plexus of the bladder, where they mate and the females lay eggs to repeat the cycle [4,5]. Adult schistosomes have an average lifespan of 3–10 years, but they may also live as long as 30–40 years in their human hosts [3–5]. The eggs are highly immunogenic and are majorly responsible for disease outcomes by triggering localized pathologic reactions within the human host [4,7,8]. Although human infection with *Schistosoma* species may cause non-specific but incapacitating systemic morbidities such as malnutrition, anemia, and impaired physical and cognitive development in children, poor birth outcomes in infected pregnant women, and neurological aberrations, *S. haematobium* is specifically responsible for urogenital pathologies, while other *Schistosoma* species majorly cause gastrointestinal complications, but also hepatosplenic enlargement, ascites, and portal hypertension in advanced cases [3,7,9,10]. Again, there is growing evidence that female urogenital schistosomiasis poses an increased risk of HIV transmission and/or progression [11–13].

Taking a leap towards the beginning of the end human schistosomiasis requires an integrated control approach that cuts across both the vector and the human cycles. Current strategy in the fight against the disease co-implements ongoing preventive chemotherapy through mass drug administration (MDA), with complementary public-health interventions. This approach, as defined by WHO/AFRO, is known as PHASE—preventive chemotherapy, health education, access to clean water, sanitation improvement, and environmental snail control and focal mollusciciding [14]. Recent efforts made to evaluate the degree of importance of snail control in schistosomiasis elimination [15–18] clearly showed that sustainable snail control is pivotal in achieving targeted disease elimination. This is especially true in the present era of highly challenging anti-schistosome vaccine development, as well as the monochemotherapeutic availability of praziquantel and its feared resistance by schistosomes [19–21]. Strategies currently in use for controlling schistosomiasis snail vectors are: biocontrol using competitors or predators, modification of snail habitats, and application of molluscicides. These approaches, used either singly or in combination, have evidently contributed to many successful schistosomiasis control efforts in different localities and countries [15,22–27]; however, each approach is not without limitations [24]. The application of chemical molluscicides has been mostly exploited. Among other chemical molluscicidal agents, niclosamide has a long track record of being successful against snail hosts, and is often regarded as the molluscicide of choice. Nevertheless, apart from its expensiveness, toxicity of niclosamide to a variety of non-target aquatic life forms (plants, invertebrates and vertebrates including amphibians) has led to its decreased acceptability. Again, the inability of niclosamide to prevent snail recolonization, especially in large permanent water bodies, necessitates repeated applications that result in high cost [24,28–30].

In view of the present challenges facing schistosomiasis control efforts, coupled with the endorsement by the World Health Assembly Resolution 65.21 to take full advantage of non-drug-based interventions to prevent schistosomiasis transmission [31], it will be timely to adapt new strategies in order to interrupt snail-mediated schistosome transmission, and thus, forestall human infection. The use of genetic techniques to manipulate snail vectors of schistosomiasis has long been stressed as a novel biocontrol strategy with the potential to constitute an important complementary tool for transmission reduction or breaking. Embracing all the means to actualize this potential, studies unraveling the complexities of the vector biology and those exploring the molecular underpinnings of snail resistance/susceptibility to schistosome infection have been expanding in various breadths, generating many significant discoveries and raising the hope for future breakthroughs. The aim of this review is to provide a compendium of relevant findings, and discuss how transgenic snail approach may be adapted and harnessed to control human schistosomiasis.

2. Biology of Snail Resistance/Susceptibility to *Schistosoma* Infections–Major Exploits so Far

The first groundbreaking discovery on the identification of intermediate snail hosts of schistosomes was made by Miyairi and Suzuki, who observed stages of *S. japonicum* in *Oncomelania* snails in Japan in 1913 [32,33]. This was followed by the achievements of Robert Leiper, who also demonstrated the complete life cycles of *S. haematobium* and *S. mansoni* in their respective snail hosts in Egypt [34,35]. Subsequent to these watershed moments in the long history of schistosomiasis, investigations on the interactions between schistosomes and their snail vectors became kinetic. The genetic study of snail-schistosome compatibility was pioneered by Newton [36,37], who demonstrated that susceptibility of snail vectors to *Schistosoma* infections is fundamentally genetic and a heritable character. This was later underscored by other investigators who revealed that resistance character, which is acquired at the maturity phase in the adults of resistant snail stocks, is monogenic, dominant, and heritable by a simple Mendelian pattern of inheritance [38–41]. This genetic dominance of the resistance trait has been confirmed by various crossbreeding experiments in *Biomphalaria* species [42–46]. Be that as it may, Rosa et al. [45] showed that resistance in *B. tenagophila* is determined by two dominant genes. In contrast, in juvenile *B. glabrata*, resistance is a complex trait governed by a minimum of four genes, each having multiple alleles (alternative forms of the same gene) [40,47]. From these various lines of evidence, it could be understood that genetic determinism of resistance is governed by a single major locus (position of a particular gene or allele on a chromosome) to a potentially high number of loci, and snails with significantly increased resistance could be artificially selected in the laboratory; meanwhile, molecular markers mapped to resistance could be identified in genetic crosses.

Thus far, work has been done most extensively using the *Biomphalaria-Schistosoma* model, and has led to the nomenclature of some stocks known for resistance (e.g., pigmented BS-90 [48], black-eye 10-R2 [49], and 13-16-IR [50]) or susceptibility (e.g., the albino M-line and NMRI [51], and BB02 [52]) to *S. mansoni* infection, which are now maintained in the laboratory for research purposes. In contrast to the 10-R2 and 13-16-IR strains, however, BS-90 demonstrates unflinching resistance stability, irrespective of age (juvenile or adult), under laboratory conditions [40,53].

A major physiological determinant of snail resistance/susceptibility to infections, which is also under genetic influence, is the snail internal defense system (IDS). The IDS comprises the cellular elements (hemocytes) and the humoral (plasma) factors of the hemolymph that work independently or in concert to recognize, encapsulate, kill, and clear intruding trematodes [6,54–56]. Establishment of the *B. glabrata* embryonic (*Bge*) cell line in 1976 [57] provided an enabling avenue for investigators to delve into the molecular and cellular aspects of the complex snail immune functions against schistosomes by using an *in vitro* culture model, rather than using the whole intact animal, which could have resulted in a rudimentary understanding of the complex biological events. Moreover, major advances in *Biomphalaria* omic studies, such as the recent availability of the whole genome sequence of *B. glabrata* [58], provide a useful resource in deciphering complex functions of the snail biology that were previously obscure. Using various strain and species combinations of the *Biomphalaria-Schistosoma* model system, robust molecular studies have been carried out, leveraging various techniques to identify and characterize endogenous effector protein/gene candidates that are functional in the snail internal defense machinery against schistosomes. Table 1 below presents a synopsis of various endogenous factors that have been implicated in *Biomphalaria* resistance to schistosomes.

Table 1. Putative genes and proteins conferring *Biomphalaria* resistance to *Schistosoma* infection.

Resistance Factor	Snail spp.	Schistosoma spp.	Function	Reference(s)
40S ribosomal protein S9	B. glabrata	S. mansoni	Protein translation in hemocytes.	[59]
BgAIF	B. glabrata	S. mansoni	Modulates hemocyte activation.	[60]
BgGRN	B. glabrata	S. mansoni	Production of adherent hemocytes.	[61]
BgMIF	B. glabrata	S. mansoni	Induces hemocyte proliferation.	[62]
BgTLR	B. glabrata	S. mansoni	Parasite recognition and activation of effector functions.	[63]
Biomphalysin	B. glabrata	S. mansoni	Binds to the sporocyst surface and lyses it.	[54,64]
Cathepsin B	B. glabrata	S. mansoni	Lysis of encapsulated sporocyst.	[65]
Cathepsin L	B. glabrata	S. mansoni	Lysis of encapsulated sporocyst.	[66]
Copine 1	B. glabrata	S. mansoni	Involves in signaling processes.	[66]
CREPs	B. glabrata	S. mansoni	Pattern recognition receptors/adhesion proteins.	[67]
Cu/Zn SOD (SOD1)	B. glabrata	S. mansoni	Catalyzes the production of H_2O_2 which is cytotoxic to sporocyst.	[50,68,69]
Cystatin 2	B. glabrata	S. mansoni	Protease inhibitor.	[70,71]
Cytidine deaminase	B. glabrata	S. mansoni	Nucleobase, nucleoside, nucleotide, and nucleic acid metabolism.	[47]
Cytochrome b	B. glabrata	S. mansoni	Mitochondrial respiration.	[70]
Cytochrome C oxidase subunits	B. glabrata	S. mansoni	Mitochondrial respiration.	[70,71]
Dermatopontin2	B. glabrata	S. mansoni	Participates in hemocyte adhesion and encapsulation responses.	[59,67,70]
Elastase2	B. glabrata	S. mansoni	Lysis of encapsulated sporocyst.	[66,70]
Elongation factors 1α & 2	B. glabrata	S. mansoni	Transcription enzymes (bind t-RNA to ribosomes).	[59,67]
Endo-1,4-β-glucanase	B. glabrata	S. mansoni	Carbohydrate metabolism.	[70]
Ferritin	B. glabrata	S. mansoni	Stores and transport iron in non-toxic form.	[70,71]
FREP1, 2, 3 & 12	B. glabrata	S. mansoni	Pattern recognition receptors/adhesion proteins.	[67,70,72,73]
Fribillin	B. glabrata	S. mansoni	Participates in hemocyte adhesion and encapsulation responses.	[70]
GlcNAc↓	B. tenagophila	S. mansoni	Increases hemocyte binding to sporocyst.	[74]
GPCR kinase 2	B. glabrata	S. mansoni	Signal transduction.	[70]
Grctm6	B. glabrata	S. mansoni	Modulates cercarial shedding.	[75]
GREPs	B. glabrata	S. mansoni	Pattern recognition receptors/adhesion proteins.	[67]
GSTs	B. glabrata	S. mansoni	Prevent cellular damage to the hemocytes.	[70]
Hsp40, 60 & 70 #	B. glabrata	S. mansoni	Housekeeping cell repair activities.	[66,67,70,76–78]
Importin 7	B. glabrata	S. mansoni	Involves in signaling processes.	[66]
Inferred phagocyte oxidase	B. glabrata	S. mansoni	Production of superoxide anions.	[60]
Interleukin 1	B. glabrata	S. mansoni	Stimulates hemocyte defense response.	[79]
LPS-binding protein	B. glabrata	S. mansoni	Adhesion protein.	[67]
Matrilin	B. glabrata	S. mansoni	Participates in hemocyte adhesion and encapsulation responses.	[59,70]

Table 1. *Cont.*

Resistance Factor	Snail spp.	*Schistosoma* spp.	Function	Reference(s)
Metalloproteases	*B. glabrata*	*S. mansoni*	Tissue morphogenesis/remodeling.	[67]
MPEG 1	*B. glabrata*	*S. mansoni*	Participates in hemocyte defense responses.	[47]
Neo-calmodulin	*B. glabrata*	*S. mansoni*	Cacium signaling and homeostasis.	[67]
NF-kB	*B. glabrata*	*S. mansoni*	Downstream transcription in the TLR pathway.	[59,63,70,80]
NADH dehydrogenase subunis	*B. glabrata*	*S. mansoni*	Mitochondrial respiration.	[70]
Peroxiredoxines 1 & 4	*B. glabrata*	*S. mansoni*	Neutralize ROS and RNS that can damage cellular functions.	[60,81]
PGRP 1	*B. glabrata*	*S. mansoni*	Pattern recognition receptor.	[70]
PKC receptor	*B. glabrata*	*S. mansoni*	Signal transduction.	[47]
TEPs	*B. glabrata*	*S. mansoni*	Pattern recognition receptors/adhesion proteins.	[67]
TNF-α	*B. glabrata*	*S. mansoni*	Stimulates hemocyte defense response.	[82]

Symbols: ↓ in lower concentrations; # contrasting reports (see [67,78] for some details). Abbreviations: *BgAIF, B. glabrata* allograft inflammatory factor; *BgGRN, B. glabrata* granulin; *BgMIF, B. glabrata* macrophage migration-inhibitory factor; *BgTLR, B. glabrata* Toll-like receptor; CREP, C-type lectin-related protein; Cu/Zn SOD, copper/zinc superoxide dismutase; FREP, fibrinogen-related protein; GlcNac, N-acetyl-D-glucosamine; GPCR, G-protein coupled receptor; Grctm, Guadeloupe resistance complex transmembrane; GREP, galectin-related proteins; GSTs, glutathione-S-transferases; H_2O_2, hydrogen peroxide; Hsp, heat shock protein; LPS, lipopolysaccharide; MPEG, macrophage expressed gene; NADH, reduced nicotinamide adenine dinucleotide; NF-kB, nuclear factor kappa B; PKC, protein kinase C; PGRP, peptidoglycan recognition protein; RNS, reactive nitrogen species; ROS, reactive oxygen species; t-RNA, transfer ribonucleic acid; TEP, thioester-containing protein; TNF-α, tumor necrosis factor-alpha.

3. Transgenic Snail Methods for Schistosomiasis Control

The use of genetically engineered vectors to either suppress (reduce) or modify (replace) the natural populations of the biological vectors of some globally important infectious diseases has been a convincing concept that is now on the verge of deployment to control disease transmission. This rapidly emerging genetic control approach is distinguished from other biocontrol strategies (such as the use of natural parasitoids, predators, competitors, and infectious microbial agents), as it is mating-based, highly species-specific, and capable of being transmitted or inherited vertically [83]. In this context, suppression or elimination of natural local vector populations could be achieved by releasing transgenic vectors carrying sterile or detrimental characters into the local populations, while the population modification approach requires the release of transgenic pathogen-resistant vector strains or species. Depending on their characteristics or specific configurations, genetic methods for transgenic vector control may be self-limiting with transient persistence among subsequent vector generations unless replenished by repeated release of engineered vectors, or self-sustaining with indefinite persistence from the initial target population to the subsequent ones [83]. With revolutions in biotechnology, the use of gene drive systems (self-sustaining, selfish genetic elements that are inherited by progenies at frequencies largely exceeding those expected in Mendelian inheritance) has become an attractive method for vector control applications, as gene drivers are invasive wherever present, and so may overcome some evolutionary constraints [83,84].

As first proposed in 1958 [85], much emphasis has been placed on the use of genetic biocontrol for schistosomiasis vector control. To select a suitable transgenic vector method for schistosomiasis control however, the basics of the biology of the snail vectors must be taken into account. Although a wealth of genetic studies has been centered on the production of transgenic mosquito vectors of human diseases, biological differences between these dipterans and schistosomiasis molluscan vectors create the need for selective transgenic vector strategies for schistosomiasis control application. For example, unlike in mosquitoes where only females are capable of transmitting pathogens, *Biomphalaria* and *Bulinus* are hermaphrodites capable of self- or cross-fertilization [86], and all mating types serve as hosts for schistosomes. *Oncomelania* has separate sexes [86] but nevertheless, both sexes can also carry *S. japonicum*, only perhaps at varying degree of susceptibility [87,88]. These biological peculiarities render population reduction strategies unsuitable for genetic control of the snail hosts. This is because the newly released transgenic snails carrying harmful characters would remain susceptible to *Schistosoma* infections, therefore intensifying parasite transmission. Consequently, present focus in the genetic control of schistosomiasis vectors is set on strategies to modify the natural snail populations. According to Hubendick [85], population of the resistant strains can displace that of the susceptible ones in the field by natural selection. Although this scenario is plausible, it can be realized only through the application of self-sustaining transgenic vector systems (Figure 1).

Promoted by its advantages over other gene drive systems—such as transcription activator-like effector nucleases (TALENs) and zinc finger nucleases (ZFNs)—used in genome editing technology, and over other genetic techniques such as RNA interference (RNAi) [84,89,90], the recently-discovered CRISPR/Cas9 (clustered regularly-interspaced short palindromic repeats/CRISPR-associated protein 9) system has flowered, and is being widely used in current research trials and applications to modify genome sequences in diverse species spanning microbes, plants, animals, to even humans [89–93]. In parallel, the use of CRISPR/Cas9 to drive anti-*Schistosoma* effector genes into the genome of naturally susceptible snail strains is being envisioned, and has become an important subject in current discussions [17,75,94,95]. Fascinatingly, a proof-of-concept study [96] has demonstrated the possibility of CRISPR/Cas9-mediated gene editing in molluscs; indeed, more insights into the possible ways by which this may be achieved for schistosomiasis vector control, as well as the current and potential future challenges, will constitute a key guide for the scientific community in the appropriate fostering of this tantalizing approach in snail molecular research.

Figure 1. Transgenic snail system for field control of schistosomiasis transmission.

The three basic requirements for a CRISPR-based precise gene knock-in editing are Cas9 endonuclease, single-guide RNA (sgRNA), and repair template DNA (donor). The Cas9 enzyme combs through the genome of the host organism, acting as the 'molecular scissors' that cuts a specific DNA sequence at a genomic locus. The sgRNA (~20 nucleotides) is designed to match and target the desired DNA sequence to be deleted, while the donor DNA provides a template for genomic repair of the cleaved locus [92,97]. In the case of schistosomiasis snail vectors, Cas9-mediated introgression of refractoriness into susceptible strains will require an engineered donor DNA encoding a locus known to confer resistance. The anti-*Schistosoma* donor DNA can be tightly anchored to the Cas9/sgRNA complex, and the entire cassette is co-injected with a viral vector, such as lentivirus [98], into the early single-cell stage embryos of the snail vectors (Figure 2). In essence, the viral vector ensures safe and effective delivery of these components into the nuclei of the target cells. Suitable sites for the driver–cargo system injection may include the ovotestis of *Biomphalaria / Bulinus* snails and the ovary of female *Oncomelania* snails. In *Biomphalaria*, the ovotestis is located at the tip of the shell spire [99] and the driver–cargo system insertion into the ovotestis will be more appealing in the albino strain, as the transparency of the snail shell allows easy visibility of internal organs. Further analyses to assess targeting efficiency or screen for transgenic mutants among progenies may be done by T7 endonuclease I (T7E1) assay, restriction enzyme assay, next generation sequencing or direct PCR assay as applicable (Figure 2).

Figure 2. A schematic representation of CRISPR/Cas9 genome editing system in a snail vector of schistosome. Abbreviations: DSB, double-strand break; HDR, homology-directed repair; P1 & P2, promoters; PCR, polymerase chain reaction; RE, restriction enzyme; T7E1, T7 endonuclease I.

To date, the main genetic loci that have been identified in association with *B. glabrata* resistance to schistosome are *Sod1* and *RADres* (a restricted-site associated DNA-determined resistance locus) [50,68,69], and a *GRC* (Guadeloupe Resistance Complex) genomic region (<1 Mb) [69]. In combination with other known and yet unknown resistance genes, *Sod1* and *RADres* occupy haplotype blocks of >2 Mb genomic region [69,100]. Although putative functional gene candidates have been identified in the *GRC* region [75,95], the *Sod1* and *RADres* regions appear to demonstrate a wider spectrum of snail resistance [69]. Nevertheless, there is still a need to further narrow down these regions to the embedding causative genes, and to understand their immune stability and functions under different genetic backgrounds and environmental conditions.

4. Further Considerations

An early investigator [101] stated that the genetic factors controlling snail insusceptibility to schistosomes must first be clarified, and snail strains ferrying only refractory traits must be developed before we can gainfully engage genetic control methods. The first criterion has largely been met through relentless research unveiling resistance-determining proteins and genes. Despite these advances, current stumbling blocks involve developing snail strains that are reliably recalcitrant to schistosome infection. One major bottleneck is the highly variable strain-by-strain interaction—compatibility polymorphism—that is well-documented to occur in snail-schistosome systems [102,103]. As a consequence, developing a transgenic target for individual strain-to-strain combinations becomes cumbersome, but can be circumvented only if genetic loci with wide-spectrum resistance activities conserved across various strain-to-strain combinations could be identified and characterized. The BS-90 strain of *B. glabrata* (isolated in Salvadore, Brazil) has been bred in the laboratory for many years and has been shown to be steadily resistant; however, its relative performance in the field remains unpredictable. A tenable reason for this is that generations of the laboratory-bred strains are poor representatives of the genetic variations that actually occur in the original wild populations [103]. Another caveat in the future use of either the resistant BS-90 or transgenic snail strains is global warming, characterized by an increasing earth's average surface temperature. In sharp contrast to what was earlier known, Knight et al. [78] showed that snail resistance to schistosomes is also temperature-dependent, and even the naturally resistant BS-90 strain could be rendered susceptible at 32 °C. Other local environmental factors such as altitude, water level, soil, and vegetation may also cause differential gene expression and regulation among snails of the same species as a result of local adaptation mechanisms [104].

Organism biodiversity and signatures of interactions between other organisms and the snail vectors living in the same habitat may also impact the outcome of transgenic snail application. In an ecological milieu where natural predators [e.g., *Macrobrachium vollenhovenii* (a freshwater prawn), *Procambarus clarkia* (a freshwater crayfish), *Marisa cornuarietis* (an ampullarid snail), and cichlid fishes such as *Trematocranus placodon* and *Geophagus brasiliensis*] or competitors [e.g., thiarid snails such as *Melanoides tuberculata* and *Tarebia granifera*] of the snail vectors of schistosomiasis [4,24] exist in meaningful abundance, there is a possibility that the population of the released transgenic snails becomes reduced below levels required to displace that of the naturally susceptible vectors as a result of a more biased killing/eating of the transgenic snails (and eating of their egg masses) or deprivation of resources. When such a scenario operates, the resistance effect tapers off. Given this contingency, the release of transgenic snails may be chosen only in lieu of introducing predators or competitors of snail vectors; co-implementation of both methods in the same freshwater focus may not always complement the transgenic snail approach. In foci where populations of predators or competitors already occur in significant abundance, one-off niclosamide application prior to the release of transgenic snails may offer a more palatable approach in reducing the probability of diluted effect of the transgenic snail release. These phenomena highlight the importance of sampling water habitats for species diversity prior to, and periodically after, releasing transgenic snails.

The merits of using schistosome-resistant transgenic snails beat the limitations of other biological and environmental interventions. For instance, populations of molluscivorous fishes and prawns large enough to eat the snail vectors may rapidly diminish due to indiscriminate fishing by residents of communities where schistosomiasis is endemic, since these molluscivores are also a major source of food for humans. Moreover, introduction of competitor species of snails could greatly endanger agriculture and the ecosystem. On the other hand, environmental modifications (such as removal of vegetation on which the snail vectors feed, lining canals with cement, or draining water habitats) are very expensive and impractical for resource-constrained areas. Meanwhile, vegetation removal poses an increased risk of infection to workers who may not have protective tools [24]. Generally, however, certain issues concerning the use of gene drive systems have come into view. The most important of all include potential off-target mutations that may result in unpredictable effects, development of drive resistance in populations, fitness and competitiveness of released strains compared to wild populations, and possible difficulty in the containment, reversal, or adjustment of gene drive spread [83,84,105]. Nevertheless, it is somewhat relieving that a good number of these limitations can feasibly be overcome through the meticulous design of more specific sgRNAs, and development of reversal drive systems [84,89,91,92,97,105]. Moreover, the majority of the current issues regarding the application of gene drives for the control of disease vectors arose from studies focusing on mosquitoes, implying that some of the risk issues, such as vector dispersal beyond intended political boundaries [84], may be of lesser concern in other non-insect vector control systems. Conversely however, the significant body of research on mosquitoes may have also overcome some series of technical challenges that may remain unresolved for other disease vectors.

Should a breakthrough on the use of CRISPR-based vector control occur, the fine line between mating/reproductive biology of *Oncomelania* and that of *Bulinus* or *Biomphalaria*, as well as the varying degree of selfing among species of the hermaphroditic (*Bulinus* and *Biomphalaria*) snail vectors, will also have important implications in schistosomiasis snail control application. As shown in Figure 1, CRISPR/Cas9-driven resistance traits may spread more rapidly among successive progeny of *Oncomelania* (being a dioecious outcrossing vector) than in *Bulinus* and *Biomphalaria* snail vectors. More precisely, in the two latter snail vectors, gene drive approach may not be effective in predominantly selfing species, such as *Bulinus truncatus*, *Bulinus forskalii*, and *Biomphalaria pfeifferi*.

5. Conclusions

The prospective use of genetically manipulated vectors to stop the spread of vector-borne diseases maintains its impressiveness and is awaited by the scientific community. In fast-tracking sustainable schistosomiasis elimination, the use of CRISPR-based vector modification strategy appears fascinating and potentially effective. However, this approach is currently still underdeveloped in snail molecular research. Finding the pertinent missing pieces in our jigsaw of knowledge of schistosome/snail biology, and identifying ways to bypass potential future challenges, are requisites for achieving this promising snail control strategy. Finally, the use of schistosome-resistant transgenic snails may have the propensity to singly interrupt schistosomiasis transmission when only outcrossing vector species are present, but in foci where both predominantly selfing species and outcrossing species of *Bulinus* or *Biomphalaria* snails coexist, the integration of additional suitable snail control methods will provide a way of complementing this genetic control method for more effective outcomes.

Acknowledgments: The author would like to thank Officer Adewale Adeniyi of the Nigerian Customs Service (NCS) for his financial assistance.

References

1. World Health Organization. Schistosomiasis and soil-transmitted helminthiasis: Number of people treated in 2016. *Wkly. Epidemiol. Rec.* **2017**, *92*, 49–60.
2. World Health Organization. *Global Health Estimates Summary Tables. DALYs by Cause, Age and Sex, by WHO Region, 2000–2015*; World Health Organization: Geneva, Switzerland, 2016.
3. Colley, D.G.; Bustinduy, A.L.; Secor, W.E.; King, C.H. Human schistosomiasis. *Lancet* **2014**, *383*, 2253–2264. [CrossRef]
4. Muller, R.; Wakelin, D. *Worms and Human Disease*, 2nd ed.; CABI Publishing: Oxon, UK; New York, NY, USA, 2002; pp. 1–300.
5. Adenowo, A.B.; Oyinloye, B.E.; Ogunyinka, B.I.; Kappo, A.B. Impact of human schistosomiasis in sub-Saharan Africa. *Braz. J. Infect. Dis.* **2015**, *19*, 196–205. [CrossRef] [PubMed]
6. Famakinde, D.O. Molecular context of *Schistosoma mansoni* transmission in the molluscan environments: A mini-review. *Acta Trop.* **2017**, *176*, 98–104. [CrossRef] [PubMed]
7. Olveda, D.U.; Li, Y.; Olveda, R.M.; Lam, A.K.; Chau, T.N.P.; Harn, D.A.; Williams, G.M.; Gray, D.J.; Ross, A.G.P. Bilharzia: Pathology, diagnosis, management and control. *Trop. Med. Surg.* **2013**, *1*, 135. [CrossRef] [PubMed]
8. Colley, D.G.; Secor, W.E. Immunology of human schistosomiasis. *Parasite Immunol.* **2014**, *36*, 347–357. [CrossRef] [PubMed]
9. Friedman, J.F.; Mital, P.; Kanzaria, H.K.; Olds, G.R.; Kurtis, J.D. Schistosomiasis and pregnancy. *Trends Parasitol.* **2007**, *23*, 159–164. [CrossRef] [PubMed]
10. Salawu, O.T.; Odaibo, A.B. Maternal schistosomiasis: A growing concern in sub-Saharan Africa. *Pathog. Glob. Health* **2014**, *108*, 263–270. [CrossRef] [PubMed]
11. Kjetland, E.F.; Ndhlovu, P.D.; Gomo, E.; Mduluza, T.; Midzi, N.; Gwanzura, L.; Mason, P.R.; Sandvik, L.; Friis, H.; Gunderseen, S.G. Association between genital schistosomiasis and HIV in rural Zimbabwean women. *AIDS* **2006**, *20*, 593–600. [CrossRef] [PubMed]
12. Mbabazi, P.S.; Andan, O.; Fitzgerald, D.W.; Chitsulo, L.; Engels, D.; Downs, J.A. Examining the relationship between urogenital schistosomiasis and HIV infection. *PLoS Negl. Trop. Dis.* **2011**, *5*, e1396. [CrossRef] [PubMed]
13. Bustinduy, A.; King, C.; Scott, J.; Appleton, S.; Sousa-Figueiredo, J.C.; Betson, M.; Stothard, J.R. HIV and schistosomiasis co-infection in African children. *Lancet Infect. Dis.* **2014**, *14*, 640–649. [CrossRef]

14. Tchuenté, L.-A.T.; Rollinson, D.; Stothard, J.R.; Molyneux, D. Moving from control to elimination of schistosomiasis in sub-Saharan Africa: Time to change and adapt strategies. *Infect. Dis. Poverty* **2017**, *6*, 42. [CrossRef] [PubMed]

15. King, C.H.; Sutherland, L.J.; Bertsch, D. Systematic review and meta-analysis of the impact of chemical-based mollusciciding for control of *Schistosoma mansoni* and *S. haematobium* transmission. *PLoS Negl. Trop. Dis.* **2015**, *9*, e0004290. [CrossRef] [PubMed]

16. Lo, N.C.; Gurarie, D.; Toon, N.; Coulibaly, J.T.; Bendavid, E.; Andrews, J.R.; King, C.H. Impact and cost-effectiveness of snail control to achieve disease control targets for schistosomiasis. *Proc. Natl. Acad. Sci. USA* **2018**, *115*, E584–E591. [CrossRef] [PubMed]

17. Sokolow, S.H.; Wood, C.L.; Jones, I.J.; Lafferty, K.D.; Kuris, A.M.; Hseih, M.H.; De Loe, G.A. To reduce the global burden of human schistosomiasis, use 'old fashioned' snail control. *Trends Parasitol.* **2018**, *34*, 23–40. [CrossRef] [PubMed]

18. Sokolow, S.H.; Wood, C.L.; Jones, I.J.; Swartz, S.J.; Lopez, M.; Hseih, M.H.; Lafferty, K.D.; Kuris, A.M.; Rickards, C.; De Leo, G.A. Global assessment of schistosomiasis control over the past century shows targeting the snail intermediate host works best. *PLoS. Negl. Trop. Dis.* **2016**, *10*, e0004794. [CrossRef] [PubMed]

19. Alsaqabi, S.M.; Lofty, W.M. Praziquantel: A review. *J. Vet. Sci. Technol.* **2014**, *5*, 1000200. [CrossRef]

20. Cioli, D.; Pica-Mattoccia, L.; Basso, A.; Guidi, A. Schistosomiasis control: Praziquantel forever? *Mol. Biochem. Parasitol.* **2014**, *195*, 23–29. [CrossRef] [PubMed]

21. Tebeje, B.M.; Harvie, M.; You, H.; Loukas, A.; McManus, D.P. Schistosomiasis vaccines: Where do we stand? *Parasit. Vectors* **2016**, *9*, 528. [CrossRef] [PubMed]

22. Ebisawa, I. Epidemiology and eradication of schistosomiasis japonica in Japan. *J. Travel Med.* **1998**, *5*, 33–35. [CrossRef] [PubMed]

23. Barakat, R.M.R. Epidemiology of schistosomiasis in Egypt: Travel through time: Review. *J. Adv. Res.* **2013**, *4*, 425–432. [CrossRef] [PubMed]

24. Secor, W.E. Water-based interventions for schistosomiasis control. *Pathog. Glob. Health* **2014**, *108*, 246–254. [CrossRef] [PubMed]

25. Tlamçani, Z.; Er-Rami, M. Schistosomiasis control: Moroccan experience compared to other endemic countries. *Asian Pac. J. Trop. Dis.* **2014**, *4*, 329–332. [CrossRef]

26. King, C.H.; Bertsch, D. Historical perspective: Snail control to prevent schistosomiasis. *PLoS Negl. Trop. Dis.* **2015**, *9*, e0003657. [CrossRef] [PubMed]

27. Sun, L.P.; Wang, W.; Hong, Q.B.; Li, S.Z.; Liang, Y.S.; Yang, H.T.; Zhou, X.N. Approaches being used in the national schistosomiasis elimination programme in China: A review. *Infect. Dis. Poverty* **2017**, *6*, 55. [CrossRef] [PubMed]

28. Lardans, V.; Dissous, C. Snail control strategies for reduction of schistosomiasis transmission. *Parasitol. Today* **1998**, *14*, 413–417. [CrossRef]

29. Huang, D.; Zhen, J.; Quan, S.; Liu, M.; Liu, L. Risk assessment for niclosamide residues in water and sediments from Nan Ji Shan Island within Poyang Lake region, China. *Adv. Mat. Res.* **2013**, *721*, 608–612. [CrossRef]

30. World Health Organization. *Field Use of Molluscicides in Schistosomiasis Control Programmes: An Operational Manual for Programme Managers*; World Health Organization: Geneva, Switzerland, 2017.

31. World Health Assembly. Elimination of Schistosomiasis. In *Sixty-fifth World Health Assembly: Resolutions and Decisions*; World Health Organization: Geneva, Switzerland, 2012; pp. 36–37.

32. Miyairi, K.; Suzuki, M. On the development of *Schistosoma japonicum*. *Tokyo Med. J.* **1913**, *1836*, 1961–1965.

33. Tanaka, H.; Tsuji, M. From discovery to eradication of schistosomiasis in Japan: 1847–1996. *Int. J. Parasitol.* **1997**, *27*, 1465–1480. [CrossRef]

34. Leiper, R.T. On the relation between the terminal-spined and lateral-spined eggs of bilharzia. *Br. Med. J.* **1916**, *1*, 411. [CrossRef] [PubMed]

35. Leiper, R.T. Report on the results of the bilharzias mission in Egypt, 1915. *J. R. Army Med. Corps* **1918**, *30*, 235–260.

36. Newton, W.L. The comparative tissue reaction of two strains of *Australorbis glabratus* to infection with *Schistosoma mansoni*. *J. Parasitol.* **1952**, *38*, 362–366. [CrossRef] [PubMed]

37. Newton, W.L. The inheritance of susceptibility to infection with *Schistosoma mansoni* in *Australorbis glabratus*. *Exp. Parasitol.* **1953**, *2*, 242–257. [CrossRef]

38. Richards, C.S. Genetic studies of a molluscan vector of schistosomiasis. *Nature* **1970**, *227*, 231–241. [CrossRef]

39. Richards, C.S. Genetic factors in susceptibility of *Biomphalaria glabrata* for different strains of *Schistosoma mansoni*. *Parasitology* **1975**, *70*, 231–241. [CrossRef] [PubMed]

40. Richards, C.S. *Schistosoma mansoni*: susceptibility reversal with age in the snail host. *Exp. Parasitol.* **1977**, *42*, 165–168. [CrossRef]

41. Richards, C.S.; Knight, M.; Lewis, F.A. Genetics of *Biomphalaria glabrata* and its effects on the outcome of *Schistosoma mansoni* infection. *Parasitol. Today* **1992**, *8*, 171–174. [CrossRef]

42. Abou-El-Naga, I.F.; Eissa, M.M.; Mossallam, S.F.; El-Halim, S.I.A. Inheritance of *Schistosoma mansoni* infection incompatibility in *Biomphalaria alexandrina* snails. *Mem. do Inst. Oswaldo Cruz* **2010**, *105*, 149–154. [CrossRef]

43. Dos Santos, M.B.L.; Freitas, J.R.; Correia, M.C.R.; Coelho, P.M.Z. Susceptibility of *Biomphalaria tenagophila* hybrids to *Schistosoma mansoni*: Crossing between strains from Taim (RS), Cabo Frio (RJ), and Belo Horizonte (MG), Brasil. *Rev. Inst. de Med. Trop. São Paulo* **1979**, *21*, 281–286.

44. Knight, M.; Miller, A.N.; Patterson, C.N.; Rowe, C.G.; Michaels, G.; Carr, D.; Richards, C.S.; Lewis, F.A. The identification of markers segregating with resistance to *Schistosoma mansoni* infection in the snail *Biomphalaria glabrata*. *Proc. Natl. Acad. Sci. USA* **1999**, *96*, 1510–1515. [CrossRef] [PubMed]

45. Rosa, F.M.; Godard, A.L.B.; Azevedo, V.; Coelho, P.M.Z. *Biomphalaria tenagophila*: dominant character of the resistance to *Schistosoma mansoni* in descendants of crossbreedings between resistant (Taim, RS) and susceptible (Joinville, SC) strains. *Mem. do Inst. Oswaldo Cruz* **2005**, *100*, 19–23. [CrossRef]

46. Haggag, S.H.; El-Sherbiny, M. Molecular markers associated with resistance to *Schistosoma mansoni* infection in the *Biomphalaria glabrata* snails. *Biotechnology* **2006**, *5*, 404–412.

47. Ittiprasert, W.; Miller, A.; Myers, J.; Nene, V.; El-Sayed, N.M.; Knight, M. Identification of immediate response genes dominantly expressed in juvenile resistant and susceptible *Biomphalaria glabrata* snails upon exposure to *Schistosoma mansoni*. *Mol. Biochem. Parasitol.* **2010**, *169*, 27–39. [CrossRef] [PubMed]

48. Paraense, W.L.; Correa, L.R. Variation in susceptibility of populations of *Australorbis glabratus* to a strain of *Schistosoma mansoni*. *Rev. Inst. Med. Trop. São Paulo* **1963**, *5*, 15–22. [PubMed]

49. Richards, C.S. Susceptibility of adult *Biomphalaria glabrata* to *Schistosoma mansoni* infection. *Am. J. Trop. Med. Hyg.* **1973**, *22*, 748–756. [CrossRef] [PubMed]

50. Goodall, C.P.; Bender, R.C.; Brooks, J.K.; Bayne, C.J. *Biomphalaria glabrata* cytosolic copper/zinc superoxide dismutase (SOD1) gene: Association of SOD1 alleles with resistance/susceptibility to *Schistosoma mansoni*. *Mol. Biochem. Parasitol.* **2006**, *147*, 207–210. [CrossRef] [PubMed]

51. Newton, W.L. The establishment of a strain of *Australorbis glabratus* which combines albinism and high susceptibility to infection with *Schistosoma mansoni*. *J. Parasitol.* **1955**, *41*, 526–528. [CrossRef] [PubMed]

52. Adema, C.M.; Luo, M.Z.; Hanelt, B.; Hertel, L.A.; Marshall, J.J.; Zhang, S.M.; DeJong, R.J.; Kim, H.R.; Kudrna, D.; Wing, R.A.; et al. A bacterial artificial chromosome library for *Biomphalaria glabrata*, intermediate snail host of *Schistosoma mansoni*. *Mem. Inst. Oswaldo Cruz* **2006**, *101*, S167–S177. [CrossRef]

53. Ittiprasert, W.; Myers, J.; Odoemelam, E.C.; Raghavan, N.; Lewis, F.; Bridger, J.M.; Knight, M. Advances in the genomics and proteomics of the freshwater intermediate snail host of *Schistosoma mansoni*, *Biomphalaria glabrata*. In *Biomphalaria Snails and Larval Trematodes*; Toledo, R., Fried, B., Eds.; Springer: New York, NY, USA, 2011; pp. 191–213.

54. Pinaud, S.; Portela, J.; Duval, D.; Nowacki, F.C.; Olive, M.A.; Allienne, J.F.; Galinier, R.; Dheilly, N.M.; Kieffer-Jaquinod, S.; Mitta, G.; et al. A shift from cellular to humoral responses contributes to innate immune memory in the vector snail *Biomphalaria glabrata*. *PLoS Pathog.* **2016**, *12*, e1005361. [CrossRef] [PubMed]

55. Yoshino, T.P.; Coustau, C. Immunobiology of *Biomphalaria*–trematode interactions. In *Biomphalaria Snails and Larval Trematodes*; Toledo, R., Fried, B., Eds.; Springer: New York, NY, USA, 2011; pp. 159–189.

56. Pila, E.A.; Li, H.; Hambrook, J.R.; Wu, X.; Hanington, P. Schistosomiasis from a snail's perspective: Advances in snail immunity. *Trends Parasitol.* **2017**, *33*, 845–857. [CrossRef] [PubMed]

57. Hansen, E.L. A cell line from embryos of *Biomphalaria glabrata* (Pulmonata): Establishment and characteristics. In *Invertebrate Tissue Culture: Research Applications*; Maramorosch, K., Ed.; Academic Press: New York, NY, USA, 1976; pp. 75–97.

58.   Adema, C.M.; Hillier, L.D.W.; Jones, C.S.; Loker, E.S.; Knight, M.; Minx, P.; Oliveira, G.; Raghavan, N.; Shedlock, A.; do Amaral, L.R.; et al. Whole genome analysis of a schistosomiasis-transmitting freshwater snail. *Nat. Comm.* **2017**, *8*, 15451. [CrossRef] [PubMed]

59.   Zahoor, Z.; Lockyer, A.E.; Davies, A.J.; Kirk, R.S.; Emery, A.M.; Rollinson, D.; Jones, C.S.; Noble, L.R.; Walker, A.J. Differences in the gene expression profiles of haemocytes from schistosome-susceptible and -resistant *Biomphalaria glabrata* exposed to *Schistosoma mansoni* excretory secretory products. *PLoS ONE* **2014**, *9*, e93215. [CrossRef] [PubMed]

60.   Larson, M.K.; Bender, R.C.; Bayne, C.J. Resistance of *Biomphalaria glabrata* 13–16-R1 snails to *Schistosoma mansoni* PR1 is a function of haemocyte abundance and constitutive levels of specific transcripts in haemocytes. *Int. J. Parasitol.* **2014**, *44*, 343–353. [CrossRef] [PubMed]

61.   Pila, E.A.; Gordy, M.A.; Phillips, V.K.; Kabore, A.L.; Rudkom, S.P.; Hanington, P.C. Endogenous growth factor stimulation of hemocyte proliferation induces resistance to *Schistosoma mansoni* challenge in the snail host. *Proc. Natl. Acad. Sci. USA* **2016**, *113*, 5305–5310. [CrossRef] [PubMed]

62.   Garcia, A.B.; Pierce, R.J.; Gourbal, B.; Werkmeister, E.; Colinet, D.; Reichhart, J.; Dissous, C.; Coustau, C. Involvement of the cytokine MIF in the snail host immune response to the parasite *Schistosoma mansoni*. *PLoS Pathog.* **2010**, *6*, e1001115.

63.   Pila, E.A.; Tarrabain, M.; Kabore, A.L.; Hanington, P.C. A novel toll-like receptor (TLR) influences compatibility between the gastropod *Biomphalaria glabrata*, and the digenean trematode *Schistosoma mansoni*. *PLoS Pathog.* **2016**, *12*, e1005513. [CrossRef] [PubMed]

64.   Galinier, R.; Portela, J.; Mone, Y.; Allienne, J.F.; Henri, H.; Delbecq, S.; Mitta, G.; Gourbal, B.; Duval, D. Biomphalysin, a new β pore-forming toxin involved in *Biomphalaria glabrata* immune defense against *Schistosoma mansoni*. *PLoS Pathog.* **2013**, *9*, e1003216. [CrossRef] [PubMed]

65.   Myers, J.; Ittiprasert, N.; Raghavan, N.; Miller, A.; Knight, M. Differences in cysteine protease activity in *Schistosoma mansoni*-resistant and -susceptible *Biomphalaria glabrata* and characterization of the hepatopancreas cathepsin B fulllength cDNA. *J. Parasitol.* **2008**, *94*, 659–668. [CrossRef] [PubMed]

66.   Lockyer, A.E.; Spinks, J.; Kane, R.A.; Hoffmann, K.F.; Fitzpatrick, J.M.; Rollinson, D.; Noble, L.R.; Jones, C.S. *Biomphalaria glabrata* transcriptome: cDNA microarray profiling identifies resistant- and susceptible-specific gene expression in haemocytes from snail strains exposed to *Schistosoma mansoni*. *BMC Genomics* **2008**, *9*, 634. [CrossRef] [PubMed]

67.   Wu, X.; Dinguirard, N.; Sabat, G.; Lui, H.; Gonzalez, L.; Gehring, M.; Bickham-Wright, U.; Yoshino, T.P. Proteomic analysis of *Biomphalaria glabrata* plasma proteins with binding affinity to those expressed by early developing larval *Schistosoma mansoni*. *PLoS Pathog.* **2017**, *13*, e1006081. [CrossRef] [PubMed]

68.   Bonner, K.M.; Bayne, C.J.; Larson, M.K.; Blouin, M.S. Effects of Cu/Zn superoxide dismutase (*sod1*) genotype and genetic background on growth, reproduction and defense in *Biomphalaria glabrata*. *PLoS Negl. Trop. Dis.* **2012**, *6*, e1701. [CrossRef] [PubMed]

69.   Tennessen, J.A.; Bonner, K.M.; Bollmann, S.R.; Johnstun, J.A.; Yeh, J.Y.; Marine, M.; Tavalire, H.F.; Bayne, C.J.; Blouin, M.S. Genome-wide scan and test of candidate genes in the snail *Biomphalaria glabrata* reveal new locus influencing resistance to *Schistosoma mansoni*. *PLoSNegl. Trop. Dis.* **2015**, *9*, e0004077. [CrossRef] [PubMed]

70.   Lockyer, A.E.; Emery, A.M.; Kane, R.A.; Walker, A.J.; Mayer, C.D.; Mitta, G.; Coustau, C.; Adema, C.M.; Hanelt, B.; Rollinson, D.; et al. Early differential gene expression in haemocytes from resistant and susceptible *Biomphalaria glabrata* strains in response to *Schistosoma mansoni*. *PLoS ONE* **2012**, *7*, e51102. [CrossRef] [PubMed]

71.   Nowak, T.S.; Woodards, A.C.; Jung, Y.; Adema, C.M.; Loker, E.S. Identification of transcripts generated during the response of resistant *Biomphalaria glabrata* to *Schistosoma mansoni* infection using suppression subtractive hybridization. *J. Parasitol.* **2004**, *90*, 1034–1040. [CrossRef] [PubMed]

72.   Hanington, P.C.; Forys, M.A.; Dragoo, J.W.; Zhang, S.; Adema, C.M.; Loker, E.S. Role for a somatically diversified lectin in resistance of an invertebrate to parasite infection. *Proc. Natl. Acad. Sci. USA* **2010**, *107*, 21087–21092. [CrossRef] [PubMed]

73.   Hanington, P.C.; Forys, M.A.; Loker, E.S. A somatically diversified defense factor, FREP3, is a determinant of snail resistance to schistosome infection. *PLoS Negl. Trop. Dis.* **2012**, *6*, e1591. [CrossRef] [PubMed]

74. Martins-Souza, R.L.; Pereira, C.A.J.; Rodrigues, L.; Araújo, E.S.; Coelho, P.M.Z.; Corrêa, A., Jr.; Negrão-Corrêa, D. Participation of N-acetyl-D-glucosamine carbohydrate moieties in the recognition of *Schistosoma mansoni* sporocysts by haemocytes of *Biomphalaria tenagophila*. *Mem. Inst. Oswaldo Cruz* **2011**, *106*, 884–891. [CrossRef] [PubMed]

75. Allan, E.R.O.; Tennessen, J.A.; Bollmann, S.R.; Hanington, P.C.; Bayne, C.J.; Blouin, M.S. Schistosome infectivity in the snail, *Biomphalaria glabrata*, is partially dependent on the expression of Grctm6, a Guadeloupe Resistance Complex protein. *PLoS Negl. Trop. Dis.* **2017**, *11*, e0005362. [CrossRef] [PubMed]

76. Ittiprasert, W.; Knight, M. Reversing the resistance phenotype of the *Biomphalaria glabrata* snail host *Schistosoma mansoni* infection by temperature modulation. *PLoS Pathog.* **2012**, *8*, e1002677. [CrossRef] [PubMed]

77. Ittiprasert, W.; Nene, R.; Miller, A.; Raghavan, N.; Lewis, F.; Hodgson, J.; Knight, M. *Schistosoma mansoni* infection of juvenile *Biomphalaria glabrata* induces a differential stress response between resistant and susceptible snails. *Exp. Parasitol.* **2009**, *123*, 203–211. [CrossRef] [PubMed]

78. Knight, M.; Elhelu, O.; Smith, M.; Haugen, B.; Miller, A.; Raghavan, N.; Wellman, C.; Cousin, C.; Dixon, F.; Mann, V.; et al. Susceptibility of snails to infection with schistosomes is influenced by temperature and expression of heat shock proteins. *Epidemiology* **2015**, *5*, 1–18.

79. Granath, W.O., Jr.; Connors, V.A.; Tarleton, R.L. Interleukin 1 activity haemolymph from strains of the snail *Biomphalaria glabrata* varying in susceptibility to the human blood fluke, *Schistosoma mansoni*: Presence, differential expression, and biological function. *Cytokine* **1994**, *6*, 21–27. [CrossRef]

80. Zhang, S.M.; Coultas, K.A. Identification and characterization of five transcription factors that are associated with evolutionarily conserved immune signaling pathways in the schistosome-transmitting snail *Biomphalaria glabrata*. *Mol. Immunol.* **2011**, *48*, 1868–1881. [CrossRef] [PubMed]

81. Knight, M.; Raghavan, N.; Goodal, C.; Cousin, C.; Ittiprasert, W.; Sayed, A.; Miller, A.; Williams, D.L.; Bayne, C. *Biomphalaria glabrata* peroxiredoxin: effect of *Schistosoma mansoni* infection on differential gene regulation. *Mol. Biochem. Parasitol.* **2009**, *167*, 20–31. [CrossRef] [PubMed]

82. Ouwe-Missi-Oukem-Boyer, O.; Porchet, E.; Capron, A.; Dissous, C. Characterization of immunoreactive TNF-α molecules in the gastropod *Biomphalaria glabrata*. *Dev. Comp. Immunol.* **1994**, *18*, 211–218. [CrossRef]

83. Alphey, L. Genetic control of mosquitoes. *Annu. Rev. Emtomol.* **2014**, *59*, 205–224. [CrossRef] [PubMed]

84. Macias, V.M.; Ohm, J.R.; Rasgon, J.L. Gene drive for mosquito control: Where did it come from and where are we headed? *Int. J. Environ. Res. Public Health* **2017**, *14*, 1006. [CrossRef] [PubMed]

85. Hubendick, B. A possible method of schistosome-vector control by competition between resistant and susceptible strains. *Bull. World Health Organ.* **1958**, *18*, 1113–1116. [PubMed]

86. Rozendaal, J.A.; World Health Organization. Freshwater snails. In *Vector Control: Methods for Use by Individuals and Communities*; World Health Organization: Geneva, Switzerland, 1997; pp. 337–356.

87. Claveria, F.G.; Etges, F.J. Differential susceptibility of male and female *Oncomelania hupensis quadrasi* infected with *Schistosoma japonicum*. *Int. J. Parasitol.* **1987**, *17*, 1273–1277. [CrossRef]

88. Moose, J.W.; Williams, J.E. Infection rates of *Schistosoma japonicum* in experimentally exposed female and male oncomelanid snails. *Jan. J. Med. Sci. Biol.* **1964**, *17*, 333–334. [CrossRef]

89. Sun, D.; Gou, Z.; Liu, Y.; Zhang, Y. Progress and prospects of CRISPR/Cas systems in insects and other arthropods. *Front. Physiol.* **2017**, *8*, 608. [CrossRef] [PubMed]

90. Zhang, Z.; Zhang, Y.; Gao, F.; Han, S.; Cheah, K.S.; Tse, H.F.; Lian, Q. CRISPR/Cas9 genome-editing system in human stem cells: Current status and future prospects. *Mol. Ther. Nucleic Acids* **2017**, *9*, 230–241. [CrossRef] [PubMed]

91. Singh, V.; Braddick, D.; Dhar, P.K. Exploring the potential of genome editing CRISPR-Cas9 technology. *Gene* **2017**, *599*, 1–18. [CrossRef] [PubMed]

92. Liu, X.; Wu, S.; Xu, J.; Suin, C.; Wei, J. Application of CRISPR/Cas9 in plant biology. *Acta Pharm. Sin. B* **2017**, *7*, 292–302. [CrossRef] [PubMed]

93. Cai, L.; Fisher, A.L.; Huang, H.; Xie, Z. CRISR-mediated genome editing and human diseases. *Genes Dis.* **2016**, *3*, 244–251. [CrossRef]

94. Mouahid, G.; Rognon, A.; de Carvalho-Augusto, R.; Driguez, P.; Geyer, K.; Karinshak, S.; Luviano, N.; Mann, V.; Quack, T.; Rawlinson, K.; et al. Transplantation of schistosome sporocysts between host snails: A video guide. *Wellcome Open Res.* **2018**, *3*, 3. [CrossRef] [PubMed]

95. Tennessen, J.A.; Théron, A.; Marine, M.; Yeh, J.Y.; Rognon, A.; Blouin, M.S. Hyperdiverse gene cluster in snail host conveys resistance to human schistosome parasites. *PLoS Genet.* **2015**, *11*, e1005067. [CrossRef] [PubMed]

96. Perry, K.J.; Henry, J.Q. CRISPR/Cas9-mediated genome modification in the mollusc, *Crepidula fornicata*. *Genesis* **2015**, *53*, 237–244. [CrossRef] [PubMed]

97. Bortesi, L.; Zhu, C.; Zischewski, J.; Perez, L.; Bassié, L.; Nadi, R.; Forni, G.; Lade, S.B.; Soto, E.; Jin, X.; et al. Patterns of CRISPR/Cas9 activity in plants, animals and microbes. *Plant Biotechnol. J.* **2016**, *14*, 2203–2216. [CrossRef] [PubMed]

98. Wang, L.; Li, F.; Dang, L.; Liang, D.; Wang, C.; He, B.; Liu, J.; Li, D.; Wu, X.; Xu, X.; et al. *In vivo* delivery systems for therapeutic genome editing. *Int. J. Mol. Sci.* **2016**, *17*, 626. [CrossRef] [PubMed]

99. Jarne, P.; Pointier, J.-P.; David, P. Biosystematics of *Biomphalaria* spp. with an emphasis on *Biomphalaria glabrata*. In *Biomphalaria Snails and Larval Trematodes*; Toledo, R., Fried, B., Eds.; Springer: New York, NY, USA, 2011; pp. 1–32.

100. Blouin, M.S.; Bonner, K.M.; Cooper, B.; Amarasinghe, V.; O'Donnell, R.P.; Bayne, C.J. Three genes involved in the oxidative burst are closely linked in the genome of the snail, *Biomphalaria glabrata*. *Int. J. Parasitol.* **2013**, *43*, 51–55. [CrossRef] [PubMed]

101. Berg, C.O. Biological control of snail-borne diseases: A review. *Exp. Parasitol.* **1973**, *33*, 318–330. [CrossRef]

102. Galinier, R.; Roger, E.; Moné, Y.; Duval, D.; Portet, A.; Pinaud, S.; Chaparro, C.; Grunau, C.; Genthon, C.; Dubois, E.; et al. A multistrain approach to studying the mechanisms underlying compatibility in the interaction between *Biomphalaria glabrata* and *Schistosoma mansoni*. *PLoS Negl. Trop. Dis.* **2017**, *11*, e0005398. [CrossRef] [PubMed]

103. Mitta, G.; Adema, C.M.; Gourbal, B.; Loker, E.S.; Theron, A. Compatibility polymorphism in snail/schistosome interactions: From field to theory to molecular mechanisms. *Dev. Comp. Immunol.* **2012**, *37*, 1–8. [CrossRef] [PubMed]

104. Zhao, J.S.; Wang, A.Y.; Zhao, H.B.; Chen, Y.H. Transcriptome sequencing and differential gene expression analysis of the schistosome-transmitting snail *Oncomelania hupensis* inhabiting hilly and marshland regions. *Sci. Rep.* **2017**, *7*, 15809. [CrossRef] [PubMed]

105. Esvelt, K.M.; Smidler, A.L.; Catteruccia, F.; Church, G.M. Concerning RNA-guided gene drives for the alteration of wild population. *eLife* **2014**, *3*, e03401. [CrossRef] [PubMed]

15

Asian Schistosomiasis: Current Status and Prospects for Control Leading to Elimination

Catherine A. Gordon [1,†], Johanna Kurscheid [2,†], Gail M. Williams [3], Archie C. A. Clements [4,5], Yuesheng Li [1], Xiao-Nong Zhou [6], Jürg Utzinger [7,8], Donald P. McManus [1] and Darren J. Gray [2,*]

[1]   QIMR Berghofer Medical Research Institute, Herston, QLD 4006, Australia; Catherine.Gordon@qimrberghofer.edu.au (C.A.G.); Yuesheng.Li@qimrberghofer.edu.au (Y.L.); Don.McManus@qimrberghofer.edu.au (D.P.M.)

[2]   Department of Global Health, Research School of Population Health, Australian National University, Acton, ACT 2601, Australia; Johanna.Kurscheid@anu.edu.au

[3]   School of Public Health, University of Queensland, Herston, QLD 4006, Australia; g.williams@sph.uq.edu.au

[4]   Faculty of Health Sciences, Curtin University, Bentley, WA 6102, Australia; archie.clements@curtin.edu.au

[5]   Telethon Kids Institute, Nedlands, WA 6009, Australia

[6]   Center for Disease Control and Prevention, National Institute for Parasitic Diseases, Shanghai 200025, China; zhouxn1@chinacdc.cn

[7]   Swiss Tropical and Public Health Institute, CH-4002 Basel, Switzerland; juerg.utzinger@swisstph.ch

[8]   University of Basel, CH-4003 Basel, Switzerland

*   Correspondence: darren.gray@anu.edu.au

†   Joint first authors.

Abstract: Schistosomiasis is an infectious disease caused by helminth parasites of the genus *Schistosoma*. Worldwide, an estimated 250 million people are infected with these parasites with the majority of cases occurring in sub-Saharan Africa. Within Asia, three species of *Schistosoma* cause disease. *Schistosoma japonicum* is the most prevalent, followed by *S. mekongi* and *S. malayensis*. All three species are zoonotic, which causes concern for their control, as successful elimination not only requires management of the human definitive host, but also the animal reservoir hosts. With regard to Asian schistosomiasis, most of the published research has focused on *S. japonicum* with comparatively little attention paid to *S. mekongi* and even less focus on *S. malayensis*. In this review, we examine the three Asian schistosomes and their current status in their endemic countries: Cambodia, Lao People's Democratic Republic, Myanmar, and Thailand (*S. mekongi*); Malaysia (*S. malayensis*); and Indonesia, People's Republic of China, and the Philippines (*S. japonicum*). Prospects for control that could potentially lead to elimination are highlighted as these can inform researchers and disease control managers in other schistosomiasis-endemic areas, particularly in Africa and the Americas.

Keywords: Asia; control; elimination; epidemiology; *Schistosoma japonicum*; *Schistosoma malayensis*; *Schistosoma mekongi*; schistosomiasis

1. Introduction

Schistosomiasis is a parasitic disease caused by blood flukes of the genus *Schistosoma*. Six species of schistosomes infect humans: *Schistosoma mansoni* (occurring in Africa, South America, the Caribbean, and the Middle East), *S. haematobium* (mainly occurring in Africa and the Middle East, with recent autochthonous transmission observed in Corsica, France), *S. intercalatum* and *S. guineensis* (two rare species confined to a few countries in Central Africa), *S. japonicum* (Asia), and *S. mekongi* (Mekong Delta including Cambodia, Lao People's Democratic Republic (Lao PDR), and previously Thailand whose current status is transmission interruption) [1–3]. A seventh species, *S. malayensis*, which is thought to be closely related to *S. mekongi*, is endemic in Malaysia [4]. In this review, we focus on only those species currently occurring in Asia: *S. japonicum*, *S. mekongi*, and *S. malayensis*, which cause intestinal schistosomiasis. The three Asian schistosomes are all zoonotic, whereas the remaining species infecting humans are generally considered human-only parasites, with some notable exceptions [5–10].

Schistosomiasis has a long history in Asia with the first descriptions and reports of the disease in modern times appearing in the early 1900s, although it is thought to have been endemic for at least 400 years earlier in Japan, and at least 2200 years ago in the People's Republic of China (P.R. China) after the discovery of *S. japonicum* eggs in a mummy [11–14]. To date, Japan is the only country in Asia to have eliminated schistosomiasis, while Thailand is awaiting verification of transmission interruption by the World Health Organization (WHO) [15]. Currently, schistosomiasis is endemic in six Asian countries: P.R. China, the Philippines, Indonesia, Lao PDR, Cambodia, and Malaysia, and is emerging in a seventh—Myanmar (Figure 1) [16]. Considerable progress in control has been made in recent decades, largely through praziquantel-based preventive chemotherapy (i.e., periodic administration of praziquantel to entire at-risk populations without prior diagnosis). However, preventive chemotherapy alone is insufficient to break the transmission cycle. Lack of safe water, poor sanitation, inadequate hygiene practices, limited health education, and the presence of animal reservoirs are known barriers to the elimination of schistosomiasis from a region [17]. Old challenges remain while new ones emerge, requiring a comprehensive, multi-sectoral, and multifaceted approach across the region to control this disease, and to reach the desired goal of elimination by 2030 [17].

The aim of this review is to provide an overview of the current status of schistosomiasis in Asia, with a particular focus on endemic countries in the region and the unique challenges they face. Our review also aimed to identify current knowledge gaps and future research needs as the affected countries move toward the ultimate goal of control and elimination of this persistent and debilitating disease.

Figure 1. (A) Map of Southeast Asia showing the location of endemic areas for schistosomiasis, including a focus in central Myanmar. **(B)** Map of Myanmar highlighting the state of Rakhine.

2. Parasite Features

The genus *Schistosoma* is a group of parasitic blood flukes, or flatworms, of the class Trematoda. Unique amongst the trematode class, schistosomes have separate sexes as adults, whereas all other trematodes are hermaphrodites. The Asian schistosomes discussed in this review are considered zoonotic, unlike schistosome species occurring elsewhere, which are largely human-only excepting some hybrid forms in Africa [5,6,9,10,18], and cases of *S. mansoni* infecting non-human primates in Africa and the Caribbean, and rats in Guadeloupe and Brazil [7,8]. *S. japonicum* is the most cosmopolitan, with 46 mammalian definitive hosts identified thus far, whereas *S. mekongi* has been found in dogs, and *S. malayensis* in rodents, specifically *Rattus muelleri* [19–22] (Table 1). Pigs have been experimentally infected with *S. mekongi*, but, to date, no natural infections have been identified in these hosts [23]. Morphologically, the eggs and adults of the three species are very similar; the eggs are ovoid with a small 'nubby' lateral spine (Table 1) [24].

Table 1. A comparison of features of the three Asian schistosome species that can infect humans [4,25,26].

	Geographic Distribution	Animal Definitive Hosts	Intermediate Hosts	Eggs
S. japonicum	Indonesia, the Philippines, P. R. China	46 known mammalian hosts including water buffalo and cattle, dogs, pigs, and rodents	*Oncomelania* spp.	70–100 × 55–64 μm
S. mekongi	Cambodia, Lao PDR, Thailand	Dogs and pigs	*Neotricula* spp.	50–80 × 40–65 μm
S. malayensis	Malaysia	Rodents	*Robertsiella* spp.	53–90 × 33–62 μm

2.1. Lifecycle

The schistosome lifecycle is complex with an intermediate molluscan host, definitive host, and seven lifecycle stages involving both asexual and sexual reproductive phases (Figure 2). An in-depth understanding of social-ecological systems is required to grasp the spatial focality of schistosomiasis distributions [27].

2.1.1. S. japonicum

S. japonicum is the most prevalent of the Asian schistosomes. It is endemic in P.R. China, the Philippines, and small foci occur in Indonesia. There are 46 known mammalian definitive hosts of *S. japonicum*, although water buffalo and cattle have previously been shown to be the major reservoirs of infection [19,28,29]. *S. japonicum* was first identified in Japan in 1901, whereas the last new human case was recorded there in 1977. *S. japonicum* parasites in P.R. China and the Philippines have distinct genetic differences, resulting from geographic isolation over time. In general, the strain of *S. japonicum* in P.R. China is more virulent than the parasite in the Philippines; additional genetically variant geographic isolates are known to be present in both countries [30–32].

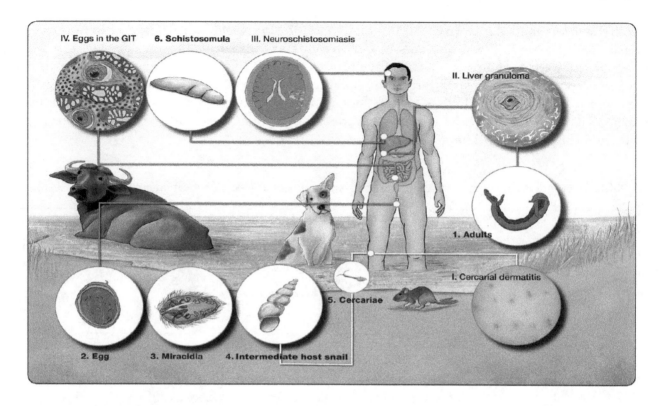

Figure 2. Schistosome lifecycle. Adult worms (**1**) reproduce sexually in the mesenteric veins surrounding the small intestine of the definitive mammalian host. Female worms deposit eggs (**2**), which are excreted in the feces. Upon contact with freshwater, the eggs hatch miracidia (**3**), which penetrate a snail intermediate host (**4**) and undergo asexual reproduction; this includes development of mother and daughter sporocysts, which produce cercariae (**5**). Cercariae exit the snail and swim around until they penetrate the skin of the mammalian definitive host, potentially causing cercarial dermatitis (**I**), shed their tail and become schistosomula (**6**). The schistosomula migrate through the body to the lungs before migrating and maturing to adult worms in the mesenteric veins. Chronic schistosomiasis occurs as the result of an immune reaction to the eggs resulting in granuloma formation in tissues where eggs are lodged. This most commonly occurs in the liver and spleen (**II**), which can result in hepatosplenomegaly and portal hypertension; in the walls of the intestine (**IV**) as eggs pass from the blood into the intestine; and less commonly in the brain (**III**), causing neuroschistosomiasis, characterized by a range of neurological symptoms. (Abbreviation: GIT, gastrointestinal tract).

2.1.2. *S. mekongi*

S. mekongi was first identified in 1857 [33]. While morphologically very similar to *S. japonicum*, *S. mekongi* differs in a number of characteristics that indicate it is a distinct species. These differences include the morphology of the testis and ovary in adult worms [34] and the eggs of *S. mekongi* are smaller and more round than those of *S. japonicum* (Table 1) [35]. Morphological differences in the miracidial stage of the two species are also apparent [35]. Early genetic studies showing electrophoretic enzyme variation indicated sequence differences between *S. japonicum* and *S. mekongi* [36].

Apart from human infection, *S. mekongi* has only been identified naturally in dogs, although there have been successful laboratory infections of pigs. The intermediate host of *S. mekongi* is *Neotricula aperta* (previously *Lithoglyphopsis aperta*), and studies have found *Oncomelania* spp. snails to be refractory to infection with *S. mekongi* [34].

2.1.3. *S. malayensis*

As with the other Asian schistosomes, *S. malayensis* is zoonotic and is primarily a parasite of the rodent *R. muelleri* (Table 1). *S. malayensis* is a sister species to *S. japonicum*, as is *S. mekongi*, to which it is more closely related [24]. Early studies identified the intermediate host of *S. malayensis* as *Robertsiella karporensis* [4,24].

2.2. Clinical Features

There are three clinical stages of schistosome infection. The initial early stage, a second 'silent' phase, also known as Katayama fever (or Katayama syndrome, named after the prefecture in Japan where it was first identified), and the third 'chronic' stage [1,37]. As the average life of an adult schistosome is 10 years and may be as long as 30 years, assuming no treatment, chronic infection can be lifelong [38,39].

The initial disease phase begins as a skin rash caused by an immune reaction to the penetrating cercariae (Figure 2, I). After penetrating the definitive host, the cercariae transform into schistosomula, which migrate to the lungs where they can cause pulmonary schistosomiasis, characterized as small nodules on a chest x-ray and a dry cough in the infected individual. After the lungs, the worms migrate to the venus plexus of the intestine, where they mature and pair up, reproducing sexually (Figure 2, 1). There is little immune response generated against the adult worms; thus, the second silent stage lasts for six to eight weeks post-infection when eggs begin to be produced. At this point, the acute Katayama fever begins, manifesting as fever, cough, rash, abdominal pain, nausea, diarrhea, and eosinophilia. Acute disease is more commonly seen in naïve persons, whereas chronic disease, the third phase, is more likely to occur in individuals resident in schistosome-endemic areas. Chronic disease occurs due to retention of eggs in the liver, spleen, and intestinal walls, and is the result of an immune response generated against the eggs, which causes granuloma formation in the various tissues (Figure 2, II and III). This can result in hepatosplenomegaly, portal hypertension, abdominal pain, and bloody diarrhea. A rarer manifestation of disease is neuroschistosomiasis (Figure 2, IV), which causes neurological symptoms, such as seizures and headaches, due to a granulomatous response against eggs in the brain, appearing as lesions on scans [40–43]. Infection in children is associated with growth stunting and intellectual disability and, in adults, with a reduced ability to work [44,45].

2.3. Diagnostics

A number of diagnostics are available, including coproparasitological examination (CopE), as well as molecular and immunological diagnostics. CopE methods rely on direct detection and visualization of parasite eggs in feces and include the Kato-Katz (KK) thick smear procedure, which is a mainstay of control programs due to the relative ease of performing the test at low cost, although it lacks sensitivity in low-intensity infections [46,47] and FLOTAC [48,49]. Other diagnostic approaches include formal-ethyl acetate sedimentation-digestion (FEA-SD) [50], the Danish Bilharziasis Laboratory (DBL) technique [51,52], and the miracidial hatching technique (MHT) [53,54], which also tests egg viability. Molecular diagnostics rely on detection of parasite DNA in clinical samples, often stool but also in urine, blood, and saliva, and include loop-mediated isothermal amplification (LAMP) [55–58], conventional polymerase chain reaction (cPCR) [59,60], real-time PCR (qPCR) [28,61–64], and digital droplet PCR (ddPCR) [65–67]. Immunological diagnostics rely on detection of circulating parasite antigens or antibodies generated against parasite antigens. Antibody detection might lack specificity and generally does not distinguish between past and current infections. A study by Cai et al., however, suggested that an immunological test combining two antigens (SjSAP4 + Sj23-LHD) may be useful for monitoring schistosomiasis control programs in the Philippines [68]. The main immunological methods include the enzyme-linked immunosorbent assay (ELISA) [69–72] and the rarely used circumoval precipitation test (COPT) [73,74]. Comprehensive reviews of the current diagnostic methods for schistosomiasis were provided by Weerakoon et al. and Utzinger et al. [58,75].

Sensitive and specific diagnostic procedures are required to monitor the success or failure of schistosomiasis control programs as well as to determine whether control efforts have resulted in elimination. However, the most sensitive diagnostics, involving molecular or immunological techniques, can be expensive and require specialized facilities and equipment and trained personnel to perform the procedures [57,76].

2.4. Treatment

Laboratory studies and clinical trials have shown that praziquantel, a pyrazinoisoquinoline derivative, is a safe and highly efficacious oral drug that is active against all schistosome species, although it is less active against juvenile schistosomes compared with adult worms and eggs [77–81]. The effective clinical praziquantel dosage regimen is 60 mg/kg orally in divided doses over one day (3 × 20 mg/kg doses 4-hourly, or 2 × 30 mg/kg either 4- or 6-hourly) for S. japonicum and S. mekongi [77,78]. Praziquantel is also the mainstay for preventive chemotherapy for morbidity control of schistosomiasis. In the Philippines, the efficacy of a single dose of 40 mg/kg vs. 60 mg/kg was compared; 40 mg/kg was effective and better tolerated and thus 40 mg/kg was adopted for preventive chemotherapy [82]. A single dose is beneficial for large-scale administration as it does not require follow up treatment as occurs with split doses. Despite the reliance on 40 mg/kg for preventive chemotherapy programs, two doses of 60 mg/kg separated by two weeks is recommended by the Philippine government in case finding, i.e., eggs identified in the stool [82].

Treatment with praziquantel does not prevent reinfection [83] and is therefore relatively ineffective at interrupting the transmission cycle. Praziquantel is principally aimed at reducing the prevalence and intensity of infection and to control morbidity over the longer term. Some concern has been expressed that praziquantel-resistant schistosomes may develop, most likely in Africa [84,85], and there is thus a pressing need to develop new anti-schistosomal drugs [86] and other non-pharmaceutical interventions.

3. Epidemiology

Due to the requirement of an intermediate host snail, schistosomiasis is a focal disease, occurring in areas where snail habitats and susceptible transmitting snails are present. This means that village-level prevalence can be very high, whereas country and province prevalence can be low. Demographic factors such as age, sex, and occupation are strongly associated with risk of infection [87,88]. Open defecation remains a common phenomenon in schistosomiasis-endemic countries and is strongly associated with transmission.

Snail habitats generally occur in still or slow moving water bodies such as streams, lakes, dammed waterways, and rice fields. The susceptible snails also have a preference for vegetation and snail control measures can include the removal of this vegetation.

3.1. Mammalian Definitive Hosts

Of the 46 known S. japonicum hosts, bovines, particularly water buffalo, are considered the most important for transmission due to the high levels of schistosome eggs they excrete into the environment [89,90] and their predisposition to natural infection. Epidemiological studies conducted in the Poyang and Dongting Lake regions of P.R. China revealed that water buffaloes account for up to 75–80% of S. japonicum infections, and hence are considered to be the most important reservoir hosts [29,89–91]. In mountainous and hilly endemic areas, water buffaloes are frequently used for ploughing rice fields and, while rodents have been considered to be important reservoirs, Van Dorssen et al. posited that this may not be the case owing to low levels of egg output and questions around egg viability [92,93]. Other potentially important animal reservoir hosts for S. japonicum in P.R. China include goats, pigs, and dogs due to their close contact with humans and water [93,94].

In Indonesia, 13 mammalian species, mostly wild animals (wild rodents, wild pigs, wild deer, wild celedus, and wild civet cats), but also cattle, water buffalo, horses, and dogs, have been identified as susceptible hosts for S. japonicum [95]. The prevalence of S. japonicum in water buffalo (known also as carabao) in the Philippines has been reported to be as high as 80%, particularly in agricultural areas, and water buffalo are thought to be a major reservoir [96]. In both the Philippines and P.R. China, there are fewer cattle than water buffalo/carabao. Cattle are more susceptible to infection than water buffalo, likely due to their more recent introduction into Asia compared with water buffalo, which have co-evolved with *S. japonicum* for much longer. Although studies suggested that water buffalo exhibit some age-acquired resistance to infection and self-cure [28,97,98], there is still uncertainty regarding this phenomenon [99].

Due to the close genetic relationship between *S. japonicum* and *S. mekongi*, bovines could act as reservoir hosts of *S. mekongi* but, to date, this has not been demonstrated. A range of potential animal hosts have been examined for *S. mekongi*, but currently dogs are the only animal species that have been confirmed as natural hosts of this species [22].

In regards to control, little has been done to target definitive hosts of *S. japonicum*, with the exception of P.R. China, which has practiced both chemotherapy of bovines and removal of the animals, facilitated by mechanization of agriculture (i.e., replacing water buffalo with tractors) [16,29,89,100,101]. Without targeting intermediate host snails, re-infection of humans after treatment can occur almost instantaneously. Animals can also contribute to rebounding infections in areas where humans have been declared free of schistosomiasis [102]. In Lao PDR, chemotherapy of dogs against *S. mekongi* has been highlighted as a priority. This has been proposed as part of community-led initiatives to eliminate schistosomiasis that combine deworming with water, sanitation, and hygiene interventions: community-led school, water, sanitation, and hygiene (CL-SWASH) activities [103].

Animal vaccines against schistosomiasis have been developed and used in controlled trials [104–107]. Whereas none of the currently developed vaccines provide 100% immune protection (0–80% worm reduction in mice and baboons [108]; 41–51% in water buffalo [109]), they do induce a significant reduction in adult worms, decreased egg output, and stunting of adults. A knockdown in adult worm fecundity alone can have a huge impact on transmission. Modeling has shown that an animal vaccine with 75% efficacy will be required to ensure long-term control of schistosomiasis [110].

3.2. Molluscan Intermediate Hosts

The intermediate snail hosts of *S. japonicum* are amphibious and belong to the genus *Oncomelania*, with species dependent on geographical location. Studies investigating the susceptibility of snails from different geographic locations to cercariae from disparate locations have produced mixed results, indicating a certain amount of genetic drift of the parasite [111,112]. Although Japan has successfully eliminated schistosomiasis, the requisite intermediate host snail species, *Oncomelania hupensis nosphora* and *O. hupensis formosana*, are still present [113].

In P.R. China, four sub-species of the intermediate host *Oncomelania hupensis* have been identified based on morphological and molecular characteristics [114–116], each with different growth rates, population genetics, and ecological niches. Control measures have been successful in reducing the populations of *O. h. guangxiensis* and *O. h. tangi* [13] leaving *O. h. hupensis* and *O. h. robertsoni* as the dominant sub-species [114]. Of these, *O. h. hupensis* is the most widely distributed [114]. Few studies have reported *S. japonicum* infection rates in *Oncomelania* snails in endemic regions of P.R. China in the last decade. One study in the marshland regions along the Yangtze River [114] examined more than 70,000 snails over a 15-year period (2001–2015) and found an overall prevalence of 0.05% with no new infections since 2007 [117]. An earlier study reported a decline from 0.88% in 2009 to zero in 2012 in Jiangling county, Hubei province [118]. According to a 2017 WHO meeting report on Asian schistosomiasis, an active sentinel surveillance program, conducted in 2016 in areas where transmission was considered interrupted or under control, also failed to identify infected snails [119]. However, the same report indicated that in two other studies undertaken in 2012 and 2017, in four and seven provinces, respectively, infected snails were found based on LAMP analysis, but no infection was recorded by microscopy, although actual infection rates for the LAMP analysis were not provided [119]. As snail infection rates continue to decline, consistent and highly sensitive diagnostic tests, such as LAMP, will be required to provide accurate information [75,120].

In the Philippines, the sole intermediate host snail for *S. japonicum* is *O. h. quadrasi*. It is amphibious but prefers an aquatic environment, such as wet soil surfaces, swamps, rice fields, ponds, and stream banks, thus making chemical snail control difficult due to the risk of contaminating the water or food source [17]. The current status of S. japonicum infection in the snail intermediate hosts in the Philippines is poorly understood. One study, conducted in Samar province, found a mean infection rate of 1.09% across 147 sites with higher infection among snails located in irrigated compared to rain-fed villages [121]. More recent data from 2013 to 2015 indicate infection rates of less than 2% in most endemic provinces, although Northern Samar was found to have a prevalence of above 12% [76].

In Indonesia, the intermediate snail host of S. japonicum is O. h. lindoensis, which is located focally around Lake Lindu. In 2011, the prevalence of infected O. h. lindoensis snails in Lindu Valley was 3.6% and 4.0% in Napu Valley, although the prevalence has fluctuated between 0 and 13.4% in Napu Valley and between 0% and 9.1% in Lindu Valley since 2005 [95]. Prevalence of infected snails in Bada Valley appears to be much lower, with a survey conducted in 2010 identifying a prevalence of only 1% (3 among 299 snails sampled) [122].

The intermediate hosts of S. mekongi are Neotricula spp., and endemic areas are closely associated with the Mekong Delta where these snails occur. The prevalence of infected snails in Lao PDR was quite low, 0.01% on the Mekong Islands [123] and 0.22% in Khong District, although the snail density was quite high [124]. Neotricula aperta snail density in Thailand decreased between 2005 and 2011 in the downstream area of the Nam Theun 2 hydroelectric dam, which began operation in 2010 [125]. A similar decrease in Oncomelania snails in low-land areas was initially seen in P.R. China after the building of the Three Gorges Dam [126]. However, snail density began to increase in 2011 after initially decreasing in the years immediately after completion of the dam in 2003. A similar trend may eventually be seen in Thailand with the Nam Theun 2 Dam.

Control of intermediate host snails is an important aspect of schistosomiasis control programs, particularly as the stage of the lifecycle occurring in snails is asexual and involves an exponential increase in parasite numbers. Snail control measures previously implemented in Asia have involved environmental modification and chemical mollusciciding. The snails live in vegetation around rivers and lakes and removal of this vegetation can lead to removal of the snails themselves. This method was used with great success in Japan in combination with mollusciciding. In Japan, the most common method of environmental modification was the use of concreting canals where the snails lived [113]. This method is more difficult to implement in areas where the snail habitats are rice fields or marshland. Early reports from Mindanao in the Philippines showed that the method of farming (weeding and ploughing) practiced in Mindanao reduced snail habitat on the rice fields, and thus snails were primarily found in swampland, at least when intensive farming was practiced [127]. Changing land use in Japan from rice crops to either housing or fruit trees, which did not require flood irrigation and thus no longer provided snail habitats, was an important feature for control.

Mollusciciding has also been used in P.R. China, Indonesia, and the Philippines, although to a limited degree in the latter two countries. Environmental contamination with chemical molluscicides is an important issue, and a number of previously used compounds have been abandoned due to these concerns and as a result of the damage they cause to the environment. In the schistosomiasis foci in Indonesia, the snail habitats occur close to the Lore Lindu National Park, which precludes the use of molluscicides [128] and environmental modification. Early molluscicides included lime, which proved inefficient, calcium cyanamide, and, later, sodium pentachlorohenate (Na-PCP), which was eventually stopped in all countries due to environmental toxicity [129]. In P.R. China, the molluscicide of choice has been niclosamide, used in two different formulations: (1) a 50% niclosamide ethanolamine salt wettable powder and (2) a 4% niclosamide ethanolamine powder [106,130]. Both formulations resulted in substantial, but not 100%, killing of snails, which meant that mollusciciding needed to be performed more than once a year.

Neotricula spp., the intermediate host snails of S. mekongi, exhibit a different ecological niche than those transmitting S. japonicum in that, rather than being present in marshlands and rice fields, these snails are primarily found in shallow areas of rivers (particularly the Mekong River) and tributaries. Thus, snail control for S. mekongi has largely been deemed infeasible [17], although ecological management of snail habitats upstream of human habitation, as occurs in P.R. China, should be explored. Instead, preventive chemotherapy, along with improved WASH is practiced. Lao PDR has previously used niclosamide for snail control, although this did not significantly impact the numbers of snails in the treatment areas [124].

3.3. Environment

The majority of environmental factors associated with *S. japonicum* transmission are related to distance to a snail habitat or those that influence snail habitats, such as the building of dams. The majority of *S. japonicum*-endemic zones are within 1 km of water bodies such as rivers, lakes, or wetlands [131,132]. Environmental factors that influence snail habitat include land cover, particularly the presence of flooded agricultural land [133,134], seasonal land surface temperature (LST), elevation, and rainfall [131].

In P.R. China, endemic areas occupy three different geographical landscapes: (1) marshland and lake areas, (2) mountainous and hilly areas, and (3) water network areas. Of these, marshland and lake areas are characteristic of the major endemic foci for *S. japonicum*, and might account for 95% of the snail habitats [17,87]. *Oncomelania* snails survive best at areas of low elevation—one of the potential environmental factors associated with high prevalence of snails in marshy areas. A study on snail habitats in mountainous and hilly areas identified a maximum elevation of 2300 m above sea level for snail survival [131]. The same study identified an ideal LST of $\geq$22.7 °C and a normalized difference vegetation index (NDVI) of $\geq$0.446 in the mountainous areas. Distance from the nearest stream was also important, as the *Oncomelania* snails are amphibious; yet, require water to survive. A distance of $\leq$1000 m from the nearest stream was found to be ideal for snail habitats [131].

As the marshy and lake areas are categorized by the presence of water bodies, more areas are available for the snails to exist. The area of these landscapes, which cover the four provinces of Hunan, Jiangxi, Anhui, and Hubei, is vast, complicating snail control in these locations [135]. Mountainous and hilly areas, located primarily in the western part of P.R. China in the provinces of Yunnan and Sichuan [131], account for approximately 5% of the remaining snail habitats [17]. The complex environmental conditions present in these areas make it difficult to control snail populations [131]. The third type of landscape are water network areas, mainly located around the Yangtze River, which account for <1% of snail habitats in endemic areas of P.R. China [17].

Local epidemic outbreaks and the geographic distribution of snail hosts are heavily influenced by flooding events caused by the Yangtze River as they facilitate snail dispersion to new localities such as rivers, lakes, and wetlands [136,137]. Large-scale water development projects [138], particularly the aforementioned Three Gorges Dam and the South-North Water Diversion project (SNWD), also influence the transmission and geographic distribution of schistosomiasis [139,140]. The SNWD plans to divert water from the Yangtze River to the North [141]. Climate prediction models have indicated that this project may result in the expansion of viable snail habitats for the main snail intermediate host *O. h. hupensis* as well as *O. h. robertsioni* and *O. h. guangxiensis* [141]. The Three Gorges Dam, begun in 2003 and completed in 2012, was built to decrease flooding events as well as to generate power. As a consequence, it has changed the ecology of the surrounding area and impacted the habitat of *Oncomelania* spp. snails. The decrease in flooding events has decreased the density of snails in some areas, although in others, the density appears unchanged, or is on the increase [126].

In the Philippines, more than 3000 bodies of water are thought to be infested with snails susceptible to *S. japonicum* infection: 80% in Mindanao, 18% in Visayas, and 2% in Luzon [76]. Endemic regions have no distinct dry season and are predominantly comprised of rice fields, where contact between humans and snails is maximized [11,82]. Environmental factors, such as close proximity to large perennial water bodies (PWB), LST, NDVI, and precipitation, influence *S. japonicum* infection prevalence differently in the three main regions of the Philippines [87]. As is the case in P.R. China, the distance from water is an important factor for snail habitats, with the prevalence of schistosomiasis in humans decreasing with distance to PWB [87]. Some differences exist between the three regions, with increased distance to PWB associated with decreased prevalence in Luzon and the Visayas, but not Mindanao, whereas LST increase only significantly associated with decreased prevalence in Luzon. Similarly increased precipitation was associated with higher prevalence in the Visayas but decreased prevalence in Mindanao [87]. A confounding factor may be the differences in average socioeconomic status between the three areas: people in Luzon tend to have higher socioeconomic status compared to schistosomiasis-endemic areas of the Visayas and Mindanao. Natural habitats of *O. h. quadrasi* include flood plains, forests, and swamps, whereas man-made habitats resulting from agricultural development are thought to be important habitats (e.g., drainage channels, roadside ditches, small canals, and drainage canals of irrigation works). These snails are generally found on banks but also occur in shallow water (depth <20 cm) [121]. *O. h. quadrasi* snails prefer areas shaded by vegetation where the temperature is relatively stable and cool.

Endemic regions of Indonesia are located in marshland areas around Lake Lindu and Napu and Bada valleys. Prevalence of *S. japonicum* in snails from this area ranged from 0 to 13.4% in the Lindu Valley and 0 to 9.1% in the Napu Valley, although human prevalence remained <1% as of 2006 [128].

S. mekongi transmission occurs in the Mekong Delta. In Khong and Mounlapamok districts in Lao PDR, 202 villages are situated along the Mekong River with 114 currently or previously endemic for schistosomiasis. The only villages with zero prevalence for *S. mekongi* are in parts of the river where the riverbed is sandy, which is not conducive to the intermediate host snail, or those villages that are more than 6 km away from the river [142].

Limited information is available regarding risk factors and snail intermediate hosts in Myanmar [16]. The current areas where schistosomiasis occurs are around Lake Inlay in Shan State, although a recent outbreak has occurred in Rakhine State on the Coast of the Bay of Bengal [143]. The wet season runs from May to October.

3.4. Transmission and Control

In P.R. China, transmission usually occurs across two distinct seasons [17], coinciding with the natural annual flooding events in the Yangtze River: firstly in April to June/July when flooding is at its peak, and secondly after the waters subside in September/October with transmission continuing until November [140]. Although environmental factors heavily influence the snail intermediate hosts, demographic factors and the presence of host reservoirs play a more significant role in human transmission of *S. japonicum*. Infection with *S. japonicum* is strongly associated with age, sex, and occupational exposure. Males aged 40 years and above who engage in fishing, farming, and herding are at greatest risk of infection [144]. Defecation into lake waters or marshlands by fishermen and grazing water buffalo facilitate the continuance of transmission.

In the Philippines, there is no distinct dry season on the main endemic islands of Leyte and Samar and the province of Mindanao. Hence, transmission is not as variable by season as in P.R. China and occurs all year round [82]. The most common crop in these endemic areas is rice, which provides contact between snails that live in the rice paddies, swamps, and streams, whereas water buffalo and cattle are used to work on the fields (Figure 3). In addition to farming, washing, and recreational use of rivers are associated with higher risk of infection (Figure 4).

Figure 3. Water buffalo (carabao) in the Philippines are tethered in rivers, rice fields, and wallows—the same areas where the intermediate snail host for *S. japonicum* is also found. (Images from the Philippines, captured by C.A.G.).

Figure 4. Washing and recreational uses of waterways are risk factors for contracting schistosomiasis. (Image from the Philippines, captured by C.A.G.).

Whereas 13 species of mammalian hosts have been identified in Indonesia, limited research has been undertaken on their involvement in transmission. Rodents of the genus *Rattus* have been suggested as the primary source of transmission, with a peak prevalence of 20% found in one endemic village [128]. Primary species thought to be involved in transmission are *R. exulans*, *R. hoffmani*, *R. chysocomus rallus*, *R. marmosurus*, and *R. celebensis* [128]. Reservations around the role that rodents can play in transmission were addressed earlier [92,93]. As in P.R. China, Indonesia experiences wet and dry seasons; hence, it is likely that schistosome transmission is also seasonal there, with increased transmission occurring in the wet season (November–March).

The transmission season for *S. mekongi* is matched with the lifecycle of the snail. During times of high water levels (2–3 m), the majority of available snails are young, while in times of low water (April–May; 10–60 mm), the snails have matured to adults capable of carrying the infection.

Peak transmission of *S. mekongi* in Cambodia occurs between February and April coinciding with peak water use for fishing [17]; whereas in Lao PDR, the main transmission season occurs in April and May.

In Malaysia, the wet season differs between the southwest where the monsoon season is May–October, and the northeast where the monsoon season runs from November to March, and the typhoon season occurs from April to November. It is therefore difficult in the absence of yearly surveys to pinpoint when transmission in Malaysia might peak, but it is certainly influenced by rainfall brought by the monsoons and typhoons.

Preventive chemotherapy with praziquantel has been the mainstay of schistosomiasis morbidity control and, in addition to targeting mammalian and snail hosts mentioned earlier, efforts to control transmission have also included programs aimed at improving WASH and health education. Until relatively recently, the role of WASH in schistosomiasis control was limited [145–148], despite the strong association of the disease with poverty and poor sanitation. In 2012, the World Health Assembly (WHA) encouraged the incorporation of WASH into control and elimination strategies [149]. Due to the transmission dynamics of schistosomiasis, WASH primarily limits environmental contamination with schistosome eggs and reduces human contact with potentially infested waters [150]. Improvements in sanitation and access to clean water have been shown to reduce the risk of schistosome infection [151], and have the added benefit of reducing infection with other parasites such as soil-transmitted helminths [146]. The impact of WASH is, however, dependent on the setting [151]. For example, access to clean water is not considered to play a significant role in endemic areas where schistosome infections are attributed to occupational or recreational contact with water as opposed to water used for drinking or for everyday activities (e.g., laundry and bathing) [151]. Traditional WASH practices, such as handwashing, have little impact on schistosome infection as the parasite eggs excreted in stools are not infective to human or animal hosts. However, water use practices involving rivers, such as bathing and washing clothes, will increase risk of contact with the infectious cercariae. Hence, much of the WASH emphasis to date has focused on sanitation and sanitary behavior. A number of programs focusing on improving access to clean water and improved sanitation outside of schistosomiasis control are ongoing throughout schistosomiasis-endemic countries in Asia [152–157].

Health education is important not only for educating the public on risk reduction measures and changing behavior, but has also been found to facilitate diagnosis, surveillance, and treatment [157]. Through health education activities and water contact studies, many high-risk behaviors and at-risk populations have been identified [158]. This has enabled health messages to be tailored to specific groups, such as school-age children swimming in freshwater and farmers and fishermen, and has largely been aimed at methods of avoiding water contact and self-protection [158]. However, it can be difficult to change behavior in some groups, such as fishermen or farmers, due to the nature of their occupations [158]. The support of local and national governments, through implementing infrastructure such as public toilets and using sanitary containers for stool on fishing boats, is therefore important in these situations [117,159]. The vehicles used for health education messages are many-fold and include audio-visual (radio, television, film, drama, traditional opera, and exhibits), print media (poems, slogans, posters, magazines, and newspaper), and other daily articles such as printed shirts, towels, fans, and umbrellas, among others [158]. Health information can also be passively disseminated through the community by students, teachers, village leaders, and parents [158]. Although health education is considered an important component of an integrated control program for schistosomiasis [160–163], it needs to be thoroughly planned, targeted, trialed, and evaluated prior to implementation [158], and needs to be sustained over a long period of time in order to maximize effectiveness [164]. To date, health education has been a major focus in P.R. China. Elsewhere, health education has generally been combined with preventive chemotherapy and has played a limited role in schistosomiasis control and elimination programs [82,165].

Research is ongoing for the development of schistosomiasis vaccines targeting humans and, unlike the African schistosomes, the zoonotic nature of the Asian schistosomes allow for the targeting of animal hosts. With bovines, particularly water buffalo/carabao confirmed as the major reservoirs of

S. japonicum, there is the rationale for the development and deployment of a transmission-blocking anti-*S. japonicum* vaccine targeting bovines [29,91,166,167]. The SjCTPI-Hsp70 vaccine is one of the most efficacious to date with an experimental efficacy of ~52% [101] and cluster-randomized controlled trials are currently being finalized to determine efficacy in natural settings. Vaccines may be the key for long-term sustainable control and elimination of schistosomiasis but research needs to be ongoing [167].

4. Current and Historical Status of Schistosomiasis in Asia

Notably, most prevalence estimates reported are based on microscopic detection of schistosome eggs in stool samples, usually using the KK thick smear technique [87,168,169]. However, numerous studies have demonstrated significantly higher prevalence when molecular detection methods have been applied on the same set of samples, with differences of up to 70% reported [28,60,63,170]. Prevalence is also largely influenced by the size of the sampled population. This is particularly relevant to the Philippines and Indonesia where funds are often limited, thus restricting the number of personnel available to interview and process collected samples. Another confounding factor, which is also common in P.R. China, is a fall in participation rates in many endemic areas, often referred to as treatment fatigue. Some communities in highly endemic areas have been participating in surveys for decades; hence, it is not surprising that these villagers have tired of the routine. In areas where prevalence has dropped significantly, the disease is no longer seen as a priority. Based on these factors, it is conceivable that the prevalence of schistosomiasis is considerably underestimated.

4.1. S. japonicum

The first reports of *S. japonicum* in P.R. China and the Philippines occurred around the same time in the early 1900s [171,172] and the epidemiology of the disease is similar in the two countries. The presence of the disease in Indonesia was first reported about three decades later, with an autochthonous infection in a 35-year-old male suffering from chronic schistosomiasis resulting in his death in 1937 [128].

4.1.1. Japan

As indicated in the species name, *S. japonicum* was once found in Japan, the last reported human case was in 1977, and elimination of schistosomiasis was declared in 1996 [17]. There were a number of endemic areas in Japan pre-elimination, including Kofu basin, Fukuoka, and Saga prefectures, which appeared to have had the highest prevalence [173]. Due to a successful control program, transmission of the parasite no longer occurs there, although the requisite intermediate host snail species, *Oncomelania nosphora*, is still present [113]. In addition to the control initiatives implemented, modernization and socioeconomic development had a large impact on elimination of this parasite in Japan. Elimination of schistosomiasis in Japan occurred pre-praziquantel and the available drug at the time, stibnal, caused severe adverse events, which resulted in low treatment compliance. Thus, most control efforts focused on targetting the snail intermediate hosts and preventing transmission to humans.

Environmental modification in the form of concreting canals, where the *Oncomelania* snails bred, began in 1938 and was the primary method used [17]. In addition, the Japanese government purchased and buried snails from people in the endemic areas. Mollusciciding using lime, which proved to be inefficient; calcium cyanamide, which proved to be more efficient; and later Na-PCP were trialed. The use of Na-PCP was eventually stopped after 13 years due to its environmental toxicity. Hot water and flamethrowers were also used to kill snails, and proved effective in small areas. In addition, geese and firefly larvae were released into endemic fields to eat snails, although these measures proved unsuccessful [129]. Land use was changed, with increased urbanization meaning that many paddy fields were converted to housing, and in other areas, crops changed from rice to fruit trees; this precluded the use of flood watering and thus no longer provided areas for snail breeding [17]. Education of farmers to prevent the use of "night soil" as fertilizer was also performed, thus limiting environmental contamination with schistosome eggs from human feces. Bovines were replaced with horses, which can act as reservoir hosts but are less efficient transmitters, and other potential reservoirs such as wild populations of mice and dogs were controlled.

4.1.2. P.R. China

In P.R. China, *S. japonicum* is predominantly found in areas along the middle and upper reaches of the Yangtze River Valley in the southern part of the country where the climate and environment are highly suitable for the propagation of *Oncomelania* snails. Endemic regions are concentrated in the lake regions and in the mountainous region in the western part of the country [131]. Until relatively recently, *S. japonicum* was endemic in 12 provinces, but due to political will and sustained efforts, primarily through snail control and preventive chemotherapy, five provinces have achieved transmission interruption. Of the remaining seven provinces, four (Sichuan, Yunnan, Jiangsu, and Hubei) achieved transmission control (prevalence <5% in humans and animals) by 2014, whereas Anhui, Jiangxi, and Hunan are still in the infection control stage (prevalence <1% in humans and animals) [174,175]. In 2012, an estimated 800,000 people were infected and 65 million people considered at risk [24]. In 2016, the number of reported cases had dropped considerably and was just over 77,000 [17]. Current human prevalence in most endemic villages is between 1% and 3% but among the high-risk population, such as those who have extensive contact with water, infection levels may still exceed 10% [17].

Control approaches in P.R. China have been extensive due to the strong commitment by the national government. Funds from a 10-year World Bank Loan Project (WBLP) implemented in the 1990s [176] were put toward control and prevention strategies for schistosomiasis, including preventive chemotherapy, snail control, and WASH interventions. The mainstay of schistosomiasis control is preventive chemotherapy with praziquantel. In P.R. China, preventive chemotherapy is primarily targeted at fishermen and boat people living within half a kilometer of schistosomiasis-infested water bodies and is administered biannually. Treatment in other high-risk populations is selective, based on the extent of water contact [16]. P.R. China is the only endemic country that also practices mass drug administration for bovines, which are treated annually. The government is replacing animals used for farming with tractors and is removing bovines [16,89,100]. Mollusciciding occurs annually and usually coincides with the onset of the transmission seasons. Ecological methods of snail control have been used in P.R. China, such as changing farming practices, submerging snail habitats, and placing black plastic film over banks post-mollusciciding [17]. P.R. China's efforts to improve WASH began during the third phase of their national schistosomiasis control program (initiated in 2004), which focused on an integrated approach to control transmission [177]. WASH interventions mainly center on fishermen and boatmen [178] in the Poyang and Donting Lake regions and include supplying tap water and stool containers and building latrines close to boat anchoring points [159,179]. Health education has been an integral component of P.R. China's schistosomiasis control program since its inception in the 1950s [164].

4.1.3. Philippines

In the Philippines, *S. japonicum* is distributed throughout all three major island groups (Luzon, Mindanao, and Visayas), although the majority of cases occur in Mindanao and the Visayas [87,180] (Figure 1). Schistosomiasis is currently endemic in 28 of the country's 80 provinces, mostly in Mindanao, with more than 12 million people estimated to be at risk and 2.5 million directly exposed [76]. Distribution of *S. japonicum* is more widespread in the Visayas compared to Luzon and Mindanao, where it is more focal [87]. Among endemic provinces, 10 are considered highly endemic (prevalence >5%), six moderately (1–4.9%), and 12 low or close to elimination levels (<1%) [76]. Prevalence studies conducted since 2000 indicate infection levels vary based on location. In 2000, Acosta et al. reported a prevalence of 60% in adolescent and young adults (aged 15–30 years) in three villages in Leyte [181]. In 2005, a cross-sectional survey in Western Samar Province reported a prevalence range of 0.7% to 47% [182], which is similar to that reported by Ross et al. in 2012 from Northern Samar [96].

A nationwide prevalence study in 2015 identified infection levels >5% in one province, 1–5% in 12 provinces, and less than 1% in 14 provinces [87]. However, a diagnostic study conducted in 2014 in Northern Samar compared the prevalence determined using the gold standard KK method against qPCR results and found a discrepancy of nearly 70% (23% for KK vs. 90% for qPCR) [64], demonstrating the need for more sensitive diagnostic methods to determine true prevalence.

The Philippines experienced a period of success in controlling schistosomiasis after the launch of the Philippines Health Development Project (PHDP) in 1991, which was financially backed by a World Bank loan. The focus shifted to active case finding and mass drug administration with praziquantel; WASH interventions and snail control were included as additional measures. Drug coverage of the target population was reported to be 100% during the 1990s [76]. However, the prevalence of *S. japonicum* increased after the cessation of the program due to a lack of financial support; inadequate resources from the government also led to a diminished capacity to control schistosomiasis in the Philippines compared to P.R. China, where the government has strongly supported control efforts for over 50 years [17,183,184]. Due to insufficient funds to support the continuation of mass examination and treatment of at-risk populations, the Department of Health in the Philippines moved to targeting only high-prevalence endemic areas with mass drug administration [17,183].

In the Philippines, niclosamide has been banned for use in snail control under the Clean Water Act [17]. So, while mollusciciding has been performed in the past, special exemption would be needed for future use. A combination of methods employed in Japan was trialed on Bohol Island in the Philippines, focusing on grass cutting in swamps, followed by mollusciciding. Land reformation from swamps to rice fields, combined with mass drug administration, was effective in reducing prevalence to less than 1% [17]. In general, snail control measures successfully used in P.R. China have not been applicable to the Philippines due to differences in ecology and habitat of the local intermediate host snails [11]. Historically, environmental modification has been used in the Philippines to decrease snail habitats [127,185,186]. This rarely occurs now, and the mainstay of control in the Philippines is preventive chemotherapy with praziquantel [187]; yet, there is low compliance in taking the drug due to a variety of reasons, such as poor community engagement and fear of adverse events, which reduces the effectiveness of this intervention [82,188–191]. A cross-sectional survey undertaken in 2015 in Northern Samar, an area with high prevalence of schistosomiasis, reported treatment coverage of only 27% [28,190].

The success of P.R. China's efforts since after the launch of the WBLP compared to the Philippines is largely attributable to the Chinese targeting both human and animals for chemotherapy as opposed to humans only in the Philippines, which ultimately proved to be far less effective [183]. The Philippines is currently undertaking measures to address the issue of *S. japonicum* infection in animals by strengthening veterinary health teams in priority areas through capacity building and operational research and moving toward implementation of WASH programs, as outlined during the 17th Meeting of the Regional Program Review Group on Neglected Tropical Diseases in the Western Pacific (175). These efforts are laudable and it can be anticipated that WASH will feature more prominently in the Philippines than in the past [187]. Lessons from early efforts (before the advent and wide use of praziquantel) to improve sanitation should be considered [82,96].

4.1.4. Indonesia

In contrast to P.R. China and the Philippines, schistosomiasis in Indonesia is endemic in three comparatively small, isolated highland regions surrounding Lore Lindu National Park in central Sulawesi. These areas include marshes around Lake Lindu, particularly in the villages of Anca, Langko, Tomado, and Puro'o; Napu Valley [11] located 30–50 km southeast of Lake Lindu; and the more recently identified focus of Bada Valley [95]. Although the prevalence of *S. japonicum* has fluctuated over the last decade, prevalence tends to be higher in Napu Valley and overall appears to demonstrate an upward trend. Up to 2005, control efforts had decreased prevalence from 37% to 1% or less in Napu and Lindu valleys, but in the period from 2008 to 2011, prevalence varied between 0.3%

and 4.8% in Napu and 0.8% to 3.2% in Lindu [95]. When Badu was first recognized as a new endemic area in 2008, prevalence was 0.5%, which later increased to 5.9% in 2010 [122].

Schistosomiasis control strategies set by the National Objectives for Health (NOH) directive for 2011–2016 varied based on the degree of endemicity, but overall took a multifaceted approach. Control objectives included mass drug administration coverage of 85% of the entire population in high endemic areas, active selective treatment in moderate endemic areas, and passive selective treatment in low endemic areas. Preventive chemotherapy has been supplemented with strategies that also focused on treating domestic animals, snail control, health education, improving water, and sanitation, and monitoring and evaluation and capacity building [76] in an effort to meet the 2020 elimination goal set by the Indonesian Ministry of Health [192]. Although Indonesia has made great strides in reducing the prevalence of schistosomiasis, control and prevention efforts have been inhibited by a lack of coordination and collaboration between the Ministry of Health and other ministries, as well as insufficient financial and human resources. The lack of funds dedicated to surveillance and control by the Ministry of Health may, in part, be due to the limited area and population affected by the disease or as a result of the decentralized and autonomous government system in Indonesia [193].

4.1.5. Myanmar

Myanmar has been previously thought to be non-endemic for schistosomiasis, although there have been some historical unconfirmed reports of the presence of both *S. japonicum* and *S. mekongi* [16]. Recent studies have indicated that schistosomiasis has been emerging/re-emerging around Lake Inlay in central Myanmar [194]. Serological analysis of patient samples between 2012 and 2013 identified a prevalence of 23.8% ($n = 315$), whereas 302 cases were identified between 2016 and 2018 [16,195]. The WHO has been involved in supporting efforts to diagnose and treat infections in Myanmar, providing praziquantel, KK thick smear equipment, and urine tests [194]. Recently, molecular diagnostics determined a *S. mekongi* prevalence of 3.9% ($n = 205$) in the Bago Region of Myanmar [196,197].

A recent schistosomiasis outbreak occurred in Rakhine State with >400 confirmed cases and >800 suspected cases as of August 2018 [143]. Rakhine is the site of unrest due to political strife with Rohingya refugees and is also one of the poorest in terms of socioeconomic status in Myanmar, with a high number of households without access to clean water and proper sanitation [198]. This outbreak is occurring outside the area where schistosomiasis has previously been identified (Figure 1B). A technical team from the WHO and Myanmar Health and Sports Ministry have been to the area and suggested a special control team to carry out activities aimed at treating and preventing infection including health education in schools, diagnostics, treatment, and snail mapping [143]. The schistosome and snail species responsible for this current outbreak have not yet been identified.

It is not immediately clear from published reports if *S. japonicum* has been definitively diagnosed in Myanmar. Until the status of schistosomiasis is further clarified, ideally by molecular methods with which *S. mekongi* has already been confirmed, we rely on early reports that suggest both species are present [196,197].

4.2. S. mekongi

4.2.1. Cambodia

The first case of schistosomiasis occurring in Cambodia was identified in 1968 in Eastern Cambodia and was seemingly confined to Vietnamese fishermen living in raft houses. Prevalence among children was higher (14–22%) than in adults (7–10%) [199]. At present, there are an estimated 80,000 people at risk of infection in Cambodia [142].

Control of schistosomiasis in Cambodia has been impacted by political unrest and upheaval through the 1970s and 1980s [200]. It was not until 1993 that control programs targeting schistosomiasis commenced. At the onset of the control program, drug compliance was low due to the treatment not being free. Subsequently, mass drug administration was provided free of charge [200]. This approach has been the mainstay of control in Cambodia for the last 20 years and, in 2016, the schistosome prevalence determined by the KK thick smear technique was 0%. In addition to preventive chemotherapy, CL-WASH programs were implemented in endemic villages in 2016. Facilitators were initially trained in CL-WASH, who then helped lead community-based training when education on schistosomiasis transmission was provided and linked to sanitation and hygiene habitats. In each community, CL-WASH teams, composed of volunteers from each community as well as a facilitator, conducted surveys on village households to determine the provision of sanitation and the level of malnutrition [201]. Initial surveys found that >60% of households did not have toilets and many still practiced open defecation. Survey results were mapped and presented to the community members who discussed how their behaviors led to schistosome infection (and other parasitic worm and intestinal protozoa infections) and how infection could be prevented with the development and implementation of CL-WASH plans. These plans included the building and use of latrines in villages [201]. Elimination was planned for 2017, although this was reliant on more sensitive diagnostic tools being employed, an increase in sentinel site surveillance, and increased use of CL-WASH in endemic areas [202].

4.2.2. Thailand

The first case of *S. mekongi*, described as a *S. japonicum*-like infection, was reported in 1950 in Thailand [199]. This 'patient zero' was a Thai native and thus it is likely this was an autochthonous case. Further investigations identified an endemic region and susceptible intermediate host snail in southern Thailand. In 1964, further cases were identified in northern Thailand. Animals including water buffalo, cattle, dogs, cats, pigs, and rats were also surveyed in the endemic areas but none were positive at that time [199]. Thailand is currently in transmission interruption, waiting on investigation and ratification by the WHO [203].

4.2.3. Lao PDR

Lao PDR followed Thailand in the identification of *S. mekongi* in 1957 in a patient who had been living in Paris for nine years, but had spent the first nine years of life in Lao PDR [34,199]. This observation indicated that the adult worms can live for many years. The patient was admitted with what was thought to be cirrhosis of the liver; a liver biopsy revealed the presence of a *S. japonicum*-like egg. It was not until 1966 that a second case was identified in Lao PDR and, in 1969, an epidemiological survey determined a prevalence of 14.4% ($n = 72$) on Khong Island. As with *S. japonicum*, hepatosplenomegaly was associated with infection [34,199,204]. On Khong Island, the parasite was first found in animals, specifically in a dog [34].

A study examining the prevalence of a range of parasites in islands of the Mekong in Lao PDR performed in 2011 determined a prevalence of 22.2% ($n = 994$) in humans and 14.7% ($n = 68$) in dogs for *S. mekongi* [123]. The infected snail prevalence was very low with 0.01% ($n = 29,583$) of collected snails being positive [123]. More recent cases have been identified in returning travelers who visited these historically endemic areas, including a Belgian visitor to Khong Island in 2013 and a French woman who was exposed to freshwater habitats in southern Lao PDR [205,206]. These cases indicate that transmission is ongoing.

Mass drug administration in Lao PDR was first carried out yearly from 1989 to 1998. In the first year of the program, only selective chemotherapy was practiced but this was expanded in subsequent years [200]. Before the onset of this preventive chemotherapy-based program, there were an estimated 11,000 cases with a further 60,000 deemed to be at risk of infection. By 1999, the prevalence was significantly reduced, but after cessation of yearly mass drug administration, the prevalence rebounded to pre-intervention levels. Hence, mass drug administration was recommenced in 2007 with financial support from WHO [202]. CL-WASH was implemented in 10 villages in 2016, to be expanded to all endemic villages by 2020 [202].

4.2.4. Myanmar

See Section 4.1.5. for Myanmar under *S. japonicum*.

4.3. *S. malayensis*

Malaysia

Schistosomiasis resembling *S. japonicum* was first identified in Malaysia in 1973 during an autopsy [199]. Previous schistosome infections identified in Malaysia were *S. japonicum* in foreign nationals from P.R. China and Singapore [207]. A review of autopsy materials between 1967 and 1975 uncovered a further nine cases of *S. japonicum*-malaysia (later classified as *S. malayensis* in 1988) [199,207]. No animal infections, snail hosts, or new human cases in the areas that the infected deceased came from could be identified [199]. The strain that caused schistosomiasis in these cases was thought to be different from the Mekong schistosome [199], and likely represents the first case of *S. malayensis*.

Until 1978, all cases of *S. malayensis* were identified in patients who were deceased with schistosomiasis identified in autopsies, although not as the reported cause of death [207,208]. In general, cases of *S. malayensis* have been aboriginal Malaysians (Orang Asli) living in rural areas and patients were either previously or concurrently co-infected with other infectious diseases. The first case identified in a living patient occurred in Selangor State and the patient presented with hepatosplenomegaly [207,208].

In the meantime, *S. malayensis* has only been recorded sporadically in humans, with few recent accounts of infected individuals. The most recent identification of infection in humans was reported in a pathology report of an individual in 2011 [209]. In this case, histology slides of the liver identified liver granulomas, although schistosomiasis had not been diagnosed prior to the death of the patient [209].

5. Concluding Remarks

Multi-component, intersectoral, and integrated control approaches provide a promising path forward for the elimination of schistosomiasis in Asia. Behavioral changes that prevent infection, such as avoiding the practice of open defecation and contact of open freshwater bodies in endemic areas, are necessary. However, without accompanying infrastructure, such as toilets provided in WASH programs, these behaviors will continue. Combined with chemotherapy of both humans and reservoir hosts (e.g., water buffalo), snail control, animal vaccination, health education, and WASH targeting multiple points in the schistosome life cycle will significantly impact the prevalence and re-infection of schistosomiasis. The success achieved in P.R. China in schistosomiasis control and elimination is due to the commitment and support of the Chinese government, including the removal of water buffalo—a major reservoir host in P.R. China—from endemic areas, thus effectively removing them from the transmission cycle. Without such governmental support, sustaining control programs is difficult, particularly those that include more than preventive chemotherapy and require considerable resources to implement, such as required for CL-WASH. There is a niche role for health education that is missing from many schistosomiasis control programs, as knowledge remains limited about the parasite and which behaviors lead to infection in endemic populations.

Limited data are available on prevalence for *S. mekongi*, particularly for *S. malayensis*, the number of human cases, and the role played by animal reservoirs in transmission. Thus, assessing the true importance of schistosomiasis in the countries where these two schistosome species are endemic is difficult.

The true *S. japonicum* prevalence is conceivably underestimated, both in P.R. China and the Philippines, due to the lack of sensitive diagnostics used in control programs. While P.R. China closes in on elimination targets, the use of sensitive diagnostics will be important to determine whether elimination has indeed occurred and to prevent re-bounding infections after treatment and the cessation of the control program. A recent study in P.R. China found a human prevalence <1% by the MHT but 11% by qPCR [63]. Although the majority of the cases detected by qPCR were light-intensity infections, they do present a significant number of individuals who were not identified by widely used diagnostic methods, and who could contribute to resurgence after interventions cease. Limited case finding and prevalence studies have been performed in either country by their national control programs. Another limitation is the lack of snail prevalence surveys performed in many of the schistosome-endemic countries.

Future challenges for schistosomiasis control and elimination include climate change and the potential spread of the disease to new areas [141,210–212]. Europe has, for example, seen a return of autochthonous schistosomiasis cases, although this may initially be due to human migration from endemic areas [213]. Increases in temperature due to climate change will shift the tropical zone, the band in which schistosomiasis currently occurs. In P.R. China, this may lead to a shift in endemic areas further North in the country as the climate changes, and with the implementation of the SNWD project.

Acknowledgments: The authors would like to thank Andrew Bedford from the Research School of Population Health at the Australian National University, and Tal Bavli and Madeleine Flynn from the Graphics Department at QIMR Berghofer Medical Research Institute for their assistance in producing the figures used in this manuscript.

References

1. McManus, D.P.; Dunne, D.W.; Sacko, M.; Utzinger, J.; Vennervald, B.J.; Zhou, X.N. Schistosomiasis. *Nat. Rev. Dis. Primers* **2018**, *4*, 13. [CrossRef] [PubMed]

2. Boissier, J.; Grech-Angelini, S.; Webster, B.L.; Allienne, J.F.; Huyse, T.; Mas-Coma, S.; Toulza, E.; Barre-Cardi, H.; Rollinson, D.; Kincaid-Smith, J.; et al. Outbreak of urogenital schistosomiasis in Corsica (France): An epidemiological case study. *Lancet Infect. Dis.* **2016**, *16*, 971–979. [CrossRef]

3. Tchuem Tchuente, L.A.; Southgate, V.R.; Jourdane, J.; Webster, B.L.; Vercruysse, J. *Schistosoma intercalatum*: An endangered species in Cameroon? *Trends Parasitol.* **2003**, *19*, 389–393. [CrossRef]

4. Greer, G.J.; Ow-Yang, C.K.; Yong, H.-S. *Schistosoma malayensis* n. sp.: A *Schistosoma japonicum*-complex schistosome from Peninsular Malaysia. *J. Parasitol.* **1988**, *74*, 471–480. [CrossRef] [PubMed]

5. Webster, B.L.; Diaw, O.T.; Seye, M.M.; Webster, J.P.; Rollinson, D. Introgressive hybridization of *Schistosoma haematobium* group species in Senegal: Species barrier break down between ruminant and human schistosomes. *PLoS Negl. Trop. Dis.* **2013**, *7*, e2110. [CrossRef] [PubMed]

6. Leger, E.; Webster, J.P. Hybridizations within the genus *Schistosoma*: Implications for evolution, epidemiology and control. *Parasitology* **2017**, *144*, 65–80. [CrossRef] [PubMed]

7. Kebede, T.; Negash, Y.; Erko, B. *Schistosoma mansoni* infection in human and nonhuman primates in selected areas of Oromia Regional State, Ethiopia. *J. Vector Borne Dis.* **2018**, *55*, 116–121. [CrossRef] [PubMed]

8. Alarcón de Noya, B.; Pointier, J.P.; Colmenares, C.; Théron, A.; Balzan, C.; Cesari, I.M.; González, S.; Noya, O. Natural *Schistosoma mansoni* infection in wild rats from Guadeloupe: Parasitological and immunological aspects. *Acta Trop.* **1997**, *68*, 11–21. [CrossRef]

9. Huyse, T.; Van den Broeck, F.; Hellemans, B.; Volckaert, F.A.M.; Polman, K. Hybridisation between the two major African schistosome species of humans. *Int. J. Parasitol.* **2013**, *43*, 687–689. [CrossRef] [PubMed]

10. Leger, E.; Garba, A.; Hamidou, A.A.; Webster, B.L.; Pennance, T.; Rollinson, D.; Webster, J.P. Introgressed animal schistosomes *Schistosoma curassoni* and *S. bovis* naturally infecting humans. *Emerg. Infect. Dis.* **2016**, *22*, 2212–2214. [CrossRef] [PubMed]

11. Zhou, X.N.; Bergquist, R.; Leonardo, L.; Yang, G.J.; Yang, K.; Sudomo, M.; Olveda, R. Schistosomiasis japonica: Control and research needs. *Adv. Parasitol.* **2010**, *72*, 145–178. [PubMed]

12. Kajihara, N.; Hirayama, K. The war against a regional disease in Japan: A history of the eradication of schistosomiasis japonica. *Trop. Med. Health* **2011**, *39*, 3–44. [PubMed]

13. Ross, A.G.P.; Sleigh, A.C.; Li, Y.; Davis, G.M.; Williams, G.; Jiang, Z.; Feng, Z.; McManus, D.P. Schistosomiasis in the People's Republic of China: Prospects and challenges for the 21st century. *Clin. Microbiol. Rev.* **2001**, *14*, 270–279. [CrossRef] [PubMed]

14. Mao, S.P.; Shao, B.R. Schistosomiasis control in the People's Republic of China. *Am. J. Trop. Med. Hyg.* **1982**, *31*, 92–99. [CrossRef] [PubMed]

15. Rollinson, D.; Knopp, S.; Levitz, S.; Stothard, J.R.; Tchuem Tchuenté, L.-A.; Garba, A.; Mohammed, K.A.; Schur, N.; Person, B.; Colley, D.G.; et al. Time to set the agenda for schistosomiasis elimination. *Acta Trop.* **2013**, *128*, 423–440. [CrossRef] [PubMed]

16. Soe, H.Z.; Oo, C.C.; Myat, T.O.; Maung, N.S. Detection of *Schistosoma* antibodies and exploration of associated factors among local residents around Inlay Lake, Southern Shan State, Myanmar. *Infect. Dis. Poverty* **2017**, *6*, 3. [CrossRef] [PubMed]

17. WHO. Expert consultation to accelerate elimination of Asian schistosomiasis. In *Meeting Report WHO*; WHO: Shanghai, China, 2017.

18. Cameron, T.W.M. A new definitive host for *Schistosoma mansoni*. *J. Helminthol.* **1928**, *6*, 219–222. [CrossRef]

19. He, Y.; Salafsky, B.; Ramaswamy, K. Host-parasite relationships of *Schistosoma japonicum* in mammalian hosts. *Trends Parasitol.* **2001**, *17*, 320–324. [CrossRef]

20. Ho, Y.H.; He, Y.X. On the host specificity of *Schistosoma japonicum*. *Chin. Med. J.* **1963**, *82*, 403–414.

21. Bustinduy, A.L.; King, C.H. 52—Schistosomiasis A2—Farrar, Jeremy. In *Manson's Tropical Infectious Diseases*, 23th ed.; Hotez, P.J., Junghanss, T., Kang, G., Lalloo, D., White, N.J., Eds.; W.B. Saunders: London, UK, 2014.

22. Matsumoto, J.; Muth, S.; Socheat, D.; Matsuda, H. The first reported cases of canine schistosomiasis mekongi in Cambodia. *Southeast Asian J. Trop. Med. Public Health* **2002**, *33*, 458–461. [PubMed]

23. Strandgaard, H.; Johansen, M.V.; Pholsena, K.; Teixayavong, K.; Christensen, N.O. The pig as a host for *Schistosoma mekongi* in Laos. *J. Parasitol.* **2001**, *87*, 708–709. [CrossRef]

24. Blair, D.; van Herwerden, L.; Hirai, H.; Taguchi, T.; Habe, S.; Hirata, M.; Lai, K.; Upatham, S.; Agatsuma, T. Relationships between *Schistosoma malayensis* and other Asian schistosomes deduced from DNA sequences. *Mol. Biochem. Parasitol.* **1997**, *85*, 259–263. [CrossRef]

25. Attwood, S.W.; Cottet, M. Malacological and parasitological surveys along the Xe Bangfai and its tributaries in Khammouane Province, Lao PDR. *Hydroécol. Appl.* **2016**, *19*, 245–270. [CrossRef]

26. CDC. Schistosomiasis Infection. Available online: https://www.cdc.gov/dpdx/schistosomiasis/index.html (accessed on 2 March 2018).

27. Utzinger, J.; N'Goran, E.K.; Caffrey, C.R.; Keiser, J. From innovation to application: Social-ecological context, diagnostics, drugs and integrated control of schistosomiasis. *Acta Trop.* **2011**, *120* (Suppl. 1), S121–S137. [CrossRef] [PubMed]

28. Gordon, C.A.; Acosta, L.P.; Gobert, G.N.; Jiz, M.; Olveda, R.M.; Ross, A.G.; Gray, D.J.; Williams, G.M.; Harn, D.; Yuesheng, L.; et al. High prevalence of *Schistosoma japonicum* and *Fasciola gigantica* in bovines from Northern Samar, the Philippines. *PLoS Negl. Trop. Dis.* **2015**, *9*, e0003108. [CrossRef] [PubMed]

29. Gray, D.J.; Williams, G.M.; Li, Y.; McManus, D.P. Transmission dynamics of *Schistosoma japonicum* in the lakes and marshlands of China. *PLoS ONE* **2008**, *3*, e4058. [CrossRef] [PubMed]

30. Rudge, J.W.; Carabin, H.; Balolong, E.; Tallo, V.; Shrivastava, J.; Lu, D.B.; Basanez, M.G.; Olveda, R.; McGarvey, S.T.; Webster, J.P. Population genetics of *Schistosoma japonicum* within the Philippines suggest high levels of transmission between humans and dogs. *PLoS Negl. Trop. Dis.* **2008**, *2*, e340. [CrossRef] [PubMed]

31. Rudge, J.W.; Lu, D.-B.; Fang, G.-R.; Wang, T.-P.; Basáñez, M.-G.; Webster, J.P. Parasite genetic differentiation by habitat type and host species: Molecular epidemiology of *Schistosoma japonicum* in hilly and marshland areas of Anhui Province, China. *Mol. Ecol.* **2009**, *18*, 2134–2147. [CrossRef] [PubMed]

32. Rudge, J.W.; Webster, J.P.; Lu, D.-B.; Wang, T.-P.; Fang, G.-R.; Basáñez, M.-G. Identifying host species driving transmission of schistosomiasis japonica, a multihost parasite system, in China. *Proc. Natl. Acad. Sci. USA* **2013**, *110*, 11457–11462. [CrossRef] [PubMed]

33. Attwood, S.W.; Fatih, F.A.; Upatham, E.S. DNA-sequence variation among *Schistosoma mekongi* populations and related taxa: Phylogeography and the current distribution of Asian schistosomiasis. *PLoS Negl. Trop. Dis.* **2008**, *2*, e200. [CrossRef] [PubMed]

34. Sornmani, S.; Kitikoon, V.; Thirachantra, S.; Harinasuta, C. Epidemiology of mekong schistosomiasis. *Malacol. Rev.* **1980**, (Suppl. 2), 9–18.

35. Kitikoon, V. Comparison of eggs and miracidia of *Schistosoma mekongi* and *S. japonicum*. *Malacol. Rev.* **1980**, (Suppl. 2), 93–103.

36. Fletcher, M.; Woodruff, D.S.; LoVerde, P.T. Genetic differentiation between *Schistosoma mekongi* and *S. japonicum*: An electrophoretic study. *Malacol. Rev.* **1980**, *2*, 113–122.

37. Ross, A.G.; Vickers, D.; Olds, G.R.; Shah, S.M.; McManus, D.P. Katayama syndrome. *Lancet Infect. Dis.* **2007**, *7*, 218–224. [CrossRef]

38. Gryseels, B. Schistosomiasis. *Infect. Dis. Clin. N. Am.* **2012**, *26*, 383–397. [CrossRef] [PubMed]

39. Gryseels, B.; Polman, K.; Clerinx, J.; Kestens, L. Human schistosomiasis. *Lancet* **2006**, *368*, 1106–1118. [CrossRef]

40. Li, Y.; Ross, A.G.; Hou, X.; Lou, Z.; McManus, D.P. Oriental schistosomiasis with neurological complications: Case report. *Ann. Clin. Microbiol. Antimicrob.* **2011**, *10*, 5. [CrossRef] [PubMed]

41. Kane, C.A.; Most, H. Schistosomiasis of the central nervous system: Experiences in world war II and a review of the literature. *Arch. Neurol. Psychiatry* **1948**, *59*, 141–183. [CrossRef] [PubMed]

42. Ferrari, T.C.A.; Moreira, P.R.R. Neuroschistosomiasis: Clinical symptoms and pathogenesis. *Lancet Neurol.* **2011**, *10*, 853–864. [CrossRef]

43. Liu, H.; Lim, C.C.; Feng, X.; Yao, Z.; Chen, Y.; Sun, H.; Chen, X. MRI in cerebral schistosomiasis: Characteristic nodular enhancement in 33 patients. *Am. J. Roentgenol.* **2008**, *191*, 582–588. [CrossRef] [PubMed]

44. Stecher, C.W.; Sacko, M.; Madsen, H.; Wilson, S.; Wejse, C.; Keita, A.D.; Landoure, A.; Traore, M.S.; Kallestrup, P.; Petersen, E.; et al. Anemia and growth retardation associated with *Schistosoma haematobium* infection in Mali: A possible subtle impact of a neglected tropical disease. *Trans. R. Soc. Trop. Med. Hyg.* **2017**, *111*, 144–153. [CrossRef] [PubMed]

45. WHO. Schistosomiasis: Fact Sheet. Available online: http://www.who.int/mediacentre/factsheets/fs115/en/ (accessed on 20 February 2018).

46. Glinz, D.; Silué, K.D.; Knopp, S.; Lohouringnon, L.K.; Yao, K.P.; Steinmann, P.; Rinaldi, L.; Cringoli, G.; N'Goran, E.K.; Utzinger, J. Comparing diagnostic accuracy of Kato-Katz, Koga agar plate, ether-concentration, and FLOTAC for *Schistosoma mansoni* and soil-transmitted helminths. *PLoS Negl. Trop. Dis.* **2010**, *4*, e754. [CrossRef] [PubMed]

47. Habtamu, K.; Degarege, A.; Ye-Ebiyo, Y.; Erko, B. Comparison of the Kato-Katz and FLOTAC techniques for the diagnosis of soil-transmitted helminth infections. *Parasitol. Int.* **2011**, *60*, 398–402. [CrossRef] [PubMed]

48. Cringoli, G. FLOTAC, a novel apparatus for a multivalent faecal egg count technique. *Parassitologica* **2006**, *48*, 381–384.

49. Cringoli, G.; Rinaldi, L.; Maurelli, M.P.; Utzinger, J. FLOTAC: New multivalent techniques for qualitative and quantitative copromicroscopic diagnosis of parasites in animals and humans. *Nat. Protoc.* **2010**, *5*, 503–515. [CrossRef] [PubMed]

50. Xu, B.; Gordon, C.A.; Hu, W.; McManus, D.P.; Chen, H.; Gray, D.J.; Ju, C.; Zeng, X.; Gobert, G.N.; Ge, J.; et al. A novel procedure for precise quantification of *Schistosoma japonicum* eggs in bovine feces. *PLoS Negl. Trop. Dis.* **2012**, *6*, e1885. [CrossRef]

51. Lier, T.; Johansen, M.V.; Hjelmevoll, S.O.; Vennervald, B.J.; Simonsen, G.S. Real-time PCR for detection of low intensity *Schistosoma japonicum* infections in a pig model. *Acta Trop.* **2008**, *105*, 74–80. [CrossRef] [PubMed]

52. Anh, N.T.; Phuong, N.T.; Ha, G.H.; Thu, L.T.; Johansen, M.V.; Murrell, D.K.; Thamsborg, S.M. Evaluation of techniques for detection of small trematode eggs in faeces of domestic animals. *Vet. Parasitol.* **2008**, *156*, 346–349. [CrossRef] [PubMed]

53. Zhu, H.Q.; Xu, J.; Zhu, R.; Cao, C.L.; Bao, Z.P.; Yu, Q.; Zhang, L.J.; Xu, X.L.; Feng, Z.; Guo, J.G. Comparison of the miracidium hatching test and modified Kato-Katz method for detecting *Schistosoma japonicum* in low prevalence areas of China. *Southeast Asian J. Trop. Med. Public Health* **2014**, *45*, 20–25. [PubMed]

54. Jurberg, A.D.; de Oliveira, A.A.; Lenzi, H.L.; Coelho, P.M.Z. A new miracidia hatching device for diagnosing schistosomiasis. *Mem. Inst. Oswaldo Cruz* **2008**, *103*, 112–114. [CrossRef] [PubMed]

55. Xu, J.; Rong, R.; Zhang, H.Q.; Shi, C.J.; Zhu, X.Q.; Xia, C.M. Sensitive and rapid detection of *Schistosoma japonicum* DNA by loop-mediated isothermal amplification (LAMP). *Int. J. Parasitol.* **2010**, *40*, 327–331. [CrossRef] [PubMed]

56. Kumagai, T.; Furushima-Shimogawara, R.; Ohmae, H.; Wang, T.; Lu, S.; Chen, R.; Wen, L.; Ohta, N. Detection of early and single infections of *Schistosoma japonicum* in the intermediate host snail, *Oncomelania hupensis*, by PCR and loop-mediated isothermal amplification (LAMP) assay. *Am. J. Trop. Med. Hyg.* **2010**, *83*, 542–548. [CrossRef] [PubMed]

57. Gordon, C.A.; Gray, D.J.; Gobert, G.N.; McManus, D.P. DNA amplification approaches for the diagnosis of key parasitic helminth infections of humans. *Mol. Cell. Probes* **2011**, *25*, 143–152. [CrossRef] [PubMed]

58. Weerakoon, K.G.; Gobert, G.N.; Cai, P.; McManus, D.P. Advances in the diagnosis of human schistosomiasis. *Clin. Microbiol. Rev.* **2015**, *28*, 939–967. [CrossRef] [PubMed]

59. Gobert, G.N.; Chai, M.; Duke, M.; McManus, D.P. Copro-PCR based detection of *Schistosoma* eggs using mitochondrial DNA markers. *Mol. Cell. Probes* **2005**, *19*, 250–254. [CrossRef] [PubMed]

60. Gordon, C.A.; Acosta, L.P.; Gray, D.J.; Olveda, R.; Jarilla, B.; Gobert, G.N.; Ross, A.G.; McManus, D.P. High prevalence of *Schistosoma japonicum* infection in carabao from Samar province, the Philippines: Implications for transmission and control. *PLoS Negl. Trop. Dis.* **2012**, *6*, e1778. [CrossRef] [PubMed]

61. Lier, T.; Simonsen, G.S.; Haaheim, H.; Hjelmevoll, S.O.; Vennervald, B.J.; Johansen, M.V. Novel real-time PCR for detection of *Schistosoma japonicum* in stool. *Southeast Asian J. Trop. Med. Public Health* **2006**, *37*, 257–264. [PubMed]

62. Lier, T.; Simonsen, G.S.; Wang, T.; Lu, D.; Haukland, H.H.; Vennervald, B.J.; Hegstad, J.; Johansen, M.V. Real-time polymerase chain reaction for detection of low-intensity *Schistosoma japonicum* infections in China. *Am. J. Trop. Med. Hyg.* **2009**, *81*, 428–432. [CrossRef] [PubMed]

63. He, P.; Gordon, C.A.; Williams, G.M.; Yueshang, L.; Wang, Y.; Hu, J.; Gray, D.J.; Ross, A.G.; Harn, D.; McManus, D.P. Real-time PCR diagnosis of *Schistosoma japonicum* in low transmission areas of China. *Infect. Dis. Poverty* **2018**, *7*, 8. [CrossRef] [PubMed]

64. Gordon, C.A.; Acosta, L.P.; Gobert, G.N.; Olveda, R.M.; Ross, A.G.; Williams, G.M.; Gray, D.J.; Harn, D.; Li, Y.; McManus, D.P. Real-time PCR demonstrates high prevalence of *Schistosoma japonicum* in the Philippines: Implications for surveillance and control. *PLoS Negl. Trop. Dis.* **2015**, *9*, e0003483. [CrossRef] [PubMed]

65. Weerakoon, K.G.; Gordon, C.A.; Cai, P.; Gobert, G.N.; Duke, M.; Williams, G.M.; McManus, D.P. A novel duplex ddPCR assay for the diagnosis of schistosomiasis japonica: Proof of concept in an experimental mouse model. *Parasitology* **2017**, *144*, 1005–1015. [CrossRef] [PubMed]

66. Weerakoon, K.G.; Gordon, C.A.; Gobert, G.N.; Cai, P.; McManus, D.P. Optimisation of a droplet digital PCR assay for the diagnosis of *Schistosoma japonicum* infection: A duplex approach with DNA binding dye chemistry. *J. Microbiol. Methods* **2016**, *125*, 19–27. [CrossRef] [PubMed]

67. Weerakoon, K.G.; Gordon, C.A.; Williams, G.M.; Cai, P.; Gobert, G.N.; Olveda, R.M.; Ross, A.G.; Olveda, D.U.; McManus, D.P. Droplet digital PCR diagnosis of human schistosomiasis: Parasite cell-free DNA detection in diverse clinical samples. *J. Infect. Dis.* **2017**, *216*, 1611–1622. [CrossRef] [PubMed]

68. Cai, P.; Weerakoon, K.G.; Mu, Y.; Olveda, D.U.; Piao, X.; Liu, S.; Olveda, R.M.; Chen, Q.; Ross, A.G.; McManus, D.P. A parallel comparison of antigen candidates for development of an optimized serological diagnosis of chistosomiasis japonica in the Philippines. *EBioMedicine* **2017**, *24*, 237–246. [CrossRef] [PubMed]

69. Angeles, J.M.; Goto, Y.; Kirinoki, M.; Asada, M.; Leonardo, L.R.; Rivera, P.T.; Villacorte, E.A.; Inoue, N.; Chigusa, Y.; Kawazu, S. Utilization of ELISA using thioredoxin peroxidase-1 and tandem repeat proteins for diagnosis of *Schistosoma japonicum* infection among water buffaloes. *PLoS Negl. Trop. Dis.* **2012**, *6*, e1800. [CrossRef] [PubMed]

70. Dawson, E.M.; Sousa-Figueiredo, J.C.; Kabatereine, N.B.; Doenhoff, M.J.; Stothard, J.R. Intestinal schistosomiasis in pre school-aged children of Lake Albert, Uganda: Diagnostic accuracy of a rapid test for detection of anti-schistosome antibodies. *Trans. R. Soc. Trop. Med. Hyg.* **2013**, *107*, 639–647. [CrossRef] [PubMed]

71. Lin, D.; Xu, J.; Zhang, Y.; Liu, Y.; Hu, F.; Xu, X.; Li, J.; Gao, Z.; Wu, H.; Kurtis, J.; et al. Evaluation of IgG-ELISA for the diagnosis of *Schistosoma japonicum* in a high prevalence, low intensity endemic area of China. *Acta Trop.* **2008**, *107*, 128–133. [CrossRef] [PubMed]

72. Wang, W.; Li, Y.; Li, H.; Xing, Y.; Qu, G.; Dai, J.; Liang, Y. Immunodiagnostic efficacy of detection of *Schistosoma japonicum* human infections in China: A meta analysis. *Asian Pac. J. Trop. Med.* **2012**, *5*, 15–23. [CrossRef]

73. Hinz, R.; Schwarz, N.G.; Hahn, A.; Frickmann, H. Serological approaches for the diagnosis of schistosomiasis—A review. *Mol. Cell. Probes* **2017**, *31*, 2–21. [CrossRef] [PubMed]

74. Zhou, Y.B.; Zheng, H.M.; Jiang, Q.W. A diagnostic challenge for Schistosomiasis japonica in China: Consequences on praziquantel-based morbidity control. *Parasit. Vectors* **2011**, *4*, 194. [CrossRef] [PubMed]

75. Utzinger, J.; Becker, S.L.; van Lieshout, L.; van Dam, G.J.; Knopp, S. New diagnostic tools in schistosomiasis. *Clin. Microbiol. Infect.* **2015**, *21*, 529–542. [CrossRef] [PubMed]

76. Leonardo, L.; Chigusa, Y.; Kikuchi, M.; Kato-Hayashi, N.; Kawazu, S.I.; Angeles, J.M.; Fontanilla, I.K.; Tabios, I.K.; Moendeg, K.; Goto, Y.; et al. Schistosomiasis in the Philippines: Challenges and some successes in control. *Southeast Asian J. Trop. Med. Public Health* **2016**, *47*, 651–666.

77. Gray, D.J.; Ross, A.G.; Li, Y.; McManus, D.P. Diagnosis and management of schistosomiasis. *Br. Med. J.* **2011**, *342*, d2651. [CrossRef] [PubMed]

78. Utzinger, J.; Keiser, J. Schistosomiasis and soil-transmitted helminthiasis: Common drugs for treatment and control. *Expert Opin. Pharmacother.* **2004**, *5*, 263–285. [CrossRef] [PubMed]

79. Vale, N.; Gouveia, M.J.; Rinaldi, G.; Brindley, P.J.; Gärtner, F.; Correia da Costa, J.M. Praziquantel for schistosomiasis: Single-drug metabolism revisited, mode of action, and resistance. *Antimicrob. Agents Chemother.* **2017**, *61*, e02582-16. [CrossRef] [PubMed]

80. Sabah, A.A.; Fletcher, C.; Webbe, G.; Doenhoff, M.J. *Schistosoma mansoni*: Chemotherapy of infections of different ages. *Exp. Parasitol.* **1986**, *61*, 294–303. [CrossRef]

81. Utzinger, J.; Keiser, J.; Xiao, S.H.; Tanner, M.; Singer, B.H. Combination chemotherapy of schistosomiasis in laboratory studies and clinical trials. *Antimicrob. Agents Chemother.* **2003**, *47*, 1487–1495. [CrossRef] [PubMed]

82. Olveda, D.U.; Li, Y.; Olveda, R.M.; Lam, A.K.; McManus, D.P.; Chau, T.N.; Harn, D.A.; Williams, G.M.; Gray, D.J.; Ross, A.G. Bilharzia in the Philippines: Past, present, and future. *Int. J. Infect. Dis.* **2014**, *18*, 52–56. [CrossRef] [PubMed]

83. Wu, Z.; Shaoji, Z.; Pan, B.; Hu, L.; Wei, R.; Gao, Z.; Li, J.; Uwe, B. Reinfection with *Schistosoma japonicum* after treatment with praziquantel in Poyang Lake Region, China. *Southeast Asian J. Trop. Med. Public Health* **1994**, *25*, 163–169. [PubMed]

84. Wang, W.; Wang, L.; Liang, Y. Susceptibility or resistance of praziquantel in human schistosomiasis: A review. *Parasitol. Res.* **2012**, *111*, 1871–1877. [CrossRef] [PubMed]

85. Cupit, P.M.; Cunningham, C. What is the mechanism of action of praziquantel and how might resistance strike? *Future Med. Chem.* **2015**, *7*, 701–705. [CrossRef] [PubMed]

86. Bergquist, R.; Utzinger, J.; Keiser, J. Controlling schistosomiasis with praziquantel: How much longer without a viable alternative? *Infect. Dis. Poverty* **2017**, *6*, 74. [CrossRef] [PubMed]

87. Soares Magalhães, R.J.; Salamat, M.S.; Leonardo, L.; Gray, D.J.; Carabin, H.; Halton, K.; McManus, D.P.; Williams, G.M.; Rivera, P.; Saniel, O.; et al. Geographical distribution of human *Schistosoma japonicum* infection in The Philippines: Tools to support disease control and further elimination. *Int. J. Parasitol.* **2014**, *44*, 977–984. [CrossRef] [PubMed]

88. Leonardo, L.R.; Rivera, P.; Saniel, O.; Villacorte, E.; Crisostomo, B.; Hernandez, L.; Baquilod, M.; Erce, E.; Martinez, R.; Velayudhan, R. Prevalence survey of schistosomiasis in Mindanao and the Visayas, the Philippines. *Parasitol. Int.* **2008**, *57*, 246–251. [CrossRef] [PubMed]

89. Gray, D.J.; Williams, G.M.; Li, Y.; Chen, H.; Forsyth, S.J.; Li, R.S.; Barnett, A.G.; Guo, J.; Ross, A.G.; Feng, Z.; et al. A cluster-randomised intervention trial against *Schistosoma japonicum* in the People's Republic of China: Bovine and human transmission. *PLoS ONE* **2009**, *4*, e5900. [CrossRef] [PubMed]

90. Gray, D.J.; Williams, G.M.; Li, Y.; Chen, H.; Li, R.S.; Forsyth, S.J.; Barnett, A.G.; Guo, J.; Feng, Z.; McManus, D.P. A cluster-randomized bovine intervention trial against *Schistosoma japonicum* in the People's Republic of China: Design and baseline results. *Am. J. Trop. Med. Hyg.* **2007**, *77*, 866–874. [CrossRef] [PubMed]

91. Gray, D.J.; Williams, G.M.; Li, Y.S.; Chen, H.G.; Forsyth, S.; Li, R.; Barnett, A.; Guo, J.G.; Ross, A.; Feng, Z.; et al. The role of bovines in human *Schistosoma japonicum* infection in the People's Republic China. *Am. J. Trop. Med. Hyg.* **2009**, *81*, 1046.

92. Carlton, E.J.; Bates, M.N.; Zhong, B.; Seto, E.Y.; Spear, R.C. Evaluation of mammalian and intermediate host surveillance methods for detecting schistosomiasis reemergence in southwest China. *PLoS Negl. Trop. Dis.* **2011**, *5*, e987. [CrossRef] [PubMed]

93. Van Dorssen, C.F.; Gordon, C.A.; Li, Y.; Williams, G.M.; Wang, Y.; Luo, Z.; Gobert, G.N.; You, H.; McManus, D.P.; Gray, D.J. Rodents, goats and dogs—Their potential roles in the transmission of schistosomiasis in China. *Parasitology* **2017**, *144*, 1633–1642. [CrossRef] [PubMed]

94. Angeles, J.M.; Leonardo, L.R.; Goto, Y.; Kirinoki, M.; Villacorte, E.A.; Hakimi, H.; Moendeg, K.J.; Lee, S.; Rivera, P.T.; Inoue, N.; et al. Water buffalo as sentinel animals for schistosomiasis surveillance. *Bull. World Health Organ.* **2015**, *93*, 511–512. [CrossRef] [PubMed]

95. Satrija, F.; Ridwan, Y.; Jastal, S.; Rauf, A. Current status of schistosomiasis in Indonesia. *Acta Trop.* **2015**, *141*, 349–353. [CrossRef] [PubMed]

96. Ross, A.G.P.; Olveda, R.M.; Acosta, L.; Harn, D.A.; Chy, D.; Yuesheng, L.; Gray, D.J.; Gordon, C.A.; McManus, D.P.; Williams, G.M. Road to the elimination of schistosomiasis from Asia: The journey is far from over. *Microbes Infect.* **2013**, *15*, 858–865. [CrossRef] [PubMed]

97. Wang, T.; Zhang, S.; Wu, W.; Zhang, G.; Lu, D.; Ørnbjerg, N.; Johansen, M.V. Treatment and reinfection of water buffaloes and cattle infected with *Schistosoma japonicum* in Yangtze river valley, Anhui province, China. *J. Parasitol.* **2006**, *92*, 1088–1091. [CrossRef] [PubMed]

98. Yang, J.; Fu, Z.; Feng, X.; Shi, Y.; Yuan, C.; Liu, J.; Hong, Y.; Li, H.; Lu, K.; Lin, J. Comparison of worm development and host immune responses in natural hosts of *Schistosoma japonicum*, yellow cattle and water buffalo. *BMC Vet. Res.* **2012**, *8*, 25. [CrossRef] [PubMed]

99. Li, Y.-S.; McManus, D.P.; Lin, D.-D.; Williams, G.M.; Harn, D.A.; Ross, A.G.; Feng, Z.; Gray, D.J. The *Schistosoma japonicum* self-cure phenomenon in water buffaloes: Potential impact on the control and elimination of schistosomiasis in China. *Int. J. Parasitol.* **2014**, *44*, 167–171. [CrossRef] [PubMed]

100. Guo, J.; Li, Y.; Gray, D.J.; Hu, G.; Chen, H.; Davis, G.M.; Sleigh, A.C.; Feng, Z.; McManus, D.P.; Williams, G.M. A drug-based intervention study on the importance of buffaloes for human *Schistosoma japonicum* infection around Poyang Lake, People's Republic of China. *Am. J. Trop. Med. Hyg.* **2006**, *74*, 335–341. [CrossRef] [PubMed]

101. Zhou, Y.-B.; Liang, S.; Chen, G.-X.; Rea, C.; He, Z.-G.; Zhang, Z.-J.; Wei, J.-G.; Zhao, G.-M.; Jiang, Q.-W. An integrated strategy for transmission control of *Schistosoma japonicum* in a marshland area of China: Findings from a five-year longitudinal survey and mathematical modeling. *Am. J. Trop. Med. Hyg.* **2011**, *85*, 83–88. [CrossRef] [PubMed]

102. Liang, S.; Yang, C.; Zhong, B.; Qiu, D. Re-emerging schistosomiasis in hilly and mountainous areas of Sichuan, China. *Bull. World Health Organ.* **2006**, *84*, 139–144. [CrossRef] [PubMed]

103. WHO. NTD, WASH, Animal Health, Nutrition and Education Are Joining Forces to Eliminate Schistosomiasis in Mekong Region. Available online: http://www.wpro.who.int/mvp/ntd/ntd_wash/en/ (accessed on 12 September 2018).

104. Chen, S.B.; Ai, L.; Hu, W.; Xu, J.; Bergquist, R.; Qin, Z.Q.; Chen, J.H. New anti-*Schistosoma* approaches in the People's Republic of China: Development of diagnostics, vaccines and other new techniques belonging to the 'omics' group. *Adv. Parasitol.* **2016**, *92*, 385–408. [PubMed]

105. Gray, D.J.; Li, Y.S.; Williams, G.M.; Zhao, Z.Y.; Harn, D.A.; Li, S.M.; Ren, M.Y.; Feng, Z.; Guo, F.Y.; Guo, J.G.; et al. A multi-component integrated approach for the elimination of schistosomiasis in the People's Republic of China: Design and baseline results of a 4-year cluster-randomised intervention trial. *Int. J. Parasitol.* **2014**, *44*, 659–668. [CrossRef] [PubMed]

106. Inobaya, M.T.; Olveda, R.M.; Chau, T.N.P.; Olveda, D.U.; Ross, A.G.P. Prevention and control of schistosomiasis: A current perspective. *Res. Rep. Trop. Med.* **2014**, *2014*, 65–75. [PubMed]

107. McManus, D.P.; Loukas, A. Current status of vaccines for schistosomiasis. *Clin. Microbiol. Rev.* **2008**, *21*, 225–242. [CrossRef] [PubMed]

108. Tebeje, B.M.; Harvie, M.; You, H.; Loukas, A.; McManus, D.P. Schistosomiasis vaccines: Where do we stand? *Parasit. Vectors* **2016**, *9*, 528. [CrossRef] [PubMed]

109. Da'dara, A.A.; Li, Y.S.; Xiong, T.; Zhou, J.; Williams, G.M.; McManus, D.P.; Feng, Z.; Yu, X.L.; Gray, D.J.; Harn, D.A. DNA-based vaccines protect against zoonotic schistosomiasis in water buffalo. *Vaccine* **2008**, *26*, 3617–3625. [CrossRef] [PubMed]

110. Williams, G.; Sleigh, A.C.; Li, Y.; Feng, Z.; Davis, G.M.; Chen, H.; Ross, A.G.P.; Bergquist, R.; McManus, D.P. Mathematical modelling of schistosomiasis japonica: Comparison of control strategies in the People's Republic of China. *Acta Trop.* **2002**, *82*, 253–262. [CrossRef]

111. He, Y.; Guo, Y.; Ni, C.; Xia, F.; Liu, H.; Yu, Q. Compatibility between *Onomelania hupensis* and different isolates of *Schistosoma japonicum* in China. *Southeast Asian J. Trop. Med. Public Health* **1991**, *22*, 245–254. [PubMed]

112. Wang, X.Q.; Mao, S.P. Comparison of morphology, pathogenicity and drug response among three isolates of *Schistosoma japonicum* in the mainland of China. *Ann. Parasitol. Hum. Comp.* **1989**, *64*, 110–119. [CrossRef] [PubMed]

113. Kirinoki, M.; Hu, M.; Yokoi, H.; Kawai, S.; Terrado, R.; Ilagan, E.; Chigusa, Y.; Sasaki, Y.; Matsuda, H. Comparative studies on susceptibilities of two different Japanese isolates of *Oncomelania nosophora* to three strains of *Schistosoma japonicum* originating from Japan, China, and the Philippines. *Parasitology* **2005**, *130*, 531–537. [CrossRef] [PubMed]

114. Zhao, Q.P.; Jiang, M.S.; Littlewood, D.T.; Nie, P. Distinct genetic diversity of *Oncomelania hupensis*, intermediate host of *Schistosoma japonicum* in mainland China as revealed by ITS sequences. *PLoS Negl. Trop. Dis.* **2010**, *4*, e611. [CrossRef] [PubMed]

115. Guan, W.; Li, S.Z.; Abe, E.M.; Webster, B.L.; Rollinson, D.; Zhou, X.N. The genetic diversity and geographical separation study of *Oncomelania hupensis* populations in mainland China using microsatellite loci. *Parasit. Vectors* **2016**, *9*, 28. [CrossRef] [PubMed]

116. Li, S.Z.; Wang, Y.X.; Yang, K.; Liu, Q.; Wang, Q.; Zhang, Y.; Wu, X.H.; Guo, J.G.; Bergquist, R.; Zhou, X.N. Landscape genetics: The correlation of spatial and genetic distances of *Oncomelania hupensis*, the intermediate host snail of *Schistosoma japonicum* in mainland China. *Geospat. Health* **2009**, *3*, 221–231. [CrossRef] [PubMed]

117. Sun, L.P.; Wang, W.; Zuo, Y.P.; Zhang, Z.Q.; Hong, Q.B.; Yang, G.J.; Zhu, H.R.; Liang, Y.S.; Yang, H.T. An integrated environmental improvement of marshlands: Impact on control and elimination of schistosomiasis in marshland regions along the Yangtze River, China. *Infect. Dis. Poverty* **2017**, *6*, 72. [CrossRef] [PubMed]

118. Xia, S.; Xue, J.B.; Zhang, X.; Hu, H.H.; Abe, E.M.; Rollinson, D.; Bergquist, R.; Zhou, Y.; Li, S.Z.; Zhou, X.N. Pattern analysis of schistosomiasis prevalence by exploring predictive modeling in Jiangling County, Hubei Province, P.R. China. *Infect. Dis. Poverty* **2017**, *6*, 91. [CrossRef] [PubMed]

119. WHO. *Expert Consultation to Accelerate Elimination of Asian Schistosomiasis, Shanghai, People's Republic of China, 22–23 May 2017: Meeting Report*; WHO Regional Office for the Western Pacific: Manila, Philippines, 2017; p. 18.

120. Knopp, S.; Corstjens, P.L.; Koukounari, A.; Cercamondi, C.I.; Ame, S.M.; Ali, S.M.; de Dood, C.J.; Mohammed, K.A.; Utzinger, J.; Rollinson, D.; et al. Sensitivity and specificity of a urine circulating anodic antigen test for the diagnosis of *Schistosoma haematobium* in low endemic settings. *PLoS Negl. Trop. Dis.* **2015**, *9*, e0003752. [CrossRef] [PubMed]

121. Madsen, H.; Carabin, H.; Balolong, D.; Tallo, V.L.; Olveda, R.; Yuan, M.; McGarvey, S.T. Prevalence of *Schistosoma japonicum* infection of *Oncomelania quadrasi* snail colonies in 50 irrigated and rain-fed villages of Samar Province, the Philippines. *Acta Trop.* **2008**, *105*, 235–241. [CrossRef] [PubMed]

122. Sumarni, S. The new endemic area of *Schistosoma japonicum* in Bada Highland Western Lore subdistrict, District of Poso, Central Sulawesi Province. *Trop. Med. J.* **2011**, *1*, 1–12.

123. Vonghachack, Y.; Odermatt, P.; Taisayyavong, K.; Phounsavath, S.; Akkhavong, K.; Sayasone, S. Transmission of *Opisthorchis viverrini, Schistosoma mekongi* and soil-transmitted helminthes on the Mekong Islands, Southern Lao PDR. *Infect. Dis. Poverty* **2017**, *6*, 131. [CrossRef] [PubMed]

124. Attwood, S.W. Schistosomiasis in the Mekong Region: Epidemiology and phylogeography. *Adv. Parasitol.* **2001**, *50*, 87–152. [PubMed]

125. Attwood, S.W.; Upatham, E.S. Observations on *Neotricula aperta* (Gastropoda: Pomatiopsidae) population densities in Thailand and central Laos: Implications for the spread of Mekong schistosomiasis. *Parasit. Vectors* **2012**, *5*, 126. [CrossRef] [PubMed]

126. Wu, J.Y.; Zhou, Y.B.; Chen, Y.; Liang, S.; Li, L.H.; Zheng, S.B.; Zhu, S.P.; Ren, G.H.; Song, X.X.; Jiang, Q.W. Three Gorges Dam: Impact of water level changes on the density of schistosome-transmitting snail *Oncomelania hupensis* in Dongting Lake area, China. *PLoS Negl. Trop. Dis.* **2015**, *9*, e0003882. [CrossRef] [PubMed]

127. Pesigan, T.P.; Hairston, N.G.; Jauregui, J.J.; Garcia, E.G.; Santos, A.T.; Santos, B.C.; Besa, A.A. Studies on *Schistosoma japonicum* infection in the Philippines. 2. The molluscan host. *Bull. World Health Organ.* **1958**, *18*, 481–578. [PubMed]

128. Garjito, T.A.; Sudomo, M.; Dahlan, M.; Nurwidayati, A. Schistosomiasis in Indonesia: Past and present. *Parasitol. Int.* **2008**, *57*, 277–280. [CrossRef] [PubMed]

129. Minai, M.; Hosaka, Y.; Ohta, N. Historical view of schistosomiasis japonica in Japan: Implementation and evaluation of disease-control strategies in Yamanashi Prefecture. *Parasitol. Int.* **2003**, *52*, 321–326. [CrossRef]

130. Yang, G.-J.; Li, W.; Sun, L.-P.; Wu, F.; Yang, K.; Huang, Y.-X.; Zhou, X.-N. Molluscicidal efficacies of different formulations of niclosamide: Result of meta-analysis of Chinese literature. *Parasit. Vectors* **2010**, *3*, 84. [CrossRef] [PubMed]

131. Zhu, H.R.; Liu, L.; Zhou, X.N.; Yang, G.J. Ecological model to predict potential habitats of *Oncomelania hupensis*, the intermediate host of *Schistosoma japonicum* in the mountainous regions, China. *PLoS Negl. Trop. Dis.* **2015**, *9*, e0004028. [CrossRef] [PubMed]

132. Chen, Z.; Zhou, X.N.; Yang, K.; Wang, X.H.; Yao, Z.Q.; Wang, T.P.; Yang, G.J.; Yang, Y.J.; Zhang, S.Q.; Wang, J.; et al. Strategy formulation for schistosomiasis japonica control in different environmental settings supported by spatial analysis: A case study from China. *Geospat. Health* **2007**, *1*, 223–231. [CrossRef] [PubMed]

133. Hu, Y.; Zhang, Z.; Chen, Y.; Wang, Z.; Gao, J.; Tao, B.; Jiang, Q.; Jiang, Q. Spatial pattern of schistosomiasis in Xingzi, Jiangxi Province, China: The effects of environmental factors. *Parasit. Vectors* **2013**, *6*, 214. [CrossRef] [PubMed]

134. Hu, Y.; Li, R.; Bergquist, R.; Lynn, H.; Gao, F.; Wang, Q.; Zhang, S.; Sun, L.; Zhang, Z.; Jiang, Q. Spatio-temporal transmission and environmental determinants of schistosomiasis japonica in Anhui Province, China. *PLoS Negl. Trop. Dis.* **2015**, *9*, e0003470. [CrossRef] [PubMed]

135. Li, Y.S.; Sleigh, A.C.; Ross, A.G.P.; Williams, G.; Tanner, M.; McManus, D.P. Epidemiology of *Schistosoma japonicum* in China: Morbidity and strategies for control in the Dongting Lake region. *Int. J. Parasitol.* **2000**, *30*, 273–281. [CrossRef]

136. Yang, K.; Li, L.; Huang, Y.; Zhang, J.; Wu, F.; Hang, D.; Steinmann, P.; Liang, Y. Spatio-temporal analysis to identify determinants of *Oncomelania hupensis* infection with *Schistosoma japonicum* in Jiangsu province, China. *Parasit. Vectors* **2013**, *6*, 138. [CrossRef] [PubMed]

137. Zhou, X.N.; Yang, G.J.; Yang, K.; Wang, X.H.; Hong, Q.B.; Sun, L.P.; Malone, J.B.; Kristensen, T.K.; Bergquist, N.R.; Utzinger, J. Potential impact of climate change on schistosomiasis transmission in China. *Am. J. Trop. Med. Hyg.* **2008**, *78*, 188–194. [CrossRef] [PubMed]

138. Li, Y.S.; Raso, G.; Zhao, Z.Y.; He, Y.K.; Ellis, M.K.; McManus, D.P. Large water management projects and schistosomiasis control, Dongting Lake region, China. *Emerg. Infect. Dis.* **2007**, *13*, 973–979. [CrossRef] [PubMed]

139. Gray, D.J.; Thrift, A.P.; Williams, G.M.; Zheng, F.; Li, Y.-S.; Guo, J.; Chen, H.; Wang, T.; Xu, X.J.; Zhu, R.; et al. Five-year longitudinal assessment of the downstream impact on schistosomiasis transmission following closure of the Three Gorges Dam. *PLoS Negl. Trop. Dis.* **2012**, *6*, e1588. [CrossRef]

140. McManus, D.P.; Gray, D.J.; Li, Y.; Feng, Z.; Williams, G.M.; Stewart, D.; Rey-Ladino, J.; Ross, A.G. Schistosomiasis in the People's Republic of China: The era of the Three Gorges Dam. *Clin. Microbiol. Rev.* **2010**, *23*, 442–466. [CrossRef] [PubMed]

141. Zhu, G.; Fan, J.; Peterson, A.T. *Schistosoma japonicum* transmission risk maps at present and under climate change in mainland China. *PLoS Negl. Trop. Dis.* **2017**, *11*, e0006021. [CrossRef] [PubMed]

142. Zhou, X.; Bergquist, R.; Leonardo, L.R.; Olveda, R. Schistosomiasis: The Disease and Its Control. 2008. Available online: https://www.researchgate.net/publication/242285494_Schistosomiasis_The_Disease_and_its_Control (accessed on 7 January 2019).

143. Nyein, N. WHO's Field Visit Reports over 400 Schistosomiasis Cases in Rakhine State. Available online: http://www.moi.gov.mm/moi:eng/?q=news/14/11/2018/id-14720 (accessed on 7 January 2019).

144. Raso, G.; Li, Y.S.; Zhao, Z.Y.; Balen, J.; Williams, G.M.; McManus, D.P. Spatial distribution of human *Schistosoma japonicum* infections in the Dongting Lake Region, China. *PLoS ONE* **2009**, *4*, e6947. [CrossRef] [PubMed]

145. Ziegelbauer, K.; Speich, B.; Mäusezahl, D.; Bos, R.; Keiser, J.; Utzinger, J. Effect of sanitation on soil-transmitted helminth infection: Systematic review and meta-analysis. *PLoS Med.* **2012**, *9*, e1001162. [CrossRef] [PubMed]

146. Strunz, E.C.; Addiss, D.G.; Stocks, M.E.; Ogden, S.; Utzinger, J.; Freeman, M.C. Water, sanitation, hygiene, and soil-transmitted helminth infection: A systematic review and meta-analysis. *PLoS Med.* **2014**, *11*, e1001620. [CrossRef] [PubMed]

147. Campbell, S.J.; Savage, G.B.; Gray, D.J.; Atkinson, J.M.; Magalhães, R.J.S.; Nery, S.V.; McCarthy, J.S.; Velleman, Y.; Wicken, J.H.; Traub, R.J.; et al. Water, sanitation, and hygiene (WASH): A critical component for sustainable soil-transmitted helminth and schistosomiasis control. *PLoS Negl. Trop. Dis.* **2014**, *8*, e2651. [CrossRef] [PubMed]

148. Campbell, S.J.; Biritwum, N.K.; Woods, G.; Velleman, Y.; Fleming, F.; Stothard, J.R. Tailoring water, sanitation, and hygiene (WASH) targets for soil-transmitted helminthiasis and schistosomiasis control. *Trends Parasitol.* **2018**, *34*, 53–63. [CrossRef] [PubMed]

149. WHO. *Sixty Fifth World Health Assembly: Elimination of Schistosimasis*; WHO: Geneva, Switzerland, 2012.

150. Secor, W.E. Water-based interventions for schistosomiasis control. *Pathog. Glob. Health* **2014**, *108*, 246–254. [CrossRef] [PubMed]

151. Grimes, J.E.T.; Croll, D.; Harrison, W.E.; Utzinger, J.; Freeman, M.C.; Templeton, M.R. The roles of water, sanitation and hygiene in reducing schistosomiasis: A review. *Parasit. Vectors* **2015**, *8*, 156. [CrossRef] [PubMed]

152. WHO. Sanitation, Drinking-Water and Health: Achievements and Challenges Ahead. Available online: http://www.who.int/iris/handle/10665/260222 (accessed on 19 October 2018).

153. USAID. Water, Sanitation and Hygiene in Indonesia. Available online: https://www.usaid.gov/actingonthecall/stories/indonesia-wash (accessed on 19 October 2018).

154. UNICEF. Water, Sanitation and Hygiene: Philippines. Available online: https://www.unicef.org/philippines/wes_21334.html (accessed on 19 October 2018).

155. WGF. Goal Wash Project in the Philippines. Available online: http://www.watergovernance.org/resources/goal-wash-project-philippines/ (accessed on 19 October 2018).

156. UN. *Sanitation, Drinking-Water and Hygiene Status Overview: Indonesia*; UN-Water Global Analysis and Assessment of Sanitation and Drinking-Water: Geneva, Switzerland, 2015.

157. Camon, C.B. *Implementation of Water, Sanitation and Hygiene (WASH) in Public Schools: A Citizen Participatory Audit*; Department of Education: Cagayan de Oro City, Philippines, 2017.

158. Chen, L.; Zhong, B.; Xu, J.; Li, R.Z.; Cao, C.L. Health education as an important component in the national schistosomiasis control programme in the People's Republic of China. *Adv. Parasitol.* **2016**, *92*, 307–339. [PubMed]

159. Wang, L.; Chen, H.; Guo, J.; Zeng, X.; Hong, X.; Xiong, J.; Wu, X.; Wang, X.; Wang, L.; Xia, G.; et al. A strategy to control transmission of *Schistosoma japonicum* in China. *N. Engl. J. Med.* **2009**, *360*, 121–128. [CrossRef] [PubMed]

160. Guo, J.G.; Cao, C.L.; Hu, G.H.; Lin, H.; Li, D.; Zhu, R.; Xu, J. The role of 'passive chemotherapy' plus health education for schistosomiasis control in China during maintenance and consolidation phase. *Acta Trop.* **2005**, *96*, 177–183. [CrossRef] [PubMed]

161. Hu, G.H.; Hu, J.; Song, K.Y.; Lin, D.D.; Zhang, J.; Cao, C.L.; Xu, J.; Li, D.; Jiang, W.S. The role of health education and health promotion in the control of schistosomiasis: Experiences from a 12-year intervention study in the Poyang Lake area. *Acta Trop.* **2005**, *96*, 232–241. [CrossRef] [PubMed]

162. Kloos, H. Human behavior, health education and schistosomiasis control: A review. *Soc. Sci. Med.* **1995**, *40*, 1497–1511. [CrossRef]

163. McManus, D.P.; Bieri, F.A.; Li, Y.S.; Williams, G.M.; Yuan, L.P.; Henglin, Y.; Du, Z.W.; Clements, A.C.A.; Steinmann, P.; Raso, G.; et al. Health education and the control of intestinal worm infections in China: A new vision. *Parasit. Vectors* **2014**, *7*, 344. [CrossRef] [PubMed]

164. Zhou, L.Y.; Deng, Y.; Steinmann, P.; Yang, K. The effects of health education on schistosomiasis japonica prevalence and relevant knowledge in the People's Republic of China: A systematic review and meta-analysis. *Parasitol. Int.* **2013**, *62*, 150–156. [CrossRef] [PubMed]

165. Muth, S.; Sayasone, S.; Odermatt-Biays, S.; Phompida, S.; Duong, S.; Odermatt, P. *Schistosoma mekongi* in Cambodia and Lao People's Democratic Republic. *Adv. Parasitol.* **2010**, *72*, 179–203. [PubMed]

166. McManus, D.P.; Gray, D.J.; Ross, A.G.; Williams, G.M.; He, H.B.; Li, Y.S. Schistosomiasis research in the Dongting Lake region and its impact on local and national treatment and control in China. *PLoS Negl. Trop. Dis.* **2011**, *5*, e1053. [CrossRef] [PubMed]

167. Molehin, A.J.; Rojo, J.U.; Siddiqui, S.Z.; Gray, S.A.; Carter, D.; Siddiqui, A.A. Development of a schistosomiasis vaccine. *Expert Rev. Vac.* **2016**, *15*, 619–627. [CrossRef] [PubMed]

168. Rim, H.-J.; Chai, J.-Y.; Min, D.-Y.; Cho, S.; Eom, K.S.; Hong, S.; Sohn, W.; Yong, T.; Deodato, G.; Standgaard, H.; et al. Prevalence of intestinal parasite infections on a national scale among primary schoolchildren in Laos. *Parasitol. Res.* **2003**, *91*, 267–272. [CrossRef] [PubMed]

169. Hu, Y.; Li, S.; Xia, C.; Chen, Y.; Lynn, H.; Zhang, T.; Xiong, C.; Chen, G.; He, Z.; Zhang, Z. Assessment of the national schistosomiasis control program in a typical region along the Yangtze River, China. *Int. J. Parasitol.* **2017**, *47*, 21–29. [CrossRef] [PubMed]

170. Wu, H.; Qin, Y.; Chu, K.; Meng, R.; Liu, Y.; McGarvey, S.T.; Olveda, R.; Acosta, L.P.; Ji, M.; Fernandez, T.; et al. High prevalence of *Schistosoma japonicum* infection in water buffaloes in the Philippines assessed by real-time polymerase chain reaction. *Am. J. Trop. Med. Hyg.* **2010**, *82*, 646–652. [CrossRef] [PubMed]

171. Logan, O.T. A case of dysentery in Hunan province, caused by the trematode, *Schistosoma japonicum*. *Chin. Med. J.* **1905**, *19*, 243–245.

172. Wooley, P.G. The occurrence of *Schistosoma japonicum* Vel Cattol in the Philippines. *Philipp. J. Sci.* **1906**, *1*, 83–90.

173. Okabe, K. *Progress of Medical Parasitology in Japan*; Meguro Parasitology Museum: Tokyo, Japan, 1964; Volume 1.

174. Lei, Z.L.; Zheng, H.; Zhang, L.J.; Zhu, R.; Xu, Z.M.; Xu, J.; Fu, Q.; Wang, Q.; Li, S.Z.; Zhou, X.N. Endemic status of schistosomiasis in People's Republic of China in 2013. *Chin. J. Schistosomiasis Control* **2014**, *26*, 591–597.

175. WHO. *Elimination of Schistosomiasis from Low-Transmission Areas: Report of a WHO Informal Consultation*; WHO: Geneva, Switzerland, 2008.

176. Yuan, H.; Jiagang, G.; Bergquist, R.; Tanner, M.; Xianyi, C.; Huanzeng, W. The 1992–1999 World Bank Schistosomiasis research initiative in China: Outcome and perspectives. *Parasitol. Int.* **2000**, *49*, 195–207. [CrossRef]

177. Collins, C.; Xu, J.; Tang, S. Schistosomiasis control and the health system in P.R. China. *Infect. Dis. Poverty* **2012**, *1*, 8. [CrossRef] [PubMed]

178. Sun, L.P.; Wang, W.; Hong, Q.B.; Li, S.Z.; Liang, Y.S.; Yang, H.T.; Zhou, X.N. Approaches being used in the national schistosomiasis elimination programme in China: A review. *Infect. Dis. Poverty* **2017**, *6*, 55. [CrossRef] [PubMed]

179. Wang, L.D.; Guo, J.G.; Wu, X.H.; Chen, H.G.; Wang, T.P.; Zhu, S.P.; Zhang, Z.H.; Steinmann, P.; Yang, G.J.; Wang, S.P.; et al. China's new strategy to block *Schistosoma japonicum* transmission: Experiences and impact beyond schistosomiasis. *Trop. Med. Int. Health* **2009**, *14*, 1475–1483. [CrossRef] [PubMed]

180. Leonardo, L.R.; Rivera, P.; Saniel, O.; Villacorte, E.; Labanan, M.A.; Crisostomo, B.; Hernandez, L.; Baquilod, M.; Erce, E.; Martinez, R.; et al. A national baseline prevalence survey of schistosomiasis in the Philippines using stratified two-step systematic cluster sampling design. *J. Trop. Med.* **2012**, *2012*, 936128. [CrossRef] [PubMed]

181. Acosta, L.P.; Aligui, G.D.L.; Tiu, W.U.; McManus, D.P.; Olveda, R.M. Immune correlate study on human *Schistosoma japonicum* in a well-defined population in Leyte, Philippines: I. Assessment of 'resistance' versus 'susceptibility' to *S. japonicum* infection. *Acta Trop.* **2002**, *84*, 127–136. [CrossRef]

182. Tarafder, M.R.; Balolong, E., Jr.; Carabin, H.; Bélisle, P.; Tallo, V.; Joseph, L.; Alday, P.; Gonzales, R.O.; Riley, S.; Olveda, R.; et al. A cross-sectional study of the prevalence of intensity of infection with *Schistosoma japonicum* in 50 irrigated and rain-fed villages in Samar Province, the Philippines. *BMC Public Health* **2006**, *6*, 61. [CrossRef] [PubMed]

183. Inobaya, M.T.; Olveda, R.M.; Tallo, V.; McManus, D.P.; Williams, G.M.; Harn, D.A.; Li, Y.; Chau, T.N.P.; Olveda, D.U.; Ross, A.G. Schistosomiasis mass drug administration in the Philippines: Lessons learnt and the global implications. *Microbes Infect.* **2015**, *17*, 6–15. [CrossRef] [PubMed]

184. Xu, J.; Steinman, P.; Maybe, D.; Zhou, X.N.; Lv, S.; Li, S.Z.; Peeling, R. Evolution of the national schistosomiasis control programmes in the People's Republic of China. *Adv. Parasitol.* **2016**, *92*, 1–38. [PubMed]

185. Pesigan, T.P.; Farooq, M.; Hairston, N.G.; Jauregui, J.J.; Garcia, E.G.; Santos, A.T.; Santos, B.C.; Besa, A.A. Studies on *Schistosoma japonicum* infection in the Philippines: 3. Preliminary control experiments. *Bull. World Health Organ.* **1958**, *19*, 223–261. [PubMed]

186. Pesigan, T.P.; Hairston, N.G. The effect of snail control on the prevalence of *Schistosoma japonicum* infection in the Philippines. *Bull. World Health Organ.* **1961**, *25*, 479–482. [PubMed]

187. DOH. Schistosomiasis Control Program. Available online: http://www.doh.gov.ph/content/schistosomiasis-control-program.html (accessed on 1 September 2014).

188. Leonardo, L.R.; Acosta, L.P.; Olveda, R.M.; Aligui, G.D.L. Difficulties and strategies in the control of schistosomiasis in the Philippines. *Acta Trop.* **2002**, *82*, 295–299. [CrossRef]

189. Tallo, V.L.; Carabian, H.; Alday, P.P.; Balolong, E., Jr.; Olveda, R.M.; McGarvey, S.T. Is mass treatment the appropriate schistosomiasis elimination strategy? *Bull. World Health Organ.* **2008**, *86*, 765–771. [CrossRef] [PubMed]

190. Inobaya, M.T.; Chau, T.N.; Ng, S.-K.; MacDougall, C.; Olveda, R.M.; Tallo, V.L.; Landicho, J.M.; Malacad, C.M.; Aligato, M.F.; Guevarra, J.B.; et al. Mass drug administration and the sustainable control of schistosomiasis: An evaluation of treatment compliance in the rural Philippines. *Parasit. Vectors* **2018**, *11*, 441. [CrossRef] [PubMed]

191. Inobaya, M.T.; Chau, T.N.; Ng, S.K.; MacDougall, C.; Olveda, R.M.; Tallo, V.L.; Landicho, J.M.; Malacad, C.M.; Aligato, M.F.; Guevarra, J.R.; et al. Mass drug administration the sustainable control of schistosomiasis: Community health workers are vital for global elimination efforts. *Int. J. Infect. Dis.* **2018**, *66*, 14–21. [CrossRef] [PubMed]

192. WHO. *Neglected Tropical Diseases in Indonesia: An Integrated Plan of Action 2011–2015*; Ministry of Health Indonesia: Jakarta, Indonesia, 2010.

193. Nasution, A. Government Decentralization Program in Indonesia. Available online: https://www.adb.org/publications/government-decentralization-program-indonesia (accessed on 17 September 2018).

194. WHO. *Schistosomiasis: An Emerging Public Health Problem*; WHO: Geneva, Switzerland, 2018.

195. MoH. Freshwater Snail Parasite that Infects about Schistosomiasis Cases Attended the Professional Union. Available online: http://mohs.gov.mm/ (accessed on 12 December 2018).

196. Han, K.; Wai, K.; Htun, M.W.; Aye, K.; Latt, A.; Chi Aung San, N.; Phyo, A.; Xu, J.; Li, S.-Z.; Zhou, X.-N.; et al. Molecular Verification of Schistosoma mekongi Infection in ShweKyin Township; Myanmar, 2017. In Proceedings of the 16th Annual Workshop of Regional Network on Asian Schistosomiasis and other Zoonotic Helminths (RNAS+), Yangon, Myanmar, 26–28 October 2016.

197. Wai, K.T.; Han, K.T.; Oo, T. Intensifying responsiveness towards neglected intestinal helminth infections in a resource-constrained setting. *Trop. Med. Health* **2017**, *45*, 12. [CrossRef] [PubMed]

198. Gupta, S. *Development in Times of Transition: The Socio-Econommic Status of Rakhine State*; Livelihoods and Food Security Trust (LIFT) Fund: Rakhine, Myanmar, 2018.

199. Harinasuta, C. Introduction: Schistosomiasis in Asia. *Malacol. Rev.* **1980**, *2*, 431–438.

200. Urbani, C.; Sinoun, M.; Socheat, D.; Pholsena, K.; Strandgaard, H.; Odermatt, P.; Hatz, C. Epidemiology and control of mekongi schistosomiasis. *Acta Trop.* **2002**, *82*, 157–168. [CrossRef]

201. WHO. Communities Drive Elimination of Schistosomiasis through Improving Water, Sanitation and Hygiene in Cambodia and the Lao People's Democratic Republic. Available online: http://www.wpro.who.int/mvp/ntd/cl_swash/en/ (accessed on 12 September 2018).

202. WHO. *Seventeenth Meeting of the Regional Programme Review Group on Neglected Tropical Diseases in the Western Pacific*; WHO: Manila, Philippines, 2017.

203. IAMAT. Thailand General Health Risks: Schistosomiasis. Available online: https://www.iamat.org/country/thailand/risk/schistosomiasis (accessed on 29 January 2019).

204. Sornmani, S.; Vivatanasesth, P.; Thirachantra, S. Clinical study of Mekong schistosomiasis at Khong Island, Southern Laos. *Malacol. Rev.* **1980**, *7*, 270–281.

205. Campa, P.; Develoux, M.; Belkadi, G.; Magne, D.; Lame, C.; Carayon, M.-J.; Girard, P.-M. Chronic *Schistosoma mekongi* in a traveler—A case report and review of the literature. *J. Travel Med.* **2014**, *21*, 361–363. [CrossRef] [PubMed]

206. Clerinx, J.; Cnops, L.; Huyse, T.; Tannich, E.; Van Esbroeck, M. Diagnostic issues of acute schistosomiasis with *Schistosoma mekongi* in a traveler: A case report. *J. Travel Med.* **2013**, *20*, 322–325. [CrossRef] [PubMed]

207. Chuah, C.; Gobert, G.N.; Latif, B.; Heo, C.C.; Leow, C.Y. Schistosomiasis in Malaysia: A review. *Acta Trop.* **2019**, *190*, 137–143. [CrossRef] [PubMed]

208. Murugasu, R.; Wang, F.; Dissanaike, A.S. *Schistosoma japonicum*-type infection in Malaysia—Report of the first living case. *Trans. R. Soc. Trop. Med. Hyg.* **1978**, *72*, 389–391. [CrossRef]

209. Latif, B.; Heo, C.C.; Razuin, R.; Shamalaa, D.V.; Tappe, D. Autochthonous human schistosomiasis, Malaysia. *Emerg. Infect. Dis.* **2013**, *19*, 1340–1341. [CrossRef] [PubMed]

210. Gordon, C.A.; McManus, D.P.; Jones, M.K.; Gray, D.J.; Gobert, G.N. The increase of exotic zoonotic helminth infections: The impact of urbanization, climate change and globalization. *Adv. Parasitol.* **2016**, *91*, 311–397. [PubMed]

211. McCreesh, N.; Nikulin, G.; Booth, M. Predicting the effects of climate change on *Schistosoma mansoni* transmission in eastern Africa. *Parasit. Vectors* **2015**, *8*, 4. [CrossRef] [PubMed]

212. Stensgaard, A.S.; Vounatsou, P.; Sengupta, M.E.; Utzinger, J. Schistosomes, snails and climate change: Current trends and future expectations. *Acta Trop.* **2019**, *190*, 257–268. [CrossRef] [PubMed]

213. Boissier, J.; Moné, H.; Mitta, G.; Bargues, M.D.; Molyneux, D.; Mas-Coma, S. Schistosomiasis reaches Europe. *Lancet Infect. Dis.* **2015**, *15*, 757–758. [CrossRef]

Permissions

All chapters in this book were first published by MDPI; hereby published with permission under the Creative Commons Attribution License or equivalent. Every chapter published in this book has been scrutinized by our experts. Their significance has been extensively debated. The topics covered herein carry significant findings which will fuel the growth of the discipline. They may even be implemented as practical applications or may be referred to as a beginning point for another development.

The contributors of this book come from diverse backgrounds, making this book a truly international effort. This book will bring forth new frontiers with its revolutionizing research information and detailed analysis of the nascent developments around the world.

We would like to thank all the contributing authors for lending their expertise to make the book truly unique. They have played a crucial role in the development of this book. Without their invaluable contributions this book wouldn't have been possible. They have made vital efforts to compile up to date information on the varied aspects of this subject to make this book a valuable addition to the collection of many professionals and students.

This book was conceptualized with the vision of imparting up-to-date information and advanced data in this field. To ensure the same, a matchless editorial board was set up. Every individual on the board went through rigorous rounds of assessment to prove their worth. After which they invested a large part of their time researching and compiling the most relevant data for our readers.

The editorial board has been involved in producing this book since its inception. They have spent rigorous hours researching and exploring the diverse topics which have resulted in the successful publishing of this book. They have passed on their knowledge of decades through this book. To expedite this challenging task, the publisher supported the team at every step. A small team of assistant editors was also appointed to further simplify the editing procedure and attain best results for the readers.

Apart from the editorial board, the designing team has also invested a significant amount of their time in understanding the subject and creating the most relevant covers. They scrutinized every image to scout for the most suitable representation of the subject and create an appropriate cover for the book.

The publishing team has been an ardent support to the editorial, designing and production team. Their endless efforts to recruit the best for this project, has resulted in the accomplishment of this book. They are a veteran in the field of academics and their pool of knowledge is as vast as their experience in printing. Their expertise and guidance has proved useful at every step. Their uncompromising quality standards have made this book an exceptional effort. Their encouragement from time to time has been an inspiration for everyone.

The publisher and the editorial board hope that this book will prove to be a valuable piece of knowledge for researchers, students, practitioners and scholars across the globe.

List of Contributors

Genming Zhao, Na He, Zhijie Zhang and Hongchang Yuan
Department of Epidemiology, School of Public Health, Fudan University, 130 Dong'an Road, Shanghai 200032, China

Linhan Li, Yibiao Zhou, Dongjian Yang, Ya Yang, Yu Yang and Qingwu Jiang
Department of Epidemiology, School of Public Health, Fudan University, 130 Dong'an Road, Shanghai 200032, China
Key Laboratory of Public Health Safety, Ministry of Education, 130 Dong'an Road, Shanghai 200032, China
Center of Tropical Disease Research, 130 Dong'an Road, Shanghai 200032, China

Tianping Wang and Shiqing Zhang
Institute for the Prevention and Control of Schistosomiasis in Anhui Province, 337 Wuhu Road, Hefei 230061, China

Gengxin Chen
Guichi Antischistosomiasis Station, West Qiupu Road, Chizhou 247100, China

Yue Chen
School of Epidemiology and Public Health, University of Ottawa, 600 Peter Morand, Ottawa, ON K1G 5Z3, Canada

Ganna Saelens and Sarah Gabriël
Department of Veterinary Public Health and Food Safety, Faculty of Veterinary Medicine, Ghent University, Merelbeke B-9820, Belgium

Jacques F. Mavoungou and Aubin A. Koumba
Research Institute in Tropical Ecology, National Center for Scientific and Technological Research, Libreville BP 13354, Gabon

Modeste Mabicka Mamfoumbi, Jean R. Mourou and Marielle K. Bouyou Akotet
Department of Parasitology-Mycology, Faculty of Medicine, University of Health Sciences of Libreville, Libreville BP 4009, Gabon

Julienne Atsame
Control Program of Parasitic Diseases, Libreville BP 2434, Gabon

Rodrigue Mintsa Nguema
Research Institute in Tropical Ecology, National Center for Scientific and Technological Research, Libreville BP 13354, Gabon
Department of Parasitology-Mycology, Faculty of Medicine, University of Health Sciences of Libreville, Libreville BP 4009, Gabon
Control Program of Parasitic Diseases, Libreville BP 2434, Gabon

Krystina Mengue Me Ngou-Milama
Control Program of Parasitic Diseases, Libreville BP 2434, Gabon
National Laboratory of Public Health, Libreville BP 10736, Gabon

Mariama Sani Lamine, Abdoulaye Diarra and Ghislaine Nkone Asseko
Word Health Organization Country Office Gabon, Libreville BP 820, Gabon

Hélène Moné and Gabriel Mouahid
IHPE, Univ Montpellier, CNRS, UM, IFREMER, Univ Perpignan Via Domitia, Perpignan F-66860, France

Eniola M. Abe, Yun-Hai Guo, Haimo Shen and Jing-Bo Xue
National Institute of Parasitic Diseases (NIPD), Chinese Centre for Disease Control and Prevention, Shanghai 200025, China

Jing Xu and Shi-Zhu Li
National Institute of Parasitic Diseases (NIPD), Chinese Centre for Disease Control and Prevention, Shanghai 200025, China
Key Laboratory of Parasite and Vector Biology, Ministry of Health; National Institute of Parasitic Diseases, Chinese Center for Disease Control and Prevention, Shanghai 200025, China

Masceline J. Mutsaka-Makuvaza and Nicholas Midzi
Department of Medical Microbiology, College of Health Sciences, University of Zimbabwe, Harare 00263, Zimbabwe

Mohamed R. Habib
Medical Malacology Laboratory, Theodor Bilharz Research Institute, Giza 12411, Egypt

Hala Elmorshedy
College of Medicine, Princess Nourah bint Abdulrahman University, Riyadh 11671, Saudi Arabia
Department of Tropical Health, High Institute of Public Health, Alexandria University, Alexandria 21561, Egypt

Virak Khieu, Sinuon Muth and Rekol Huy
National Center for Parasitology, Entomology and Malaria Control, Ministry of Health, Phnom Penh 12100, Cambodia

Somphou Sayasone
Lao Tropical and Public Health Institute, Vientiane 01030, Laos

Masashi Kirinoki and Hiroshi Ohmae
School of Medicine, Dokkyo Medical University, Mibu, Shimotsuga, Tochigi 321-0293, Japan

Sakhone Laymanivong
Centre for Malariology, Parasitology and Entomology, Vientiane 01000, Laos

Thipphavanh Chanthapaseuth
World Health Organization, Vientiane Office, Vientiane 01160, Laos

Aya Yajima
World Health Organization, Western Pacific Regional Office, Manila 1000, Philippines

Rattanaxay Phetsouvanh
Department of Communicable Disease Control, Ministry of Health, Vientiane 01130, Laos

Robert Bergquist
Department of Epidemiology and Public Health, Swiss Tropical and Public Health Institute, Switzerland
Ingerod, SE-454 94 Brastad, Sweden

Peter Odermatt
Department of Epidemiology and Public Health, Swiss Tropical and Public Health Institute, Switzerland
University of Basel, Switzerland

Miriam Tendler, Marília S. Almeida, Monica M. Vilar, Patrícia M. Pinto and Gabriel Limaverde-Sousa
FIOCRUZ — Instituto Oswaldo Cruz, Laboratório de Esquistossomose Experimental, Av. Brasil, 4365, Manguinhos, Rio de Janeiro 21045-900, Brazil

Catherine A. Gordon
Molecular Parasitology Laboratory, Infectious Diseases Division, QIMR Berghofer Medical Research Institute, Brisbane 4006, Australia

Kosala G. Weerakoon
Molecular Parasitology Laboratory, Infectious Diseases Division, QIMR Berghofer Medical Research Institute, Brisbane 4006, Australia
School of Public Health, University of Queensland, Brisbane 4006, Australia
Department of Parasitology, Faculty of Medicine and Allied Sciences, Rajarata University of Sri Lanka, Saliyapura 50008, Sri Lanka

Callie J. Weber, Joseph Hargan-Calvopiña, Katy M. Graef, Cathyryne K. Manner and Jennifer Dent
BIO Ventures for Global Health, 2101 Fourth Avenue, Suite 1950, Seattle, WA 98121, USA

Hong You, Pengfei Cai, Biniam Mathewos Tebeje, Yuesheng Li and Donald P. McManus
Molecular Parasitology Laboratory, QIMR Berghofer Medical Research Institute, Brisbane, QLD 4006, Australia

Zhi-Qiang Qin, Ting Feng, Shan Lv, Ying-Jun Qian, Li-Juan Zhang, Yin-Long Li and Chao Lv
Key Laboratory of Parasite and Vector Biology, Ministry of Health; National Institute of Parasitic Diseases, Chinese Center for Disease Control and Prevention, Shanghai 200025, China

Guo-Jing Yang
Department of Epidemiology and Public Health, Swiss Tropical and Public Health Institute, Socinstrasse 57, CH-4002 Basel, Switzerland
University of Basel, CH-4002 Basel, Switzerland

Stefanie J. Krauth
Institute for Biodiversity, Animal Health and Comparative Medicine, University of Glasgow, Glasgow G12 8QQ, UK

Julie Balen
School of Health and Related Research, University of Sheffield, Sheffield S1 4DA, UK

Geoffrey N. Gobert
School of Biological Sciences, Queen's University Belfast, Belfast BT9 7BL, UK

Poppy H. L. Lamberton
Institute for Biodiversity, Animal Health and Comparative Medicine, University of Glasgow, Glasgow G12 8QQ, UK
Wellcome Centre for Molecular Parasitology, University of Glasgow, Glasgow G12 8QQ, UK

Damilare O. Famakinde
Department of Medical Microbiology and Parasitology, College of Medicine, University of Lagos, Idi-Araba, Surulere, Lagos 100254, Nigeria

Johanna Kurscheid and Darren J. Gray
Department of Global Health, Research School of Population Health, Australian National University, Acton, ACT 2601, Australia

Gail M. Williams
School of Public Health, University of Queensland, Herston, QLD 4006, Australia

Archie C. A. Clements
Faculty of Health Sciences, Curtin University, Bentley, WA 6102, Australia
Telethon Kids Institute, Nedlands, WA 6009, Australia

Xiao-Nong Zhou
Center for Disease Control and Prevention, National Institute for Parasitic Diseases, Shanghai 200025, China
National Institute of Parasitic Diseases (NIPD), Chinese Centre for Disease Control and Prevention, Shanghai 200025, China
Key Laboratory of Parasite and Vector Biology, Ministry of Health; National Institute of Parasitic Diseases, Chinese Center for Disease Control and Prevention, Shanghai 200025, China

Jürg Utzinger
Swiss Tropical and Public Health Institute, CH-4002 Basel, Switzerland
University of Basel, CH-4003 Basel, Switzerland

Index

Printed in the USA
CPSIA information can be obtained
at www.ICGtesting.com
JSHW051509111223
53612JS00005B/70